Digital Academe

Dramatic advances in information and communication technologies (ICTs) such as the Internet and Web may lead to fundamental changes to the structure of higher education and the ways in which it is delivered. Some commentators believe these new media will facilitate the emergence of effective new models of electronic learning, seriously challenging the dominance of the traditional institutions of academia. Others see the automation of higher education as a management strategy that will destroy jobs and undermine quality.

Digital Academe draws together contributions from leading international practitioners, educationalists and researchers to offer informed perspectives on developments and options in distance education and distributed learning. The contributions provide the reader with a survey of current innovations, and the opportunities and challenges in higher education arising from the new ICTs. They span national boundaries and reach beyond the research community to the heart of issues of policy and practice around the world.

Digital Academe will be of value to educators, policy makers, journalists, parents and the public at large. Students at both undergraduate and postgraduate levels will find material of relevance to courses in communication, information studies, sociology, public policy, education, instructional technologies, new media and information and communications technologies. The large number of educational practitioners and academics in diverse disciplines whose careers are being shaped by these developments will gain new insights about developments in online education and scholarship.

William H. Dutton is Director of the Oxford Internet Institute, a Fellow of Balliol College and Professor of Internet Studies at the University of Oxford. **Brian D. Loader** is Director of the Community Informatics Research and Applications Unit (CIRA) based at the University of Teesside, UK.

Digital Academe

The new media and institutions
of higher education and learning

**Edited by William H. Dutton
and Brian D. Loader**

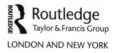

Routledge
Taylor & Francis Group

LONDON AND NEW YORK

First published 2002
by Routledge
11 New Fetter Lane, London EC4P 4EE

Simultaneously published in the USA and Canada
by Routledge
29 West 35th Street, New York, NY 10001

Routledge is an imprint of the Taylor & Francis Group

Typeset in Times by Taylor & Francis Books Ltd
Printed and bound in Great Britain by TJ International Ltd, Padstow,
Cornwall

British Library Cataloguing in Publication Data
A catalogue record for this book is available from the British Library

Library of Congress Cataloging in Publication Data
A catalog record for this book has been requested

ISBN 0–415–26224–0 (hbk)
ISBN 0–415–26225–9 (pbk)

Dedicated to

Michael Young

1916–2002

Founder of the Open University and social entrepreneur

Contents

List of illustrations   xi
Notes on contributors   xii
Foreword by Asa Briggs   xvi
Preface   xx
Acknowledgments   xxiii
List of abbreviations and acronyms   xxvi
List of relevant Web sites   xxix

**Introduction: new media and institutions of higher education
and learning**   **1**
WILLIAM H. DUTTON AND BRIAN D. LOADER

PART I
**Audiences for new media in higher education: students,
teachers and administrators as consumers and users of ICTs**   **33**

1 **Technology and the future of the university: a sober view**   **35**
A. MICHAEL NOLL

2 **Defining moments: the tension between richness and reach**   **39**
TREVOR HAYWOOD

3 **Making the case online: Harvard Business School multimedia**   **50**
SYLVIA SENSIPER

4 Targeting working professionals: the case of a Master of Arts
   in Gerontology   56
   EDWARD SCHNEIDER, MARIA HENKE AND CARL RENOLD

5 Students' difficulties in a Web-based distance education course:
   an ethnographic study   62
   NORIKO HARA AND ROB KLING

PART II
Reconfiguring institutional arrangements: the production of
higher education   85

6 A new game in town: competitive higher education in American
   research universities   87
   LLOYD ARMSTRONG

7 Jones International University™: A pioneering virtual
   university   116
   PAMELA S. PEASE

8 The Open University of Catalonia: A European virtual
   university initiative   121
   EMMA KISELYOVA

9 Distance learning through highly-interactive tutorials   128
   ALFRED BORK

10 Promoting scholarship through design   135
   TAMARA SUMNER

11 Infrastructure and institutional change in the networked
   university   152
   PHILIP E. AGRE

PART III
Utilizing new ICTs and organizational forms in higher education 167

12 Competition and collaboration in online distance learning 169
WALTER S. BAER

13 Distance education provision by universities: how institutional contexts affect choices 185
OLIVER BOYD-BARRETT

14 The Virtual University of Applied Sciences: a flagship German project 206
ROSE M M WAGNER

15 Virtual learning and the network society 215
MARTIN HARRIS

16 The informational view of the university 232
NEIL POLLOCK

PART IV
Governing digital academe: management and policy responses 251

17 'Information Society' as theory or ideology: a critical perspective on technology, education and employment in the Information Age 253
NICHOLAS GARNHAM

18 New information technologies and the restructuring of higher education: the constitutional view 268
SANDRA BRAMAN

19 New media and distance education: EU and US perspectives   **290**
    ALAIN DUMORT

20 The virtual university is ... the university made concrete?   **301**
    JAMES CORNFORD

21 Enhancing discourse on new technology within higher
    education   **318**
    MICHELE H. JACKSON AND STEPHEN D. MCDOWELL

22 Toward a digital academe: guiding principles for innovations
    in online education   **328**
    WILLIAM H. DUTTON ET AL.

    Bibliography   336
    Index   358

Illustrations

Figures

10.1	JIME's document interface	143
10.2	Outline of a review debate on the 'Originality and Importance of Ideas'	144
10.3	Lifecycle of an article under review in JIME	145
20.1	Models of universities as organizations	307

Tables

0.1	The interrelated roles ICTs can play in learning and education	4
0.2	The diversity of electronic learning environments: who does what where?	5
8.1	Universitat Oberta de Catalunya: history and organizational background	122
12.1	Firm as traditional technology vendor	173
12.2	Firm as provider of technology, administrative services and marketing	174
12.3	Firm and academic institution share content development	175
12.4	Firm as provider of all components, with some academic contributions	177
13.1	Six models of distance education	187
15.1	Resolving the productivity-innovation dilemma: four models of virtualization	223

Contributors

Philip E. Agre is an associate professor in the Department of Information Studies at the University of California, Los Angeles.

Lloyd Armstrong is Professor of Physics, and Provost and Senior Vice President for Academic Affairs at the University of Southern California, Los Angeles.

Walter S. Baer is at the Rand Corporation in Santa Monica, California where he has directed research in a wide variety of areas related to information and communication technologies.

Alfred Bork is an Emeritus Professor of information and computer science at the University of California, Irvine, where he has pioneered the development of computer-based systems, focusing on tutorial learning systems.

Oliver Boyd-Barrett is Professor of Communication at California State University Polytechnic, Pomona. Prior to joining CSU, he worked at the Open University in the UK for twenty-five years and also directed a distance education initiative at the University of Leicester.

Sandra Braman is the Reese Phifer Professor of Telecommunication in the Department of Telecommunication and Film at the University of Alabama, USA.

(Lord) Asa Briggs was Vice-chancellor of Sussex University (1967–76), Provost of Worcester College, Oxford (1976–91) and the first Chancellor of the UK's Open University. He won the Marconi Medal in 1975 for his work on the history of broadcasting.

James Cornford is a researcher at Newcastle University's Centre for Urban and Regional Development Studies (CURDS). His research is focused on the implications of information and communication technologies for the development of cities and regions.

Alain Dumort wrote his chapter as a Fellow from the European Union and Associate Professor at the School of International Relations, University of Southern California. He joined the European Commission in 1991 as chief economist in telecommunication and was head of new media for education and training from 1996 to 1999. He has been Head of Communication since 2000.

William H. Dutton is Professor of Internet Studies at the University of Oxford, where he is Director of the Oxford Internet Institute and a Fellow in Balliol College.

Nicholas Garnham is Professor of Media Studies at the University of Westminster. He founded the European Communications Policy Research Conference and is a senior editor of *Media, Culture and Society*.

Noriko Hara is Assistant Professor of Information Science in the School of Library and Information Science (SLIS) at Indiana University.

Martin Harris is a senior lecturer at the Department of Accounting, Finance and Management at the University of Essex, UK.

Trevor Haywood is an Emeritus Professor of Human Information Systems, University of Central England, Birmingham, UK.

Maria Henke is the program manager for the online division of the University of Southern California's Ethel Percy Andrus Gerontology Center.

Michele H. Jackson is an assistant professor in the Department of Communication at the University of Colorado, Boulder, where her work focuses on the organizational and social implications of new communication technologies.

Emma Kiselyova is an administrator in the International Office of the Open University of Catalonia, a virtual university headquartered in Barcelona, Spain. Formerly a researcher at the University of California, Berkeley, she conducted studies on the Russian Internet.

Rob Kling is a professor in SLIS at Indiana University, USA, where he directs the Center for Social Informatics, edits *The Information Society* journal, and conducts research about new information and communication technologies and social change.

Brian D. Loader is Director of the Community Informatics Research and Applications Unit (CIRA) based at the University of Teesside, UK. He is also General Editor of the international journal *Information, Communication and Society* (Routledge) and a member of the EU working group on ICTs, Social Movements and Citizens.

Stephen D. McDowell is an associate professor in the Department of Communication at Florida State University, conducting research on the political economy of telecommunications.

A. Michael Noll is a professor and past dean at the Annenberg School for Communication at the University of Southern California, USA, where he teaches courses on technology to students in the social sciences and humanities.

Pamela S. Pease has worked in distance education before taking her doctorate in communication from the Annenberg School for Communication. She is the President of Jones International University and was responsible for achieving accreditation of the first virtual university in the United States. In 1999, the United States Distance Learning Association recognized her with the award of Most Outstanding Achievement by an Individual in Higher Education.

Neil Pollock is a senior research associate at Newcastle University's School of Management. Previously, he conducted research under the Economic and Social Research Council's (UK) Virtual Society? Programme. More recently, he has held an ESRC award to study a University's Student Management System.

Carl Renold is a faculty member of the University of Southern California's Ethel Percy Andrus Gerontology Center.

Edward Schneider is Dean of the Andrus School of Gerontology at the University of Southern California, where he launched its online Masters of Arts in Gerontology.

Sylvia Sensiper worked as the multimedia producer at the Harvard Business School from 1998–9. She has a PhD in Public Policy and Social Research from the University of California, Los Angeles and a Masters in Visual Anthropology from USC.

Tamara Sumner is an assistant professor at the University of Colorado at Boulder, with a joint appointment in the Department of Computer Science and the Institute of Cognitive Science.

Rose M M Wagner is a professor of communication and media science at the University of Applied Sciences in Leipzig, Germany, the Hochschule für Technik, Wirtschaft und Kultur (HTWK). Her main research interests are in the social shaping of technology, cross-cultural communication and ICTs in public administration.

Foreword

Asa Briggs

I greatly appreciate being asked to write a forward to this lively and in many places provocative book. It is forum-based, and I can give it no greater praise than to say that it has made me feel, after reading its many chapters, that I wish I had been present at the forum. Fortunately, the book carries with it the drive to continue debate. The contributors offer first thoughts: and the thoughts – and the insights – will not be the last. People will be far better informed for reading this, and many of them will want to read more. The issues – and it is, above all, a book about issues – are very sharply posed. There are more choices than there are prescriptions.

Having been involved with many university institutions in many different countries, large and small, old and new, 'traditional' and 'innovatory', confident and troubled, I know how difficult it is to generalize. I note that many of the contributors to the book draw on their own specific experiences. I wish, however, that some of them had concerned themselves rather more with comparisons and contrasts in their own learning experiences. Now that I myself am largely de-institutionalized, such comparisons and contrasts in learning, teaching, researching and managing stand out in my mind. I am aware too of the advantages of de-institutionalization. I have seldom found that single institutions learn much from comparisons and contrasts with other institutions even when their histories get written. Now that they are more competitive and at the same time are being drawn into bigger consortia, they may at last be forced to do so, as many of their faculty members and managers always have been.

The focus of this book is rightly on 'learning processes' rather than on educational structures, and thanks to its editors, who have had contrasting if converging experiences, the framework of the book is sturdily constructed. The editors explain very clearly in their introduction how and why they have divided the book into four parts. As they observe, 'four interlinked processes of producing, using, consuming and governing information and communication technologies' comprise the 'pivotal elements' in their conceptual framework. Each of the contributors whom they have assembled has something to say about at least one of these processes. Some lead boldly with all four – and with the context in which they operate as well. At their best, the contributors raise issues rather than simply tell stories, as I guess they were told to do before the forum, but the stories of pioneering new institutions, like Jones International University, accredited by consensus with unbelievable speed, are fascinating in themselves.

It is when institutions are new, anticipating the future rather than recalling the past, that it is the easiest, while also most necessary, to have a complete overview of the whole institution as it is and it is projected to be. There has to be vision then as well as planning. By contrast, old institutions, however proud they may be of their heritage, usually see only through the past and, for all their layers of experience, often darkly. They are, however, of course, face-to-face. Nevertheless, as many contributors to this book demonstrate, changes are taking place in old institutions, some of them exciting, as they move through what is a changing, often rapidly changing, economic, political, social and cultural context.

The twenty-first century pressures on universities of all kinds are strong, and although for economic and political reasons there is often more emphasis inside them on restraints rather than on opportunities, this itself can add to the sense of challenge. Yet the pressures cannot be ignored, and they are political as well as financial. Some of the contributors to this volume are uneasy about claims being made by politicians that new information and communication technologies will solve all problems, and readers of this volume – and I hope that they will include politicians – cannot ignore without peril what these contributors have to say about current university scenarios in which they are actors, not audience. In education as in health – a comparison occasionally made in this book – it is the actors who have to perform the play, whether they are dealing with students or with patients. Both, indeed, are now usually referred to as consumers and they cannot, and should not, be brushed aside. There are some politicians deeply committed to ICTs, however, on both sides of the Atlantic, and they should not be ignored.

Many of the contributors to this volume are keen to give guidance, and there is occasionally a didactic touch to some of the contributions, in itself as recognizable a phenomenon as 'hype'. Yet all the contributors appear to appreciate that, whatever is happening to the learning process, the introduction of information and communication technologies has special significance in opening up access to higher education. Applicants of all ages now examine Web sites and make comparisons of their own. Economics quickly comes in, however, as both public and private providers know. Distance education and distributed learning are not cheap, and so, while the greatest allure of information and communication technologies is their potential, through tele-access, to broaden ways into higher education, there are always financial impediments. There is always too the alarming spectre of a broadening and deepening 'digital gap' which may perpetuate rather than eliminate economic, social and cultural inequalities, national and international. However promising international university networks and consortia may be for faculty and students in higher education, policy makers must inevitably concern themselves, whatever answers they give, with broad social implications, not least when they use the terminology of 'majorities' and 'minorities', rather than 'masses' and 'elites'.

Meanwhile, four other general characteristics seem to me to be relevant. First, information and communication technologies are 'enhancing the visibility of the classroom', as, it should be added, television did during the 1960s. Now, it is not only particular universities that from time to time and for various reasons are placed in the spotlight. Annual 'league lables' in Britain compare universities (and schools) on almost every count, often drawing on insecure statistics. Second, universities and schools are still 'gatekeepers'. Indeed, their role is increasingly important when we talk not of highways but of paths, the metaphor usually chosen in this book. If a university chooses one enterprise course or management system over another, its students will have access to different educational resources from other universities. I personally do not mind this since I intensely dislike university standardization. Reliance on one standard set of electronic 'courseware' is as educationally dissatisfying as reliance on one printed textbook.

Third, for good or ill, the main emphasis in the provision of information and communication technologies will necessarily be on entertainment, dwarfing the provision on education. Of the old trinity 'information, education, entertainment', written into the rules regulating British broadcasting, it is entertainment, judged on ratings in the United States, that always wins, as it does when broadcasting gives way to the Internet, and with personal choice there are few, if any, rules. The use of the ugly, hybrid word 'edutainment' is off-putting in itself. Children as well as university students must be brought into the picture, given that education is a process and not merely an institutional sector. Before beginning the learning process in schools, children learn through children's programmes on television, not all of them specifically for children, or through what is accessible on the Internet. What happens pre-school or in parallel to school can never be left out of the analysis of what comes next, whether or not what comes next is university education.

The fourth of my relevant general considerations is that it is through patterns of organisation and management, as much as through modes of teaching and learning, that information and communication technologies are already influencing, and in the future will influence more, universities and schools as institutions. The editors rightly quote Manuel Castells (2001), who, writing not of universities but of 'all kinds of business', stressed that: 'e-business is not the kind of business that is exclusively conducted on-line, but a new form of conducting business'. It will become increasingly difficult, whatever the pull of nostalgia, to manage universities (and schools) totally differently from other institutions.

On all these issues the editors of this book seek to be wise as well as informed and communicative. A foreword should not echo what will be read later, but rather suggest why what comes later should be read. Yet I want to underline in my own conclusion what the editors say in their introduction. 'The idea of a knowledge society is [and I substitute 'is' for their 'could even be'] misleading if policy makers conclude that ICTs create knowledge, rather than reconfigure access to knowledge and expertise. It is more likely [and I would add more important] that ICT initiatives will be balanced with other educational priorities.' There are many paths leading into the future, not one.

Asa Briggs
Lewes, Sussex
February 2002

Preface

The founders of modern universities built institutional structures and practices around the centrality of libraries in providing teachers, researchers and students with access to books and manuscripts. The revolution in information and communication technologies (ICTs) has changed how people can gain access to information in ways that have shaken the foundations not only of the library, but also of higher education and learning more generally. For better or worse, all sectors of higher education and learning are likely to use ICTs in ways that reconfigure access to information, people, services and technology itself, for instance when students go to the Internet instead of the library, or e-mail their professors rather than visit their offices. The new media can enhance programs in distance education. But it is still an open question as to whether they will be designed and used in ways that enhance the learning activities of individuals, classrooms, the library and colleges and universities as a whole.

Since the late 1800s, colleges and universities have offered opportunities for students to take courses from a distance, initially using the postal service. Since then, remote courses have used nearly every new medium, including the telephone, radio, television, CD-ROMs and the wide range of wired and wireless new communications multimedia. An example of such developments is the UK's Open University (OU), one of the world's leading organizations offering opportunities for mature students to study and take degree-level courses from their homes.

However, nothing in this arena stands still. Today, the Web and other ICT advances have led universities and companies to launch online educational initiatives that have implications well beyond distance education. Over time, the success of key initiatives are enabling the restructuring of higher educational institutions and practices in ways that might support, undermine or restructure traditional campus-based institutions of higher education and blur the boundaries between remote and campus-based practices and institutions.

These initiatives include new universities, such as the Globalwide Network Academy (GNA), one of the first online universities with no physical center providing courses over the Internet, the US Army's Virtual University (eARMYU) and Jones International University (JIU), the first fully accredited virtual university. In the UK the Higher Education Funding Council of England (HEFCE) announced the launch of the e-University initiative in March 2001 "designed to give UK higher education the capacity to compete globally with the major virtual and corporate universities being developed in the United States and elsewhere" (www.hefce.ac.uk/Partners/euniv/). Established universities involved in distance education, such as the OU and Duke's Fuqua School of Business, have also extended their scope and used new ICTs to complement existing offerings. In parallel, traditional campus-based universities have launched initiatives in distributed learning designed to make use of multimedia networks, for example to complement and enrich classroom instruction, as well as enabling students to reach professors and other students outside of the classroom via a multitude of online, e-mail and other electronic channels.

Advances in ICTs, like the Web, enable new forms of access to information, including the ability to search, filter and obtain multimedia information; to participate in drills and practice skills with immediate, personalized feedback; and to visualize processes and learn-by-doing in ever more realistic simulated environments. They also permit access to people, for example by networking students, teachers and outside experts. But the role of ICTs extends beyond the classroom to facilitating routine transactions, such as applying for admission, registering for courses and obtaining counseling, course evaluations and other educational services. These advances are making ICTs more central to the infrastructure of all kinds of educational institutions, including the campus-based 'wired university' and 'virtual classroom'.

There is a growing, urgent debate about the form and pedagogical consequences of alternative approaches to online higher education, such as whether higher education is indeed moving from institution-centered to more student-centered learning and whether the role of faculty is changing. The broad range of expert contributions in this book seeks to illuminate this debate by critically examining developments in distance education and distributed learning. The case studies and comparative analyses presented here highlight the main trends in these areas enabled by advances in ICTs. This provides a basis for understanding the major driving forces behind these initiatives and assessing their implications for the learning process and the institutions and practices of higher education.

A major theme running through this volume is that the value of ICTs to higher education is not predetermined by features of the new media. Many aspects of new media do enable educators to complement and strengthen both distance education programs and existing campus-based educational institutions, enhancing their efficiency and enabling them to reach larger numbers of students. And the involvement of the multimedia industry and many new information providers is reconfiguring access to higher education, such as by blurring distinctions between the producers and users of educational content. However, what will ultimately determine how campus-based and distance education change in the coming decades is how students, teachers, administrators and policy makers respond to 'virtual universities' and the other new-media initiatives that compete with traditional approaches to mainstream higher education.

There are many possible outcomes to these developments. For example, electronic-learning (*e-learning*) could remain peripheral, creating a two-tier system. Or, perhaps, ICTs could support the rise of a select group of global elite-branded universities that offer access and accreditation via the Internet and a network of satellite institutions. The pages of this volume indicate the myriad ways in which the new media open up higher education to these and many other plausible scenarios – seen within the human and institutional contexts that shape the actual outcomes.

Acknowledgments

The origin of this book was an international conference on 'New Media in Higher Education and Learning', organized in 1999 under the auspices of the journal, *Information, Communication and Society* (*iCS*), published by Taylor & Francis/Routledge (www.infosoc.co.uk). The preparation and conduct of this conference convinced us that there was an unmet need for a more empirical and analytical treatment of the debate over the impact of new information and communication technologies on universities and higher education more generally.

The editors organized the original conference and journal symposium with the support and co-operation of the Annenberg School for Communication at the University of Southern California (USC), USA; the Community Informatics Research and Applications Unit (CIRA) of the University of Teesside, UK; the Getty Center; and the publisher Taylor & Francis/Routledge. The conference was held on the USC campus in Los Angeles, California, on behalf of *iCS* on 27–30 October 1999. The last day's sessions were held at the Getty Center in Los Angeles. We are grateful to our colleagues within each of these collaborating institutions for providing the support to launch this book.

The core of the book is based on papers that evolved out of presentations to this conference. Early versions of most chapters were published either in a special issue of *iCS* (vol. 3, no. 4) or in other recent issues of the *iCS* journal. These have been updated where necessary. Other chapters have been specially written for the book to enhance its international range of examples and informed analyses.

We thank the contributors to this volume for participating in our original forum, preparing manuscripts for *iCS* and then revising and up-dating their work for this special collection. We are also very grateful to Malcolm Peltu, whose editorial skills and patience were critical to the quality and timeliness of this publication. Special thanks go to Helen Pickering, Deputy Vice-chancellor at Teesside University, for stimulating our early thinking about a conference on this subject within the convivial environment of an English hostelry. Our thanks also to Claire Taylor of CIRA, who helped us with compiling the combined references and assembling the manuscripts for our publisher. The timeliness of this volume owes much to the imminent birth of Claire's child. Our colleagues at the publisher, Taylor & Francis/Routledge, have provided excellent support – from the provision of constructive peer reviews of our original proposal to the timely and high-quality preparation of our final manuscript. And we would also like to thank our partners and children for their understanding and support of our work.

William H. Dutton, Los Angeles, USA

Brian D. Loader, Swainby, UK

January 2002

The editors wish to thank Taylor & Francis/Routledge for permission to reprint in whole or in part, the following articles, which have been revised and updated for this book:

Chapter 1 source: A. Michael Noll (2000) 'Technology and the future of the university: a sober view', *Information, Communication and Society*, 3:4, 645–7.

Chapter 2 source: Trevor Haywood (2000) 'Defining moments: the tension between richness and reach', *Information, Communication and Society*, 3:4, 648–54.

Chapter 3 source: Sylvia Sensiper (2000) 'Making the case online: Harvard Business School multimedia', *Information, Communication and Society*, 3:4, 616–21.

Chapter 4 source: Edward Schneider, Maria Henke and Carl Renold (2000) 'Targeting working professionals: the master's of arts in gerontology', *Information, Communication and Society*, 3:4, 622–6.

Chapter 5 source: Noriko Hara and Rob Kling (2000) 'Student distress in Web-based distance education', *Information, Communication and Society*, 3:4, 557–79.

Chapter 6 source: Lloyd Armstrong (2001) 'A new game in town: competitive higher education', *Information, Communication and Society*, 4:4, 479–506.

Chapter 7 source: Pamela Pease (2000) 'The virtual university: Jones International University™', *Information, Communication and Society*, 3:4, 627–8.

Chapter 8 is original to this volume.

Chapter 9 source: Alfred Bork (2000) 'Highly interactive tutorial distance learning', *Information, Communication and Society*, 3:4, 639–44.

Chapter 10 source: Tamara Sumner (2000) 'Promoting scholarship through design: a scholarly Web-journal', *Information, Communication and Society*, 3:4, 597–615.

Chapter 11 source: Phil Agre (2000) 'Infrastructure and institutional change in the networked university', *Information, Communication and Society*, 3:4, 494–507.

Chapter 12 source: Walter Baer (2000) 'Competition and collaboration in online distance learning', *Information, Communication and Society*, 3:4, 457–73.

Chapter 13 source: Oliver Boyd-Barrett (2000) 'Distance education provision by universities: how institutional contexts affect choices', *Information, Communication and Society*, 3:4, 474–93.

Chapter 14 is original to this volume.

Chapter 15 source: Martin Harris (2000) 'Virtual learning and the network society', *Information, Communication and Society*, 3:4, 580–96.

Chapter 16 source: Neil Pollock (2000) 'The Virtual University as "timely and accurate information"', *Information, Communication and Society*, 3:3, 349–65.

Chapter 17 source: Nicholas Garnham (2000), '"Information Society" as theory or ideology', *Information, Communication and Society*, 3, 2, 139–52.

Chapter 18 source: Sandra Braman (2000) 'The constitutional context: universities, new information technologies, and the US Supreme Court', *Information, Communication and Society*, 3:4, 526–45.

Chapter 19 source: Alain Dumort (2000) 'New media and distance education: an EU–US perspective', *Information, Communication and Society*, 3:4, 546–56.

Chapter 20 source: James Cornford (2000) 'The virtual university is … the university made concrete?', *Information, Communication and Society*, 3:4, 508–25.

Chapter 21 source: Michele H. Jackson and Stephen D. McDowell (2000) 'Enhancing discourse about new media in higher education', *Information, Communication and Society*, 3:4, 629–38.

Chapter 22 is original to this volume.

Abbreviations and acronyms

AAUP	American Association of University Professors
AFT	American Federation of Teachers
AI	Artificial Intelligence
ALS	Adult Learning Services
ANT	Actor Network Theory
BBC	British Broadcasting Corporation
BMBF	Federal Ministry of Education and Research, Germany
BT	British Telecom
CalREN-2	California Research Education Network 2
CENIC	Consortium for Education Network Initiatives in California
CMA	Computer Marked Assignment
COTS	Commercial Off-The-Shelf, refers to IT products
CSILE	Computer-Supported Intentional Learning Environment
CSU	California State University
CVU	California Virtual University
D3E	Digital Document Discourse Environment
DETC	Distance Education and Training Council, USA
DfEE	Department for Education and Employment, UK (precursor of DfES)
DfES	Department for Education and Skills, UK
DMCA	Digital Millennium Copyright Act, USA
EADTU	European Association of Distance Teaching Universities
eARMYU	Army's Virtual University, USA
ECTS	European Credit Transfer System
eEurope	European Commission initiative to accelerate use of the Internet in EU

e-learning	Electronic-based learning
e-rate	Educational-rate
ERP	Enterprise Resource Planning
ESRC	Economic and Social Research Council, UK
ETMA	Electronic Tutor Marked Assignment
EU	European Union
e-U	eUniversity, UK
FUOC	Foundation Universitat Oberta de Catalunya
GNA	Global Network Academy
HBS	Harvard Business School
HE	Higher Education
HEFCE	Higher Education Funding Council of England
HEI	Higher Educational Institution
HESA	Higher Education Statistics Agency, UK
HTML	Hypertext Markup Language
ICDE	International Council for Distance Education
ICDL	International Center for Distance Learning
iCS	*Information, Communication and Society*
ICT	Information and Communication Technology
IPPR	Institute for Public Policy Research, UK
IPR	Intellectual Property Rights
ISDN	Integrated Services Digital Network
ISP	Internet Service Provider
IT	Information Technology
ITAP	Information Technology Advisory Panel, UK
JANET	Joint Academic Network, UK
JIME	*Journal of Interactive Media in Education*
JISC	Joint Information Systems Committee, UK
JIU	Jones International University
KBE	Knowledge-Building Environment
LSE	London School of Economics and Political Science
MAC	Management and Administrative Computing (system)
MAG	Master of Arts in Gerontology
NCA	North Central Association, USA
NGfL	National Grid for Learning, UK
NII	National Information Infrastructure
NREN	National Research and Education Network, USA
NSF	National Science Foundation, USA
NTU	National Technological University, USA
NYU	New York University
OU	Open University, UK

PC	Personal Computer
PBS	Public Broadcasting Service, USA
PDA	Personal Digital Assistant
RAE	Research Assessment Exercise
TMA	Tutor Marked Assignment
TQA	Teaching Quality Assessment
UBC	University of British Columbia
UC	University of California
UCLA	University of California at Los Angeles
UOC	Universitat Oberta de Catalunya (Open University of Catalonia)
URL	Uniform Resource Locator
USC	University of Southern California
UfI	University for Industry, UK
Webcam	Web camera
WGU	Western Governors University, USA
WITSA	World Information Technologies and Services Alliance
WWW	World Wide Web

Web links relevant to new media in higher education

The following are a selection of Web sites relevant to distance education and distributed learning. They have been referred to directly in this book or have been recommended by one or more contributors. This list is not comprehensive, and does not indicate an endorsement of any particular program or journal. It is aimed at providing readers useful pathways to information on the progress of online initiatives covered in this volume as well as to new developments in related research. Please note that all of the following Web addresses are preceded by http//:

eLearning programs and providers

Army's Virtual University, US	www.eArmyu.com
Athabasca University, Canada's Open University	www.athabascau.ca
Babson Interactive	www.babsoninteractive.com
Blackboard.com	www.blackboard.net
California Virtual University	www.california.edu
Canadian Virtual University	www.cvu-uvc.ca
Capella University	www.capellauniversity.edu
Cardean University	www.cardean.edu
Cenquest	www.cenquest.com
click2learn.com	www.click2learn.com
Collegelearning.com	www.Collegelearning.com
Concord Law School	www.concordlawschool.com
convene.com	www.convene.com
DeVry	www.devry.com

Duke University Fuqua School of Business	www.fuqua.duke.edu
eCollege.com	www.eCollege.com
e-University	www.hefce.ac.uk/Partners/euniv
European Association of Distance Teaching Universities (EADTU)	www.esc.ac.at/intkoop/eadtu.html
European Distance Education Network (EDEN)	www.eden.bme.hu
European University Association	www.unige.ch/eua
Excelsior College joint venture programs	www.excelsior.com
Fathom.com	www.Fathom.com
FT Knowledge	www.ftknowledge.com
Horizon	horizon.unc.edu
Hungry Minds University	www.hungrymindsuniversity.com
IBM Higher Education	www.ibm.com/us
International Council for Open and Distance Education	www.icde.org
International Distance Learning Course Finder	www.dlcoursefinder.com
Jones International University	jiu-web-a.jonesinternational.edu
Keller Graduate School of Management	www.keller.edu
Leicester University	www.le.ac.uk
LifelongLearning.com	www.LifelongLearning.com
London Business School	www.london.edu
MindEdge	www.mindedge.com
National Technological University	www.ntu.edu
Northeastern University Online	www.vcampus.com/nuol
Open University	www.open.ac.uk
Open University of Catalonia (UOC)	www.uoc.es

Park University Distance Learning	www.park.edu/dist/index.htm
Quisic	www.quisic.com/ps/index.htm
Southern Regional Education Board Electronic Campus	www.electroniccampus.org
Thomson Learning	www.thomsonlearning.com
UCLA Extension	www.unex.ucla.edu
UNext	www.unext.com
Universitas 21 Global	www.universitas.edu.au
University of British Columbia	det.cstudies.ubc.ca
University of Maryland University College	www.umuc.edu
University of Phoenix Online	online.uophx.edu
University of Texas System Telecampus	www.telecampus.utsystem.edu
US Distance Learning Association	www.usdla.org
VCampus Corporation	www.vcampus.com
VirtualStudent.com	www.VirtualStudent.com
WebCT.com	www.webct.com
Western Governors University	www.wgu.edu

eLearning research links

American Journal of Distance Education	www.ed.psu.edu/acsde/ajde/jour.asp
Chronicle of Higher Education: Internet Resources	chronicle.merit.edu/free/resources
Distance Education and Technology, University of British Columbia	research.cstudies.ubc.ca
Education Technology and Society	ifets.ieee.org/periodical/
Educause	www.educause.edu
Information, Communication and Society	www.infosoc.co.uk

The Information Society	www.slis.indiana.edu/TIS
International Centre for Distance Learning	icdl.open.ac.uk
International Review of Open and Distance Learning Research	www.irrodl.org
Internet Interdisciplinary Institute (IN3), Spain	www.uoc.es/in3/eng/index.htm
Journal of Asynchronous Learning Networks	www.aln.org/alnweb/journal/jaln.htm
Journal of Computer Assisted Learning	www.blackwell-science.com
Journal of Computer-Mediated Education	www.ascusc.org/jcmc
Journal of Interactive Learning Research	www.aace.org/pubs/jilr/default.htm
Journal of Interactive Media in Education	www-jime.open.ac.uk
Journal of Science Education and Technology	www.gse.harvard.edu/~etc/jset
Networked Chemistry Studies, Germany	www.vs-c.de
New Media and Society	www.new-media-and-society.com
Office of Learning Technologies, Canada	olt-bta.hrdc-drhc.gc.ca
Oxford Internet Institute	www.oii.ox.ac.uk
Pew Learning and Technology Program	www.center.rpi.edu
Virtual Society? Research Programme, UK	virtualsociety.sbs.ox.ac.uk
VIRTUS, Germany	www.virtus.uni-koeln.de

Introduction

New media and institutions of higher education and learning

William H. Dutton and Brian D. Loader

This introduction provides an overview of online education, distributed learning and electronic service delivery in higher education – the digital academe – and a framework within which the issues and debates about new media and higher education can be understood. It also highlights key themes of the contributions to this collection, which concern the factors shaping the development of new media in higher education and the impacts of technological change on the practices and institutions of this sector.

Technological challenges facing higher education and learning

Advocates for change have raised fundamental questions about the adequacy of campus-based and classroom-centric approaches to the institutions and practices of higher education and learning (Noam, 1995; Katz and Rudy, 1999; Daniel, 1998). Advances in information and communication technologies (ICTs), such as a growing range of versatile wireless media and high-speed Internet and Web applications (*The Economist*, 2001), might enable fundamental transformations in education. These parallel developments in the restructuring of business processes, but – for better or worse – these new media could have even more profound implications for the reinvention of educational institutions because of the centrality of knowledge creation, acquisition and dissemination to conceptions of the information age, the knowledge society and to the learning process.

New ICTs are an increasingly pervasive aspect of contemporary society. They have been tied by many researchers and observers to broadly-based change in social structures and practices, for example to the erosion of hierarchy, the emergence of more consumer-oriented demand for flexible learning opportunities and the rise of networked organizations (Shapiro, 1999; Castells, 2000, 2001; Rifkin, 2000; Dertouzos, 2001). In higher education, this has led to conceptions of a 'virtual university', competition for being the most technically up-to-date 'wired' university[1] and a resurgence of interest in distance education. New educational ideas like this are being heard around the world and manifested in experiments, strategic plans, online degree programs and commercial ventures in private industry, educational institutions and various public programs (Katz and Rudy, 1999).

While the production and use of new ICTs in education and throughout society has been supported by business, industry and government, there is evidence of growing 'digital divide' inequalities (Schiller, 1996; Lax, 2001), concern over the erosion of quality (Noble, 2001) and renewed doubts whether rapid ICT innovations can be sustained, as highlighted by the turn-of-the-century crash of many 'dot-com' startups. However, it would be wrong to write a requiem for online education. Just as many early forecasts were overly optimistic, many later forecasts have failed to recognize real, albeit more evolutionary, transformations occurring already in academia – where digital technology is tied to broader social, economic, cultural and political change. For example, despite the downturn in the technology sector, enrollment in online courses has continued to grow and new programs expand, from the US Army's Virtual University (eARMYU) to Duke's Fuqua School of Business (*Business Week*, 2001). The fate of a digital academe is not connected to the outcomes of dot-com startups, but depends on what emerges from the increasing application and use of ICTs across all processes central to higher education and learning, from teaching to managing institutions. Manuel Castells said it best in the context of business:

> e-Business is not the business that is exclusively conducted on-line but a new form of conducting business, all kinds of business, by, with, and on the Internet and other computer networks – with various forms of linkage with on-site production processes and physical transactions.
>
> (Castells, 2001: 102)

ICTs are becoming increasingly central in all these ways, not only in terms of how higher educational institutions accomplish their tasks, but also in relation to the nature of the products and services they provide, for instance in considering new initiatives in distance education. Mindful of the failure of many ICT innovations in the late 1990s and earlier decades, this volume focuses attention on the institutions and practices that form the context of successful, failed or still formative technical and organizational innovations, in order to deepen understanding of how people design, incorporate, adapt or reject technologies to reinforce or restructure practices and institutions (ESRC, 2001).

Four interlinked processes of producing, using, consuming and governing ICTs in higher education comprise the pivotal elements of a conceptual framework for this book (Dutton, 1996: 2–4; ESRC, 2001). Before we discuss this organizing framework more fully, the next section provides an overview of what has been called 'tele-access' (Dutton, 1999): the role of ICTs in reconfiguring access – physical and electronic – to information, people, services and technologies in higher education and learning. This next section is therefore designed to clarify the book's broad definition of 'digital academe' and is followed by an elaboration of how the digital academe can reshape tele-access.

The concept of a 'digital academe': ICTs in all aspects of higher education

Education and training are widely regarded as being key to social and economic development, as indicated by the invention of terms like the 'knowledge society', and the identification of education, science and technology as the basis for a sound industrial policy. These views are allied to a belief that investment in ICTs can nurture a virtuous cycle in which education supports innovations in the technologies, which in turn improve learning and education (Noll and Mays, 1971: 2; Freeman, 1996; Castells, 2000). For example, one of America's leading pioneers in promoting information infrastructures, former Vice-president Al Gore (1991), initially focused US government efforts on building information infrastructures for education through the National Research and Education Network (NREN). The success of networking for research, particularly on the Internet in its early forms, led the Clinton–Gore administration to promote a new generation of high-performance computing initiatives, along with the goal of connecting all classrooms to a National Information Infrastructure (NII).

This focus on education has been evident in many other advanced economies, such as in Britain where education was a central aspect of ICT policy in national policy during the early 1980s (ITAP, 1982). In 1997, the newly elected British Prime Minister, Tony Blair, promised that his government's three main priorities would be "Education.

Education. Education." The importance of ICTs in education was emphasized through the announcement of the UK National Grid for Learning (NGfL), including the policy objective of connecting all UK schools, community centers, museums and other centers of learning to the Internet (www.dfee.gov.uk/grid/).

Knowledge is a key resource. But like information it is not a new one (Drucker, 1993: 41). What is changing is how people – teachers, researchers and students – gain access to knowledge, information or expertise (Dutton, 1999). The idea of a knowledge society could even be misleading if policy makers conclude that ICTs create knowledge, rather than reconfigure access to knowledge and expertise. It is more likely that ICT initiatives will be balanced with other educational priorities if educators and politicians focus on the value of ICTs as carriers that support 'tele-access', rather than as creators of knowledge (Kay, 1991: 100; Dutton, 1999).

As already mentioned, ICTs are central to shaping the future of education, research and the sciences by changing how we get access to information, people, services and technologies themselves (Table 0.1).

Table 0.1 The interrelated roles ICTs can play in learning and education

Information access

- Searching, screening, and obtaining multimedia information
- Drill and practice with immediate, personalized feedback
- Visualizing and learning by doing

Access to people

- Networking with students, teachers, experts
- Institutional networking among administrators

Access to services

- Facilitating routine transactions, such as course registration
- Packaging and distribution of educational services
- Breaking down distinctions between producers and users

Access to technology

- Learning about ICTs through routine exposure and use
- Wiring dormitories, classrooms and offices for electronic access
- Using ICTs to improve learning and education

Source: Adapted from Dutton (1999: 205)

E-mail, multimedia communication, the Internet and other ICT-based innovations – like the printing press before – are not just new blackboards. They are changing the way we do things and also the outcomes of these processes – the very information, people, services and technologies we can access. In doing so, they can undermine or support the role of traditional gatekeepers in education such as teachers. However, they also foster new gatekeepers, such as the developers of complete electronic platforms – known as 'courseware' – and content that support learning activities, or the management of educational processes like access to digital library resources. ICTs shape who gets access to which knowledge producers and users – and blur the accepted distinctions among them.

Distance education v. distributed learning

Distance education was once distinctly different from campus-based education. However, the use of ICTs such as the Internet in higher education and learning is not only erasing this distinction, but also creating new categories (Table 0.2). Distance education programs, such as the UK's Open University (see Chapters Thirteen and Fifteen), have been based at a central facility, where teams create a variety of print and electronic materials for remote students, in collaboration with high-quality media experts, such as from the BBC. ICTs, it is argued, can be used to expand such programs into truly 'mega-universities' (Daniel, 1998).

Table 0.2 The diversity of electronic learning environments: who does what where?

		Students	
		Campus-based	*Remote*
Teachers	*Campus-based*	Classrooms (lectures, chalk-talk, e-mail, slide presentation software, online syllabi)	Distance education (e.g. Open University); Mega-Universities
	Remote	Libraries (one-many media, text books, journals, teleconferences, educational videos, instructional media)	Virtual Universities (e.g. Jones International University) with no physical center, offering online simulations and computer-based tutorial systems

ICTs are also being used to create new 'virtual universities', for instance, the Canadian Virtual University (www.cvu-uvc.ca), Jones International University (see Chapter Seven) or the Open University of Catalonia (see Chapter Eight); these utilize networks not only to reach remote students, but also to enable distributed teams of staff and teachers to create content and courses. The notion of a 'virtual' university or classroom is based essentially on this idea of ICTs eliminating the necessity for students or teachers to be physically present on a campus or in a classroom. At the extreme, some virtual university proponents believe that media like the Internet can serve the functions of the traditional university by substituting for face-to-face education and learning (Noam, 1995; Denning, 1996).

This is arguably one of the most non-traditional visions of online education enabled by ICTs, alongside that of individualized tutorial systems, which might be viewed as an extreme representation of the virtual university (see Chapter Nine). But even traditional, campus-based education is employing many of the same online media, particularly the Internet and Web to enhance course work. This enables students to get electronic access, for instance, to class readings and notes, or to contact teachers round the clock via e-mail. Students are being perceived increasingly as customers who expect easy online access to services and resources from anywhere at any time. Such access challenges the notion of campus boundaries which can act to transfigure the student–institution relationship. At the University of Teesside, for example, initiatives are under way to use this flexible approach to provide educational and learning support for mature students in their own 'off-campus' community settings. This is potentially beneficial for widening educational opportunities for those students whose personal circumstances often present barriers to conventional higher education. These include single parents, unemployed people and those requiring a more sensitive recruitment to foster higher self-esteem.

Finally, the use of books, video tapes, compact disks (CDs) and digital video discs (DVDs) in courses illustrates the most common, but often taken-for-granted, form of distance learning: the incorporation of external, teaching material and teachers into the classroom. Decades ago, Wilbur Schramm (1977: 13–14) reminded those who looked at TV as a teaching machine that: "almost all teaching is multi-media ... with an active teacher plus textbook plus much more." Extensions of this bringing in of remote expertise into the classroom include the use of multipoint video conferencing over the telephone or Internet, as a means of holding real-time distributed class sessions by networking a classroom with teachers or students at other universities (Table 0.2).

Some chapters of *Digital Academe* focus on 'distance education', others on virtual universities and others on more traditional campus-based institutions. In reading across these selections, the editors encourage you as a reader to adopt our broad definition of the many old and emerging institutional forms and practices of distance education and distributed learning, and how all are subject to change as a consequence of advances in ICTs.

Electronic services and new management paradigms

But there is more tied into a digital academe. The administration and services of higher educational institutions are also being transformed by electronic media, as other chapters of *Digital Academe* explain (see Chapters Sixteen and Twenty). From surveying the Web sites of competing universities to applying for admission to registering for classes and obtaining grades, more students will be linked to their universities over Web-based services.

It is therefore the whole environment of higher education – not just the classroom, but teaching, learning, managing and obtaining services – that is being increasingly embedded in electronic resources. This is creating an increasingly 'digital' academe. To some, this represents an unprecedented opportunity to reinvent higher education for the information age (Noam, 1995; Chapter Nine). To others, it raises the specter of increasing commercialization and the erosion of quality in higher education (Robins and Webster, 1989; Schiller, 1996: 27–41; Noble, 2001). We believe this debate can be informed and sharpened by a focus on the role of ICTs in reshaping access, using the framework adopted in this book: which orients research and analysis to the processes of consumption, production, utilization and governance of ICTs in higher education.

Reshaping tele-access in education and learning

Tele-access clarifies the primary role of ICTs in education, where they are far more than just instructional technologies. ICTs are obviously important to the storage and distribution of information, as evident in the increasing use of online journals and other electronic resources. However, ICTs are not simply a new multimedia encyclopedia. Tele-access to people, services and technology – not just information – is also of broad importance to education (Table 0.1), such as in whether or not teachers and students have access to expertise and the infra-structure of a wired university.

Access to information

The Internet has highlighted the role ICTs can play in searching, screening and obtaining electronic information and print publications, for instance in using an online catalog to find books in the library, and in supplementing other educational media, such as text books. For example, in the weeks following the 1997 landing of the Pathfinder mission on Mars, images relayed from the Sojourn rover to the Jet Propulsion Laboratory (JPL) in California were seen by millions round the world over the Internet.[2] Similarly, video of a university lecture can be put up on the Web or Webcast to enable it to be seen anywhere in the world as it occurs. Students can look through 'Webcams' – cameras linked online to be viewed by Web browsers – located anywhere, such as underwater at a coral reef to observe marine life in real time at any time, including even controlling a camera's focus. Images of September 11, 2001 in New York City and Washington DC were viewed live via the Internet around the world.

Video technology, of course, also enables events and other multi-media material to be recorded and stored for future viewing, research and teaching. For instance, many universities have replaced idiosyncratic collections of 35 mm slides of art works with access to huge distributed digital archives of images covering the history of art, permitting students to view images outside of class. Visionaries of high-speed 'broadband' networks see a day when schools can search and retrieve an increasingly wide array of high-quality multimedia materials, at low cost, through electronic networks, creating an educational video juke-box for households and schools (Gell and Cochrane, 1996).

Digital imaging can do more than simply permit more students to access multimedia documents and video from anywhere in the world. High-resolution cameras and digital enhancements can provide access to new information, such as better satellite images of the earth. One of the 'Initiatives for Access' undertaken by the British Library, for instance, was the digitization of the earliest known manuscript of Beowulf, which included images from passages of the poem that were hidden by damage that occurred in a fire in 1731 (Kenny, 1994). Digital imaging provided access to more information about the manuscript, while also making it accessible worldwide. Another example is in the study of human anatomy, where the US National

Library of Medicine's Visual Human Project has enabled worldwide access to a valuable archive of anatomically detailed, three-dimensional representations of human bodies (www.nlm.nih.gov/research/visible/ visible_human.html).

A powerful means of coping with the huge and growing volumes of electronic information has been the development of hypertext versions of course material, first on CDs, and more recently on DVDs and the Web (Rose, 2000). Researchers, teachers and students can benefit from these tools for locating information relevant to their studies. A rapidly-accumulating corpus of electronic news coverage, trade and professional magazines, scholarly journals and books has increased the importance of tools for searching electronic resources on the Internet and Web.

Learning by virtually doing: drill and simulation

Early uses of computers in education focused on the development of instructional software that emphasized drill and practice, particularly in managing repetitive exercises in the basics, such as arithmetic, spelling and grammar. Early drill and practice software generally failed to utilize the value of computers as a means for encouraging students to discover facts and ideas on their own (Miles, Rush, Turner and Bessant, 1988: 205–12). This criticism has been addressed in the best drill and practice courseware by incorporating many game-like features and colorful elements of 'discovery software', that leads students in a process of discovery rather than in repetition to support the memorization of facts. Modern multimedia ICTs permit immediate and personalized feedback that can be far more imaginative, flexible and engaging than earlier generations of computer-aided instruction. These techniques are also of value to adults, as in grammar and style checks in some word processing software.

However, educators have increasingly emphasized the value of ICTs in helping students and researchers at all levels to visualize and learn by doing. One of the leading exponents of computers in schools (Papert, 1980: viii) argued long ago that simulation is the primary advantage of the computer. Many kinds of 'virtual reality' (VR) systems have been developed, including architectural modeling and entertainment games, which create more realistic simulated environments by enabling users to feel they are immersed in a three-dimensional audio and video image of an animated scene with which they can interact.[3]

ICTs support an expanding variety of models, simulations and games that permit students to discover how a process works, instead of only reading about it (Gell and Cochrane, 1996; Schroeder, 1996). For example, flight simulators have been used in VR environments to train pilots. Simulations have been adapted to a diversity of activities, from training railroad engineers, by permitting an engineer to take a realistic drive on a route many times in varying weather conditions before actually driving a real cargo, to military training.[4] Hollywood talent has teamed with multimedia software developers to create more realistic simulations for the military, which could have spinoffs for other arenas of education and learning.[5]

An exploding variety of other models and simulations coming onto the market can be applied to education and learning. Alfred Bork (see Chapter Nine) pushes this vision further – seeing computers as a means for simulating electronically more traditional and effective forms of tutorial education, which he sees as superior to traditional one-to-many lecture formats that, he argues, characterize most uses of the Web in higher education.

Access to people: networking

Student–teacher communication, student-student dialogue and collaboration among researchers across space and time can be supported by ICTs like e-mail and course management groupware such as Blackboard (www.blackboard.com) or WebCT (www.WebCT.com). E-mail, video conferencing and other ICTs can be used to link students and specialists. Apple Computer, for instance, pioneered the use by school children of desk-top video communications to ask questions of experts, who could respond to them when they were available. This idea is reflected routinely on computer networks when individuals post questions such as: "Does anybody know about … ?" Such applications enable students at any level to access a far wider range of expertise than provided by their teachers, while raising issues over the quality of information and the credentials of 'experts' on the Web.

This communication support is also of value to institutional networking. Teachers, students and administrators can use e-mail or other ICTs to network with other schools for sharing ideas and co-ordinating joint events, projects, speakers or other resources. In higher education, inter-library loan and similar co-operative agreements on resource sharing are being facilitated and enlarged by electronic networking. As Philip Agre (Chapter Eleven) argues, many of the most important networks among researchers are remote rather than resident at one's university, making the Internet a particularly critical tool for collaboration, but also reconfiguring with whom one is likely to collaborate.

Access to services: re-engineering the management of higher education

ICTs can facilitate routine transactions and services in education, just as they can in government and business. For example, students at many universities can register for courses over any push button phone or on the Web and not have to wait in line during the days of regular registration. Such electronic services may not be as interesting and widely discussed as those tied to the provision of teaching, but they can be critically important both to the efficiency of services and in shaping the choices of students. For example, a student browsing the Web for courses or for universities to apply to, might make different selections from those students sitting down with their parents, friends or teachers. This is one reason why teachers market themselves and their courses on the Web and why universities seek to have a greater presence on the Web. Students' reactions to university Web sites are one of the most important factors shaping their decisions on where to apply, running close behind the general reputation of a university and personal visits to a campus.

Packaging information in electronic forms can also create new ways to distribute and sell educational services. Departments can subscribe to privately licensed online databases, like LexisNexis™, which facilitates electronic access to a wide range of information, from legal documents to current news coverage (www.lexis-nexis.com). A small liberal-arts college might obtain courseware from a larger research university that would enable it to increase its course offerings, such as for a new course in business, without adding new faculty. Universities can acquire enterprise course management software, such as Blackboard or WebCT, to make it easier for teachers to put their courses online and administer tests and grading. Electronic services such as these, particularly those with interactive capabilities, are changing the producers of information, and at the same time they are helping to break down distinctions between the producers and users of information, such as when the users of an electronic forum also contribute to the creation of its content.

Access to technologies: the wired and wireless campus

The routine use and integration of ICTs in the curriculum enables teachers and students to better cope with and exploit the Web and other ICT tools in their everyday life. Teachers cannot simply put students in front of a computer and expect them to learn. However, guided exposure of teachers and students can enhance awareness of ICTs, which is one important step towards learning how to understand and exploit technologies in learning and education. Some of the best education courseware is designed to enable college teachers without multimedia skills, such as in hypertext markup languages (HTML), to put their course materials online. This kind of introduction sometimes enables the teacher to see new ways of using more online applications within their courses as they learn by doing. Similarly, college students using their Internet ports to download popular music or chat with friends can gain a better sense of the potential of the Internet for gaining access to all sorts of other electronic resources. But innovation in habits and routine processes is not automatic.

A variety of initiatives are seeking to improve the proficiency of teachers and students in the use of computing, what some have called 'computer literacy'. The most widely publicized are initiatives to get computers, educational software and broadband communications into classrooms and educational institutions to support students' access to electronic technologies and resources. Most universities in the USA are expected to have student dormitories wired for Internet access and classrooms that have fixed facilities for multimedia access, from linking to the Web to showing a video, thereby creating a huge demand for new investments in equipment and staff to install and maintain the wired university. Innovations in wireless Internet access are adding a new layer of access that students will expect to be ubiquitous in due course.

At the high end, in Europe, for example, British Telecom (BT)'s Super Joint Academic Network (SuperJANET) links higher educational institutions in the UK. UK initiatives for a NGfL build on this. In the USA, the National Science Foundation (NSF) supported a variety of high-performance computing initiatives, such as the Consortium for Education Network Initiatives in California (CENIC) to design and deploy CalREN-2, an advanced network for linking state educational institutions to each other and the national high-speed information superhighway.[6] As these technologies mature, some commercial products and services have tended to shift attention from these public-led efforts and towards competing providers.

A framework for debate and analysis: the structure of this book

One central question about the role of 'new' technologies in many contexts revolves around whether they are tied to the restructuring of practices and institutions (ESRC, 2001). This book focuses on the role of ICTs in restructuring access in ways that change how students, professors, administrators, policy makers and other actors consume, produce, utilize and govern ICTs in higher education and learning. The aim is to inform theory and practice, and to contribute to research efforts focused on these four issues.[7] An understanding of these processes and the interrelationships among them can foster a more complete assessment of change and help move debate away from overly simplistic utopian-dystopian perspectives.

The book's editors have organized the contributions under each of the four headings. You will find that all of the chapters have some relationship to each of these processes, despite our identification of their central contribution. In fact, one role of new ICTs has been to diminish the distinctions between the producers and consumers of information. But all chapters contribute to an understanding of the restructuring of practices and institutions tied to the consumption, production, utilization and governance of ICTs in higher education and learning. The following sub-sections illustrate the range of questions and topics covered by these broad terms.

Consumption: conceptions of teachers and students and their reactions to ICTs (Part I)

Part I of this book focuses on consumption as it is concerned with how people incorporate, adapt, domesticate, subvert, resist and otherwise shape how ICTs fit into the lecture, classroom, college or everyday life. This leads to questions such as: How do different cultures, genders, classes and ethnic, age and disability groups use online education? Will students use the new media as a complement or as a substitute for classroom activities?

In Chapter One of this volume, Michael Noll argues that the impact of ICTs will be limited, in light of what the history of media in education has told us about the centrality of face-to-face communication in the learning process.

While Trevor Haywood (Chapter Two) is far from optimistic about new media, he questions the picture many critics of new media paint of the traditional classroom. Many classrooms, he argues, fall short of our often romantic images of teaching. This realism leads him to take a more positive and contingent perspective on the future of online education, such as using its potential 'reach' to address the growing gap in access to a traditional high-quality education. ICTs might help to reduce, rather than reinforce, socioeconomic divisions in educational opportunities.

The potential for what Haywood calls 'richness' in education is seen in Sylvia Sensiper's description (Chapter Three) of how new media can enhance an already well-regarded instructional approach like Harvard's famous case method. She not only illustrates how ICTs can enhance the richness of case presentations, creating a complementarity of old and new media, but also the potential for online access to change how students explore information in ways that are suggestive of the discovery software discussed above.

Haywood's concept of 'reach' is illustrated by Chapter Four, which provides an overview of an online professional program that focuses on working professionals. In it, Schneider, Henke and Renold make a strong case for the new media enhancing the ability of producers to target specific audiences using ICTs to better inform more people, rather than reinforce knowledge gaps. Their case study of remote professional education in the field of gerontology indicates how the growing use of ICTs in all sectors of education can influence institutions and practices such as influencing how and where students learn.

But what are the social implications of the immediacy and proximity of online access to information, people and services, for instance in relation to information overload, social isolation and collective memory? Some of these conventional expectations of the limits of online education are actually off the mark, according to Noriko Hara and Rob Kling (Chapter Five). They report on their studies of the problems students experienced in an online distance education class, alerting us to the extent that we can entertain romantic views of online as well as traditional courses. In their view, problems with the design and implementation of this particular online distance learning course tended to undermine, rather than support, learning and education. They argue that online media are far from a 'technical fix' and that effective online teaching is going to require as much training and education as do traditional approaches to teaching. Their contribution provides a more sobering view of the student, in line with Noll's admonition in Chapter One, and directs more attention to the production of online education, which is taken up by Part II.

Production: new actors and approaches to creating and delivering content (Part II)

Social, cultural and political processes shape innovations in products, services and industries, including the structure of institutions in higher education. This raises questions about production – the focus of Part II of this collection – such as: how are the business models or the competitive environments of universities changing as the primary product for exchange is information that can be replicated and redistributed round the world at virtually no cost, for instance by sharing scholarly journals and other electronic resources over the Web?

In the lead chapter of Part II, Lloyd Armstrong (Chapter Six) provides a broad overview of the changing landscape of higher education in the US. He focuses on the prospects of heightened competition among the producers of educational offerings within a broadening geographical arena. His senior position in a major private university with a strong international orientation helps him offer a particularly insightful discussion of the strategic choices that face traditional campus-based universities within this new 'winner-take-all' environment (Frank and Cook, 1996). New ICTs appear to be playing a significant role in changing this competitive environment of higher education, and creating strategic concerns, including issues over how to protect and capitalize on a reputation for quality while competing against globally-branded online providers.

One set of competitors are the new decentralized, non-hierarchical organizational forms emerging as 'virtual universities'. Pamela Pease (Chapter Seven) provides an overview of one of the first accredited virtual universities in the US, Jones International University (JIU), of which she is President. She gives us a very concrete sense of this new organizational form and its continued growth and viability. One potential for the global virtual university is to assemble teachers and students electronically to form a critical mass that will enable universities to serve more specialized audiences.

An illustration of just such a provider is offered by Emma Kiselyova (Chapter Eight), who describes another virtual university, the Open University of Catalonia (UOC), where she is an administrator. Located in Barcelona, UOC aspires to use ICTs and the Catalan language to reach a large but widely dispersed audience across the world. Like the UK's Open University, UOC combines an open admissions policy with its use of distance education.

Digital media are not simply enabling new forms of distance education. They are also challenging underlying models of education and learning, such as by creating the potential for more individualized forms of tutorial learning to be economical on a global scale. Alfred Bork (Chapter Nine) argues that the production of contemporary campus-based and distance education is dominated by a one-to-many paradigm, despite the advance of interactive Web-based media. His vision of teams producing highly-interactive tutorial learning systems is a radical departure from current practice, replacing instructors with well-designed software to eliminate the major bottleneck in reaching the larger world of students. The high initial costs of development would be compensated, he argues, by the potentially global reach of tutorial systems.

It is not simply the teaching process that is being challenged by new media. Practices and institutions of scholarly research and publication are also anchored in older media. Tamara Sumner (Chapter Ten) illustrates how the new media enable new forms of scholarly review, which promise to change the content of scholarly publication as well as the processes for its production. In the final chapter of this section, Philip Agre (Chapter Eleven) looks broadly at how the practices and institutional arrangements of universities can be re-imagined in light of new media. How are structures, ranging from the classroom to the library, changing through the use of ICT-based capabilities? What are the barriers to achieving full synergy from the network of 'invisible colleges' across the world and creating global communities of scholars and students without pulling apart the university as a geographically-localized network? This leads to the consideration of management and organizational responses to new media in higher education, the focus of Part III.

Utilization: new organizational forms designed to employ the new media (Part III)

The way technologies are used in service provision, management and work can reinforce or transform the structure, geography and processes of organizations, in which social and organizational changes are inseparable from technological change. Key related questions include: how, and with what implications, are different kinds of universities creating new structures and processes to effectively use e-learning capabilities? In the first chapter of this section, Walter Baer (Chapter Twelve) provides a powerful typology that captures the diversity of management options open to universities. There is clearly no one best way to structure the digital academe, but Boyd-Barrett (Chapter Thirteen) argues that the political-administrative context of different universities provides one important factor shaping the best way forward. Together, Baer and Boyd-Barrett present a wide range of organizational responses to incorporating new media in higher education.

One notion furthered by earlier contributions to this volume is that new forms of e-learning enable fundamental shifts in the geography of educational institutions, such as in fostering more consortia among educational institutions or new forms of 'network' – non-hierarchical – organizations. Rose Wagner (Chapter Fourteen) presents a case in point from a German experience of developing a consortium of universities – the Virtual University of Applied Sciences. She examines the social and political forces behind this new organization form, such as increased international competition from the University of Phoenix and other providers interested in an international market. She also addresses changes in production associated with such developments, for instance the increased separation of teaching and the production of content.

Networked universities are but one manifestation of a broader argument about ICTs creating a force for change across all kinds of organizations – privileging network forms of organization over more hierarchical structures (Freeman, 1996; Castells, 2000, 2001). Martin Harris (Chapter Fifteen) seeks to address this general theoretical proposition by comparing changes in the UK's Open University with proposals for a new UK educational initiative – the University for Industry. His cases lead him to challenge some critics of the virtual university as well as some theorists of new organizational forms, since he finds many avenues toward virtualization emerging from complex sets of social, policy and institutional histories.

The administrative and managerial dimensions of the way organizations are being reconfigured to take advantage of new ICTs is also addressed in Part III. Historically, teaching, research and administration of universities have been relatively separate organizational fiefdoms. But the Internet and Web are creating a common interface for students and teachers to interact with one another and the university. Will the informational by-products of online education and electronic service delivery, such as day-to-day operational and management information, enable universities to be more efficient and business-like? And what will be the effect on the institution and quality of learning and education? Neil Pollock (Chapter Sixteen) examines one traditional campus-based university's efforts to use 'timely and accurate' information to better plan and manage operations. He notes the degree to which ICTs did not simply enable more timely or accurate information, but helped foster a way of thinking about the university that placed a premium on this value.

Governance: the control and regulation of ICTs in higher education (Part IV)

Part IV focuses on governance. Studies of the governance of ICTs examine the political and social processes of control that regulate technology and balance competing values and interests, including the role of technological change in governance processes. For example, the beliefs or paradigms of individuals, such as Pollock's (Chapter Sixteen) highlighting of the value of 'timely and accurate information' govern how they respond to new technologies. In the first contribution to this section, Nicholas Garnham (Chapter Seventeen) extends this argument, challenging widely-held assumptions about the new information society. He recognizes that acceptance of an 'information society' or new 'ICT-paradigm' (Freeman, 1996) shapes our responses to technical change. However, he believes that many advocates of the information society have uncritically accepted the assumptions underpinning this new paradigm. It has become almost an ideology rather than a theory that merits continual challenge and refinement through empirical research and reflection.

A more conventional focus of governance studies has been on public policy and regulation. Public policies are both a major driving force and constraint on the diffusion of ICTs in higher education, such as in the area of intellectual property rights. Two chapters focus on this national policy context. Sandra Braman (Chapter Eighteen) reviews case law in the US Supreme Court that deals with educational institutions. One important implication of her review is the degree of latitude that the court has provided to educational institutions to create policies within their institutions, such as over intellectual property, that enable them to take new initiatives in such areas as distance education and distributed learning. For example, legal actions of private businesses and industries – from entrepreneurial teachers interested in marketing their courseware to the recording industry interested in protecting their artists – are challenging the practices of universities (Noble, 2001). Braman shows that universities join this debate, particularly in the US setting, from a strong legal position in the courts.

Generally, however, public agencies round the world have sought to stimulate and foster the development of the digital academe. Much debate surrounds what educational policies best serve the public interest in a digital society. Alain Dumort (Chapter Nineteen) draws from his experience in the European Commission and studies in the USA to provide an overview of efforts to promote distance education. Like other key leaders in policy and politics within Europe and North America, he sees distance education as a key objective for information societies, echoing the UK's commitment to education and the value of ICTs in extending educational opportunities. His chapter raises interesting questions over how different cultures (humanities v. science and engineering) and regulatory regimes (public v. for-profit) impinge on the production of online educational services. Do national or regional differences in governance and regulation of the media, such as in the area of copyright, advantage some jurisdictions over others in the emerging global marketplace? Can the regulations of national governments and institutions, for instance, keep up with the pace of change in ICTs?

Technology itself may play a role in the governance of higher education, to the extent, as James Cornford (Chapter Twenty) argues, that the digital environment of universities is making these institutions and practices more transparent and therefore more susceptible to critical scrutiny. The simple step of teachers placing their course syllabi on the Web is one example of how ICTs make the classroom more transparent to the outside world, with potentially significant implications for accountability, oversight and control. Management information systems can have similar consequences.

The implications of ICTs on higher education and learning are therefore great, but it has been one of the least closely examined arenas in the application of ICTs across different practices and institutions. Social research on the institutional implications of the revolution in ICTs is far more likely to focus on business or government, for example, than on education. Why are the humanities and the social sciences not more reflexive when their own institutional settings are under challenge? At the end of this section, Michele Jackson and Stephen McDowell (Chapter Twenty-one) explore the relative lack of discourse within higher education, and argue for nurturing more debate within colleges and universities. More strategic choices about the future of higher education and learning depend on a more informed debate about the digital academe.

The book concludes with a brief coda compiled by William Dutton, who builds on the work of a committee at the University of Southern California (Chapter Twenty-two). This shifts to a more prescriptive set of guidelines on governance to help steer ICT initiatives in higher education and learning that move towards a digital academe. These are based on the contributions to this volume and debates within academe. The editors hope these guidelines and the book as a whole will help foster the kinds of debate advocated by Jackson and McDowell (Chapter Twenty-one).

Cross-cutting themes and issues

In spanning these four general processes – consumption, production, utilization and governance – the diverse contributions to this book raise a number of integrating themes and concepts that could help shape theory and research in the study of ICTs within higher education and in other institutional settings. These include issues regarding the social shaping of ICTs as well as their impacts on institutions and practices.

Shaping the role of ICTs in learning and education

The future of new media in higher education and learning is open-ended. Debate often focuses on whether online education will fail or succeed, but the real issues in the social shaping of digital academe revolve around more specific technological and organizational designs. A number of social – political, economic and cultural – factors shaping choices on the design and organization of new media in higher education are highlighted by the contributions to this book.

Utopian (dystopian) discourse over promises and threats

Many contributions reflect the fact that discussion of ICTs in higher education and learning is marked by a pro- versus anti-technology debate that has characterized Utopian versus dystopian extremes of much discourse about the role of technology in society (Mesthene, 1969). As Ellen Rose (2000: ix) put it, on issues of computers and education, there "appears to be no reasoned middle ground". However, the prominence of this utopian–dystopian controversy in this field underscores the degree to which new media challenge traditional practices and institutions in fundamental ways. They promise (threaten) to change the way we teach and learn, and strike at the institutions built around these traditional practices (see Chapters One and Two). The changes discussed in this collection range beyond the classroom to envelop nearly all aspects of higher education, from the recruitment and registration of students to the awarding of degrees and creation of opportunities for 'life-long learning' programs.

Change in the very geography and status of educational institutions is at stake.

The strongest proponents of ICTs in learning and education, like Alfred Bork (Chapter Nine), see the potential for new media to improve learning and extend the reach of the best instruction to the world. In contrast, many critics, like Michael Noll (Chapter One), fear that the growing centrality of distance education and distributed learning could undermine quality teaching and erode the intellectual and academic climate of the university (Noble, 2001). Trevor Haywood (Chapter Two) points out that critics of online learning frequently display a romantic view of traditional classroom teaching. Nevertheless, the habits, values and traditions of higher education represent a fundamental social factor constraining innovation and muting more informed debate over policy and practice, as argued by Michele Jackson and Stephen McDowell (Chapter Twenty-one).

Early advocates of educational innovation have criticized schooling at all levels as a 'holdover' of the industrial age (Toffler, 1970; Williams, 1982: 215–26). Educational institutions are conservative. Lecture and discussion in many contemporary classrooms still follow a traditional 'chalk-talk' format, which may remain ideal for some material, such as in mathematics, where some teachers see a professor writing in chalk as a natural way to keep the right pace for students to follow the development of a solution. Many law professors, for example, pride themselves on their ability to employ a Socratic dialogue – a technique for posing questions and pursuing the implications of answers in order for students to discover, rather than being told, the answer. Those who believe in such methods are reluctant to embrace technologies that might reshape how they teach as well as what they can teach.

Yet even when individual educators embrace new technology, there are many institutional arrangements and policies in education that constrain more innovative uses of ICTs. For example, the incentive structures in most higher educational institutions continue to reward narrow definitions of scholarship, thereby failing to encourage work with new media – such as in authoring or collaborating on the development of educational software – or in reaching new audiences like life-long learners. Also, traditional approaches to copyright and intellectual property rights (IPR) have been a barrier to the production of educational material. US and British universities, for example, have often waived their rights to teaching materials produced by their faculty, but the prospect of expanded access to virtual universities might lead many universities in North America and Europe to assert such rights (see Chapter Twenty-two).

Limited technological paradigms and practices

The Internet and Web surpass the expectations of many users, who are surprised by the capability of networks to enable global access to all kinds of information. This experience has helped create a sense that major breakthroughs in education are not just possible, but already within technical reach. Yet, this collection illustrates the degree to which visions of the role of new ICTs continue to outstrip the capability of the technology. For example, advances in expert systems and artificial intelligence (AI) over many decades have fueled speculation about the development of individualized tutorial systems for learning. In some areas, the technology already seems to be in place for educators to provide successful forms of distance education and distributed learning, such as in business and professional education (Chapters Three and Four). Yet many prototypes continue to fall far short of our imaginations. In area after area, from course management software to multipoint video conferencing systems, the industry has made major technical breakthroughs that remain some distance from major market breakthroughs. Noriko Hara and Rob Kling's case study in Chapter Five of students struggling with an online distance education course provides one example; their experience has been repeated elsewhere.

The limitations of technologies are perhaps less critical than the limitations on our visions or paradigms that could guide the design and implementation of new media. This collection highlights the complex and far-reaching institutional changes implied by efforts to re-engineer higher education and learning to take fuller advantage of ICTs. Discussions of a shift from teacher-centered to student-centered learning might capture some aspects of this new paradigm, and relate to broader visions of the impact of new technology (Dertouzos, 2001), but are too simplistic and limited. As Alfred Bork (Chapter Nine) argues, ICTs are being used most often in ways that simply extend a traditional teacher-centered approach to learning, by broadcasting notes and lectures, when they could be used to enable more one-on-one tutorial approaches to learning. Noriko Hara and Rob Kling (Chapter Five) raise questions about the degree that online education is indeed student-centered.

A great deal of energy is being focused on what some have called 'Web-based pedagogy', arguing that new paradigms are needed to make effective use of ICTs in learning and education (Cole, 2000). The film projector, programmed texts, computers, radio and television, the video cassette recorder, PCs and, more recently, the Internet have yet to revolutionize learning and education in ways that proponents had forecast. Instead, each technology has been adapted to play relatively marginal roles within traditional paradigms of the educational process – putting old wine into new bottles. Traditional educational paradigms are under challenge, but no potential replacements have been widely accepted. Without a new paradigm, educators are likely to use ICTs to do things the way they have always been done, but with new and more expensive equipment. For example, many lecturers use a PC with presentation software as a high-powered overhead or 35 mm slide projector. New teaching processes can evolve, such as when teachers begin to make their presentations accessible on the Web for students to review. However, the realization that many businesses were simply emulating traditional practices with new equipment was one impetus behind Business Process Re-engineering (Dutton, 1999: 127–34). Educators may also need to redesign how they do their work in order to achieve the potential benefits of ICTs.

One paradigm is technology-driven and has no clear foundation in an approach to education and learning. Many simply urge schools at all levels to modernize their technology, which often means making them ubiquitous. Universities compete to be on the list of most 'wired' campuses (www.wiredcolleges.com). One university advocated the installation of one computer per student in their dormitories, and this has since become a norm among those institutions that can afford to compete. A problem with a technology-driven strategy is the risk of 'overscaling'. This could be as inefficient as 'underscaling', which few educational institutions can afford (Schramm, 1977).

A more educationally-anchored paradigm regards ICTs as 'teaching machines' – substitutes for teachers – as opposed to tools for teachers and students to use in some of the ways outlined above. Yesterday, television was thought to be the new teaching machine. Today it is the computer and the Internet. The interactive nature of computers give them a 'holding power' and enable them to be more self-directed than many other ICTs, such as TV (Papert, 1980). However, teachers generally find that computers do not improve the performance of most students (Cuban, 1986), who usually also need other forms of human direction. Educators have labeled this the 'fingertip effect' – the false hope that you can sit a person in front of a computer and walk away (Perkins, 1990). There is no technical fix to the problem of effective teaching of many more students than are reached by present institutions.

A more contemporary paradigm accepts the need for teachers to use ICT support to enable them to switch more towards a role of facilitator or coach, rather than lecturer or authority (Gell and Cochrane, 1996). As information and expertise is increasingly accessible over electronic networks, it is argued from this paradigm that the teacher's prime function will be to help students navigate through and interpret that wealth of knowledge. In many respects, this extends a traditional role of education in helping students 'learn how to learn' (Tehranian, 1996). But at the same time, this perspective seems to dismiss the degree to which teachers have still had to teach despite the availability of growing numbers of books, libraries, films and other instructional technologies. However, this paradigm has started to shape policy and practice in education. A risk of this approach is that teachers are encouraged to move their vital gate-keeping role to others.

Multiple models: many paths to the future of online education

Research on the social shaping of technology has been critical of tech-nologically deterministic perspectives that see ICTs in higher education moving on a predetermined path toward the one-best-way to provide online education (Williams and Edge, 1996). Walter Baer (Chapter Twelve), Martin Harris (Chapter Fifteen) and others in this book support a social shaping perspective by underscoring the many paths that can be followed by the developers of distance education and distributed learning. Efforts to systematically classify and define these variations can make a valuable contribution to policy and practice, but also show the open-ended future of a digital academe. This multi-plicity of models can represent another constraint on new developments. A major source of widespread confusion in debates over distance education and distributed learning, for example, is the degree to which individuals have different mental models and real life examples of this phenomenon.

A changing competitive environment

Historically, a lack of competition in higher education has been a brake on institutional change. However, Lloyd Armstrong (Chapter Six) and others argue that, in opening more opportunities for tele-access, ICTs have created more options and competition among schools, including from outside the traditional education sector. Computer manufacturers, software companies and media businesses see market possibilities in the provision of multimedia education to schools. Innovative private educational offerings, such as the University of Phoenix (www.phoenix.edu) online, create a long-term threat to traditional institutions, as Rose Wagner illustrates in the

German case (Chapter Fourteen). The provision of distance education by traditional universities will put them into more competition with one another for new markets. And all kinds of private industries are undertaking their own education and training programs which increasingly compete with the continuing education ambitions of technical institutes, colleges and universities.

Economic resources and constraints

Another major challenge is the degree to which ICTs can be used to 'reduce educational costs per credit hour' (Garson, 1996: 403) by cutting staff numbers and improving efficiency. Many administrators see the potential for ICTs to be used to allow fewer faculty to teach more students using business management paradigms such as the virtual organization and lesser forms of outsourcing (Baer, Chapter Twelve). However, early analyses of the assumptions underlying many proposals for downsizing, such as through online universities, suggested that the proponents often underestimate the resources necessary to produce high-quality educational materials using qualified teachers and multimedia producers (Garson, 1996).

Distance education and distributed learning are not cheap. The production and consumption of online educational options entail major new investments in such areas as courseware, expertise and wired classrooms. It is not surprising, therefore, that the momentum behind ICT initiatives in education has been countered by a view that devoting scarce resources to ICTs will seriously undermine the quality of education (Robins and Webster, 1989; Noble, 2001). Concern about over-investment in ICTs within education has been a source of growing opposition to pushing hi-tech on schools at all levels.

Conceptions of the audience – students – and their responses

Conceptions of the audience can have a major impact on the design of ICTs (Cooper and Woolgar, 1993). In education, this process is made more difficult because it is often driven by weak conceptions of the user – student – in two major ways.

First, students are often stereotyped as ready-made users of ICTs because they grow up surrounded by the technology, while teachers are perceived as being caught in the old, linear print generation. This generational stereotyping stems, in part, from studies based on observations of the interactions with computers by exceptionally bright children of well-educated parents, such as the 'child programmers' of

MIT faculty and staff (Papert, 1980; Turkle, 1984). It is also anchored in anecdotal observations by engineers and scientists whose children grow up with computers as a part of their everyday life. However, computer proficiencies and attitudes are far more varied among the young and old than portrayed by these generational stereotypes.

The way many children initially associate computers with TV might help to account for children's attraction to ICTs (Greenfield, 1984: 127–54). Early multimedia prototypes like IBM's *Ulysses* have demonstrated how hypertext multimedia could be used to help start a child's interest in literature or music that they might otherwise never explore.[8] What has been called 'edutainment' or 'infotainment' can take advantage of popular interest in video by embedding lessons in anything from soap operas to interactive computer games. However, this approach can underestimate the sophistication of children and adults as consumers of video programming. People accustomed to video arcades and flipping through dozens of TV channels – watching TV rather than a program – are not automatically captivated by 'infotainment' unless it is outstanding in content and production values, which costs.

A second way in which ICTs are challenging conceptions of the user is by the way they can 'reconfigure' relations between users and producers (Woolgar, 1996). For example, at the University of Southern California an attempt has been made to provide its alumni – graduates of the university – with better electronic access to information, such as through the use of the Internet. It became immediately apparent that ICTs permitted the alumni to be not only an audience, but also a new set of producers of information for others, contributing knowledge in their disciplines and locales to enrich a university's pool of expertise and experience. This indicates the potential obsolescence of the old paradigm, which viewed the faculty as the producers of information and students as an audience, not active participants in education. This is a gross misconception of the way in which knowledge is distributed among faculty, students and alumni.

The impacts of ICTs in learning and education

The contributions to this book also evoke a wide variety of issues and themes concerning the social, political and economic impacts of ICTs in higher education and learning. We would like to highlight a few salient themes on the impacts of ICTs in this setting, but these are by no means exhaustive.

Technical and educational convergence: blurring distance and distributed learning

In the midst of a proliferation of organizational arrangements for the creation and delivery of distance education and distributed learning there is a growing sense of converging technical approaches centered around the Internet and World Wide Web. For example, the use of Web-based information resources to enhance classroom-based instruction, such as in Sylvia Sensiper's description in Chapter Three of the Harvard case studies, could be just as valuable for use in distance education. This is one reason why educators continue to trip over the distinctions between distance education and distributed learning (the use of ICTs to complement campus-based classroom instruction) while being less able to identify the unique mix of technologies that underpin each. It seems that all strides in distributed learning, for example, are facilitating the move of universities into distance educational options. The opposite is also true. Distance-independent course offerings can supplant and compete with campus-based instruction, as when a distance education course designed for remote students of a professional gerontology program began to enroll residential students (Chapter Four).

Blurring institutional boundaries

A closely related theme directly connected to institutional change concerns the degree to which new actors are emerging, either as the sole providers of training and education, for instance stand-alone, new communication enterprises or as the partners of more traditional educational institutions, such as when universities create a fully-owned subsidiary to administer or deliver distance education courses. As Lloyd Armstrong (Chapter Six), Walter Baer (Chapter Twelve), Rose Wagner (Chapter Fourteen) and others explain, networking among educational institutions to form new entities such as educational portals and consortia are other ways in which the existing boundaries of educational institutions are being eroded or blurred in the move to exploit ICTs.

Increased competition

While competition is one aspect shaping higher education, ICTs appear to be playing an important role in creating this environment. As Armstrong (Chapter Six) argues, remote access is raising the specter of 'winner-take-all' global competition in higher education

(Frank and Cook, 1996). Universities have competed with one another for prestige, endowments, grants and students, but often within well-defined geographical and institutional boundaries. As ICTs threaten to reconfigure the geography of higher education and bring new players into the arena as both producers and consumers, competition is likely to be heightened dramatically. If the higher education marketplace becomes the network, rather than a place, universities will face new competitors and new competitive strategies in their efforts to attract the best students and faculty. What is less clear are the consequences of such hyper-competition, what Jeremy Rifkin (2000) has labeled more generally as 'hypercapitalism'. Will it, for example, lead to the demise of higher education institutions as a result of competitive failure? Will it produce a redistribution of resources away from research activities to ensure the production and delivery of high quality revenue-earning material? Will resources move from specialized courses with few students to more popular introductory courses with larger markets, or will universities see the unique expertise of their teachers as key to entering globally competitive markets, creating more access to specialized courses?

The geography of learning and education: the virtual campus

Competition is closely connected to the changing geography of learning and education. Online uses of ICTs have begun to raise more fully the promise of distance education, which since the nineteenth century has sought to provide access to classrooms for rural, working, physically disabled, mature students and others who found it difficult to be educated at a particular location at certain times. The geography of education and learning can change through such innovations as: using Webcasts in the same way videotapes have been used to make some of the most gifted teachers accessible to more students; making published work more widely available by putting it into electronic as well as print forms; or employing computer conferencing software and e-mail to enable students to communicate about specific topics with other students and instructors, between classes and without being in the same place.

That said, discussions of the virtual university often fail to recognize the importance of tacit knowledge and values that cannot be codified well and distributed over the Internet (Lamberton, 1997: 74–5). It also underestimates the degree to which learning can depend on factors that can be undermined by mediated communication, as Noll (Chapter One) and Haywood (Chapter Two) argue, such as socialization, a sense of personal obligation or accountability (Tehranian, 1996). For instance, the OU finds it critical that students attend intensive sessions on its Milton Keynes campus to support distance education. ICTs could even make the geography of education and learning more important, because the need for face-to-face communication, rather than access to information, should become even more central to the choice of an educational institution.

The culture of new media messages

Several contributions highlight a prominent theme of media studies, that the media – of which ICTs in higher education provide an example – are not value-neutral transmitters of facts. They carry the values and priorities of their producers. Alfred Bork's (Chapter Nine) discussion of the educational agenda for tutorial-based learning systems provides a vivid example. The role of ICTs in promoting 'open-access' in the UK (Chapter Thirteen) and Catalonia (Chapter Eight) is another. The very expression of the potential for online education to extend opportunities across socioeconomic and geographical divides celebrates the value western cultures place on education as a path to social mobility and social equality (Young, 1996).

Reinforcing economic divides

Many critics have raised concerns over the degree that ICTs might exacerbate rather than diminish inequalities in access to education, locally and globally (Schiller, 1996; Flecha, 1999). An inescapable theme of this book is the degree to which wealth matters in both the kinds of courses that are likely to be viable for distance education and distributed learning, and the kinds of students who are likely to be reached. The Open University's commitment to reaching everyone who wants a college education is one of a number of exceptions to a more market-oriented approach of the new push for online degree and educational programs. Corporate training programs have been among the first to exploit the delivery of online courseware. Business, management and professional degree programs appear to be the most avid early adopters of online degree programs in universities, since they can pay. The University of Phoenix, for instance, specifically dedicated its online business course delivery to those in employment and over a certain age. The promise of online and virtual education may be great for expanding global access to information, educators and other educational services, but the current reality is constrained by the importance of viable markets and the high costs of ICTs, raising genuine concerns over the reinforcement of many tiers of educational opportunity.

Virtual transparency

A theme emphasized by James Cornford (Chapter Twenty), but reinforced by most other contributors, is the degree to which the use of ICTs in education has made activities and processes, such as grading and class discussion, more visible. Opening new doors to the classroom and the university could have dramatic unanticipated consequences, such as in being a force for more standardization across classes and graders. ICTs are enhancing the visibility of the classroom (Chapter Five) and faculty-university relationships (Chapter Six), the work of educational institutions (Chapter Twenty) and scholarship, including the academic peer review process (Chapter Ten). David Noble (2001: Afterword) has argued that certain aspects of this transparency are a "violation of the privileged relationship between teachers and students". For example, course syllabi on the Web are visible to the world and not just one's students. Others, however, welcome this visibility, almost in the spirit of open sourcing by exposing one's ideas and courses to comments and criticism. Also, new course management software like Blackboard enable teachers to create electronic walls around their virtual classroom. Will this heightened visibility undermine or enhance the accountability and quality of learning, teaching and scholarship? Will this transparency be short-lived as systems enable more control over access and with what effect on the quality and accountability of the teaching? These issues raise more general concerns over gatekeeping.

Reconfiguring the gatekeepers in higher education

In a world exploding with electronic and published information, the gatekeeping role is becoming more critical than ever in determining what educational material is best for students. ICTs can shift this educational gatekeeping role in two very different ways.

On the one hand, some emerging educational technologies can give more authority to top administrators, who choose courseware developed outside the college or university that adopts it. If administrators, for example, choose one enterprise course management system over another, their students will have access to different pools of electronic resources.[9]

In contrast, the Internet could shift gatekeeping in a different way, while just as surely diminishing the teacher's role in the choice of content. Using the Web and hypertext search tools, students can follow their interests wherever they may lead, escaping the designs of a teacher as well as any author. One reason why people speak of Web 'browsers' and 'surfing' the Internet is that many users do not read anything. Instead, they scan and download images as they click from one hypertext link to another. However, logical arguments and complex problems are often best approached through sustained attention along a linear path, as is encouraged by a book or even sitting down with a blank piece of paper.

A focus on tele-access – as one aspect of any paradigm for the use of ICTs in education – can alert educators to the basic point that more information per se is not necessarily adding value to education. All educators need to be alert to how ICTs reshape tele-access, including who plays the role of gatekeeper to educational material.

The broader ecology of new media in higher education

ICTs can 'open doors to a learning society'. Students can become their own gatekeepers on the Internet or in the library. But in the classroom and in their courses, teachers need to select which doors should be opened and closed to achieve their ends. Students and educators do not need more of everything, but control over access to the best information, services and people. If educators and politicians understand ICTs as tools for tele-access, as opposed to teaching machines, they might balance their priorities better.

But the role of ICTs in learning and education will be highly dependent on the course of development in other sectors of society, such as government, private industry and the household. The boundaries of education are being eroded by new ICTs, new paradigms for education, a changing geography and revised conceptions of knowledge producers, users and gatekeepers.

Nicholas Garnham (Chapter Seventeen) warns us that decades of research on ICTs have challenged uncritical assumptions about the social implications of the coming 'information society' or 'digital age' as an inevitable force for progress. Deepening these understandings is even more important as the technologies advance, become ubiquitous and increasingly central to key social and political institutions, such as higher education.

This book provides fresh insights into an expanding range of questions about the quality of higher education and learning now and in the future. It develops a critical, interdisciplinary analysis within an integrative framework. By informing policy and practice proactively, it can assist people to shape technology, institutions and practices in higher education and learning in beneficial ways.

Notes

1   Charts are published of the most wired universities and colleges and many teachers and administrators believe these can attract or lose students and their parents who are concerned about the technological infrastructure supporting their education. See, for example, www.zdnet.com/yil/content/college and www.wiredcolleges.com.

2   JPL recorded an average of 40 to 45 million 'hits' each day, with a peak of 80 million hits on 7 July 1997 (Yates, 1997).

3   This is one project of the Integrated Media Systems Center at the University of Southern California, supported by the National Science Foundation. See: www.nsf.gov/pubs/2000/nsf00137/nsf00137t.htm.

4   This work developed in organizations like Hughes Training, later acquired by Ratheon. See L-3 Communication's Link Simulation & Training organization's overview of these systems and their history at: www.hti.com/history.html.

5   This work is being done in the Institute for Creative Technologies at the University of Southern California. See www.ict.usc.edu/about_ict.html.

6   This consortium was formed by the University of California, the California Institute of Technology, the California State University, Stanford University and the University of Southern California.

7   This framework builds on a synthesis of research on ICTs developed in Dutton (1996) and proposed for a new program of research to be supported by the UK's Economic and Social Research Council (ESRC, 2001).

8   IBM funded the production of educational hypertext treatments of Tennyson's poem *Ulysses* and the discovery of America by Columbus, produced by David Able and his associates.

9   An example is the case of Whittle Communications in the USA. Chris Whittle developed the Whittle Educational Network in 1989 to provide free equipment to schools in return for a guarantee that teenagers would watch twelve minutes of Whittle programming each day, during which time they would see news and ads targeted to their age group. In 1994 he sold Channel One to K-III Communications Corporation, which also publishes the *Weekly Reader* for students. Although Channel One was resisted by state boards of education, and generated controversy, it received numerous awards and has been adopted by thousands of US schools, reaching millions of teenagers (Dutton, 1999: 210–11).

Part I

Audiences for new media in higher education

Students, teachers and administrators as consumers and users of ICTs

1 Technology and the future of the university

A sober view

A. Michael Noll

The Introduction spoke of the growing debate on the emerging shape of higher education. Noll now takes up this challenge. He starts by cautioning against trying to understand the future by looking through the technological lens used by many of the experts who have tried to predict what will happen in the twenty-first century. In arguing that a historical perspective is essential to distinguishing the predictions which make sense from those which are nonsense, he explains why he believes this is likely to highlight major limits to the role ICTs can play in learning and education, even within the most highly resourced universities.

Is the end of the university near?

Experts who are predicting the death of the university claim that the Internet will make universities obsolete as students around the globe study and take courses, all on the Web. They say the 'Webtization' of university education will mean the end of physical universities, making all education virtual. Other experts predict that corporations will prepare, package and sell education on such a wide scale over the Internet that conventional universities will no longer be able to compete, or to survive. The corporatization of education will occur on such a wide scale that it will lead to the death of conventional educational institutions.

When thinking about what the university of the future will look like, it is important to be aware of similar dire predictions which have been made before. I am old enough to remember the prediction that computers would lead to a paperless office. Instead, computers made it far too easy to create many drafts, all usually printed on paper by the high-speed laser printer. I can recall predictions of the electronic library in which all information would be stored in digital form without the need for any paper books. This prediction has been extended to include the impending death of books in general. Yet book sales increase each year, and hardly anyone would prefer to read a book on a computer screen. The electronic newspaper was predicted to herald the demise of conventional newspapers. Here too, the prediction was far too dire.

These kinds of dire warnings seem to be publicity stunts, designed to attract the attention of the media. Outlandish speculation on the impending death of established institutions are usually successful at receiving far more attention than they deserve. Rarely do the media remember what was predicted last year, and thus no negative publicity returns to tarnish the image of the wild predictor when the predictions turn to rubbish.

Taking a historical perspective on the future of education

We all know the tremendous pace of computer technology over the past forty years, and thus we are tempted to believe the claims that similar revolutionary change will occur to educational institutions. But a saner approach to making predictions of the future is to look back forty years to see what has happened in the intervening years. This historical perspective can then be used to make more realistic extrapolations to the future. When this is done for universities, we see that very little has changed. The classroom is still the dominant technique for teaching, although computers and the Web are much used by students for research and to register for courses.

What then of distance education and the predictions that the conventional classroom will soon disappear? In fact, distance education is a very old idea. Correspondence schools have existed throughout the twentieth century. Tele-education through two-way video, and one-way video with an interactive audio return, has been available for decades and is still used by many engineering schools.

Students have studied with each other over the telephone for decades, and today use e-mail for similar purposes. The Internet is a great supplement to the library, but its use for research makes students lazy and much material is missed because it is not available over the Web, perhaps because it is too old or simply has not been entered. Students routinely complain to me about too much emphasis on the Web and state their desire to have access to physical books and reference materials.

Whenever I ask my students whether they want to take courses over the Web, they respond very negatively. Students do not seem to want Web-based courses! Students prefer the classroom and the personal interactions with other students. This is not to say that there are special circumstances for distance education over the Web, for example, for students who are far too busy to attend physically. But this is a small market, already satisfied by correspondence schools and others specializing in distance education.

The university is – and always has been – a physical place where students, scholars, and teachers come together. The university that creates a rich environment to facilitate interactions, both in and outside the formal classroom, will indeed flourish in the future. It is the university that emphasizes distance education and the Web that will die, because of the cold, impersonal nature of such education.

Changes that might be tied to the use of the Web

There have been some changes, though, because of the Web. A few years ago, nearly all of our graduate students found out about our school through the use of college guides. Today, nearly all have instead used the Internet and the Web to find out about the school and its academic programs. The Web is a tremendous marketing tool. It can be used to create a package of instantly-available material to help a prospective student decide where to apply, including faculty biographies, program descriptions, information about graduates, course syllabi, faculty publications and live Webcam views of the campus. Even the material needed to submit an application is available over the Web.

In the future, the Web could have a negative impact on the university bookstore. Each term, the university's bookstore asks me to give it a list of the books required for my courses. Filling out this form takes time with no rewards to me. All too often, the bookstore forgets to order the books. Students are discovering the use of the Web to search for a cheap price and then have the books shipped directly to them, thereby avoiding the bookstore. I too have joined this new approach and am no longer filling out the bookstore's form. Instead, I give the students a list of the books along with the suggestion that they search the Web for the best price and delivery schedule to meet their needs, in addition to checking the university's bookstore.

The university's bookstore prepares course readers, consisting of copies of all the required readings for the course. The bookstore is making a business in obtaining permissions from the copyright owners, paying royalties and printing the readers. Here too, the Web could facilitate much change. Many publications are available over the Web, either for free or for a nominal charge. All the faculty would need to do is prepare a list of the readings along with the appropriate URLs on the Web. Indeed, it is the university bookstore that would seem to have a dim future!

2   Defining moments

The tension between richness and reach

Trevor Haywood

Traditional and distance-education approaches have distinctive benefits when they are well implemented. In this chapter, Haywood highlights the trade-offs that will need to be made between what he calls the 'defining moments' in each approach: a 'richness' in educational experience nurtured in spatially-based institutions, and the 'reach' and convenience of distance learning. He explores the actual nature of these defining moments and argues for a realistic appraisal of the past in order to allow for the development of policies and practices that successfully mix the best of traditional and new-media approaches.

'Fluid' and 'fixed' educational experiences

Most students, parents and academics are likely to agree – give or take a few whistles and bells – that the traditional defining moments of a university or college education encompass a mixture of 'fixed' and 'fluid' experiences. The fixed moments embrace (at their best) student attendance at lectures and seminars under the tutelage of excellent teachers, who set demanding assignments that they later discuss to draw out connections and links, which enrich and accelerate the acquisition of knowledge and understanding. The portfolio of higher education moments also include valuable but more fluid encounters (at their best):

* time for reflection and sharing discoveries with peers;
* the pleasure of life in a community that is generally insulated from worldly cares and which may never be experienced again;

- the formation of friendships that could form the basis of a personal network in later life;
- a *curriculum vitae* that proclaims understandable values and credentials.

Distance learning, however it is accomplished, does not deliver this mix. By its very nature, it questions the authority and relevance of the spatially-located collegiate experience, with closeness to faculty and fellow students at its core. The coincidence of new delivery mechanisms, particularly the Internet, the high cost of higher education (for students, parents and the state), ever busier lives and the increased demand for vocational qualifications, has re-invigorated the debate over what constitutes the defining moments of the higher education experience. The once unquestioned case for spatially-located higher education has come under greater scrutiny as policy makers begin to take the alternatives more seriously than they have ever done before.

Richness in the traditional educational experience

The social, as compared to the personal, return on investment in higher education is a serious question, but it is one that has always been difficult to quantify. However, the richness that derives from the fluid experience of traditional higher education is generally seen as benefiting the individual rather than society at large. This may be a narrow way of looking at a return on higher education investment, in that the fluid experiences may spin off all kinds of benefits to do with citizenship, such as communication skills and learning to co-operate with others. However, as more and more providers of distance higher education emerge, using all the technologies at hand, it will be students rather than academics who define the kind of 'fixed and fluid' richness package that they need, or are willing to pay for.

Those providers of higher education that operate primarily in distance mode, such as the UK's Open University (see Boyd-Barrett, Chapter Thirteen, and Harris, Chapter Fifteen) and the accredited Jones (cyber) International University in the USA (see Pease, Chapter Seven), clearly ground their operations in facilitating knowledge acquisition by individuals without the costly infrastructure necessary to create the 'fluid' richness so valued in spatially-based higher education. The student pays for and gets the 'fixed' package; the 'fluid' element is them getting on with the rest of their life.

Of course, the defining moments of traditional higher education, as set out above, have never been uniformly achieved (hence the qualification 'at their best'). It is still possible to experience a reasonable port-folio of fixed and fluid moments in some private or elite institutions. However, in the public institutions, which the bulk of students attend, things have been creaking badly since the mid-1970s. In the UK, for example, public respect for universities is at an all time low, as exemplified in an article by a respected journalist (Humphrys, 2001) which attacked British universities as "a world of pretence and disillusion and corruption of purpose". This populist and sweeping piece prompted sixteen letters of support, cataloguing a range of perceived sins and omissions in university higher education. The article, and many of the respondents, focused on how institutions were exaggerating pass rates to secure funding, still saw vocational education as second class, and now only paid lip service to academic standards. Similar views are shared by many in the UK academy, but they seem powerless to change the direction of the wave.

Understanding the need for change in higher education

Many general perceptions of publicly-funded higher education are thus now more about nostalgia than reality. Many academics, still cocooned in ways that they protest they are not, tend to dwell on idyllic memories of fixed and fluid moments long lost in the push for an 'economic' mass higher education. They are torn in many directions, but they have to face the harsh truth that students encounter a wide range of experiences in traditional higher education institutions, that – at the poorer end of the spectrum – scream out for reformation. It is important to recognize that all is not rosy in existing delivery systems before condemning alternative scenarios out of hand.

One criticism of David Noble's (1998) 'Digital Diploma Mills' is his implicit assumption that a 'universal richness' exists within the traditional modes of delivery. I have no doubt that, in some higher education environments, in some subjects, a well-constructed Web-based program would not only substitute for, but be superior to what many students have received through traditional modes. Many first year undergraduate courses in universities are already defined by text books with lectures, 'at their best', adding a slightly different perspective to a set book and, at their worst, just repeating their contents in the form of printed handouts or overhead slides. In such situations, it should not surprise us that publishers regard higher education as just another part of their value chain.

The possibility that many first year undergraduate courses could eventually be taught over distance, using Web-based texts and occasional tutorial support, is not difficult to imagine. The "raw and precious jewel that, with wisdom, could be polished to a proud shine", taken from 'Tuesdays with Morrie' and quoted by Noble (1998), is still too often left to polish itself, while faculty polish up their status in other ways than teaching. How many first year classes on any given day in the USA are being taught by doctoral students rather than experienced teachers?

Although sharing some of his concerns about the dubious deals with commercial entities being done by some universities, I believe that Noble over-estimates the value of lecture-based learning and under-estimates the capacity of academics to develop in response to new modes of delivery. The academics at the Open University (OU) prepare their materials in teams creating innovative courses that are celebrated for their quality by the UK's quality assurance system and by other systems around the world. They don't get angst-ridden over the fact that administrators then mail them off to students without their further input.

Many organizations, when looking to define the environment they operate in, still end up defining it in their own well-honed image despite the changes they clearly see going on around them. Over the years, academics have defined their environment as a place where students want and need to attend lectures in a particular kind of location, and structured according to particular conventions, which are sacrosanct. But to many observers and students, these conventions have begun to look more like the pillars supporting a certain kind of life-style, rather than a responsive student-centered edifice.

UK universities, for instance, are burdened by a seemingly unmovable geology of procedural ritual with regard to examination assessment, course validation and course monitoring that makes most US universities look anarchic – all in the name of maintaining a chimerical equality of standards. These rituals gobble up the time of academics and give employment to thousands of unproductive administrators, who have become skilled at laying down sterile sediment at the expense of serving the core mission.

While these rituals keep internal structures busy grooming themselves, and retain processes whose purpose has long been forgotten, students have been meeting the real world. Many students in full-time education are now awash with worldly cares – including student loans, poor accommodation and part-time working – and their contact with tutors is only rarely 'close'. The prized insulation from external pressures necessary to fuel time for deep reflection has all but evaporated, and the pressure to get certification (for a job), rather than an education (for life), has diluted much of the idealism that they and their tutors once shared.

The value of 'reach' in distance education

The intimacy of tutorial education in the UK is all but dead and the quality of the pervasive lecture-based delivery system is highly variable. Coincident with this, many new social and economic factors are influencing what students want from higher education. Many students buy into distance education (however it is packaged) because they want convenience (reach) above all else. They accept that, although it will never replicate the perceived richness of an institution-based experience at the 'best' institutions, it will not differ much from the richness they would have gained in many of the rest. Older students consciously reject the need for collegiate richness because, at that stage in their life, they do not value it and feel that the richness they desire is that which will come from within themselves after an appropriate course of tuition. The richness they value is represented by greater confidence, improved self-discipline, the acquisition of new strands of knowledge, greater promotional prospects and an improved ability to perform in the world. These desires involve a view of education as a part of 'real' life rather than an activity distinct and separate from it.

It is common for mature students, those either catching up or adding to their portfolio, to trade academic community for convenience in order to run learning, family life and continued employment in parallel. This is not new, but the student numbers likely to be involved in the future will be new (given the rising demand for higher education all over the world). Hence the need to evaluate new approaches to richness and reach that satisfy much larger numbers, without the sophistry that too often attends the celebration of spatially-located higher education.

Most distance-learning schemes around the world build in summer schools, regional group meetings and occasional one-to-one tutorial support, as an antidote to student isolation. These 'real space' events give students the opportunity to discuss course materials with others, to identify both individual and common worries and to tap into the wisdom of a tutor in a face-to-face encounter. The success of these 'intensive' gatherings to supplement remote contact suggests that we may have always over-estimated the importance of 'full-time' spatially-based higher education and that well-orchestrated face-to-face 'richness' in small doses can work well. Such an argument might suggest that the focus and concentration encouraged by the self-discipline of home-based learning, uninterrupted by the non-academic temptations of collegiate life, offers a powerful richness of its own that only requires occasional refreshment from other sources.

The OU has clearly demonstrated that reach (various forms of high-quality learning materials delivered over distance) supported by the occasional richness of summer schools and group meetings works well for many students. However, it is important to remember that the OU has had over three decades to learn from its mistakes, and to grow unprecedented knowledge (albeit in one cultural milieu) about the processes involved in delivering a high-quality education, at low cost, over space. It has also leveraged its advantages of scale intelligently to release tremendous relative powers from its faculty. It would be foolish to imagine that institutions getting into distance education via whatever mix of mailbox, real space and ICT delivery can emulate this kind of success within a span of five to six years.

Distinguishing between 'hard' and 'soft' technologies

Web-based learning is being added to the portfolio of tools used to reach students both within traditional universities and in purely 'distance-based' higher education operations and, like the application of all new technologies, it will have its share of successes and failures. The B3002 project (see Hara and Kling, Chapter Five), albeit small scale, confirmed that managing the human factor (e.g. unexpected illness, teaching by a foreign-born PhD candidate, message overload, lack of non-verbal information or failure to return assignments on time), however it operates, is still the key. And while many of the frustrations experienced by students doing B3002 could easily be replicated on any day in any traditional university, the frustrations were exaggerated by lack of access to a person in real space. Much of this is not new. We already know a lot about Web failures in our day-to-day use of it for other purposes, and it is not difficult to see how, without assiduous attention to detail, these failures could be replicated in distance-learning environments. The key to making distance learning work is excellent materials and excellent infrastructure; what Sir John Daniel (1999c), a former Vice-chancellor of the Open University, calls the 'hard and soft' technologies.

The 'hard' stuff includes the ICTs that are changing all the time. Given their velocities of change, any frozen Polaroid definition of 'best' ICT is likely to be temporary. The 'soft' stuff includes the processes, approaches, sets of rules and models of organization that emerge out of the body of knowledge created by running and evaluating distance-learning programs. The latter are more important in a purely distance-learning enterprise because so much of the actual delivery relies on the efficient administration of the programs that have been created by academic teams.

To get both the hard and soft bits working well, traditional higher education providers have been tempted to enter partnerships with commercial entities. As with all ICT choices, the only criteria for seeking commercial partners must be 'fitness for purpose'. Define your purpose and the core values that you will never compromise, and the choice of both available technologies and commercial partners almost becomes self-selecting. Reconciling the age-old suspicions that exist between academics and administrators in traditional higher education institutions, in order to agree and secure these values before any deals are made, is crucial to the long-term success of any campus-based distance programme. These suspicions are often deep rooted and, from the academic point of view, are associated with declining trust and discretion and memories of the almost irreconcilable differences in their respective priorities. With the classroom at the center of their lives, academics often feel frustrated by the demands of administrators who know so little about the alchemy of those treasured spaces. One unsung feature of successful distance education is its insistence on partnerships and teamwork between academics and administrators, which clearly recognize the strengths of each without the distorting mirror of the classroom between them.

Students will soon come to recognize whether a distance-learning program embraces fitness for purpose. For instance, the once largely passive student body in the UK is slowly waking up in the early twenty-first century as more and more of them contribute directly to the cost of their higher education. Along with other consumers, they are benefiting from the proliferation of printed and Web-based guides that are reducing the asymmetry of information that used to make it so difficult for them to make informed choices. On the Web, students can make all kinds of comparisons between university programs, and not many of them will base their choice on only one factor.

Searching for effective new blends of traditional and distance higher education

By 2001, distance-based options utilizing multimedia were not attractive enough to younger students in Europe and the USA. Despite financial and other difficulties, they still aspire to the assumed richness of a campus-based education. But continuing changes in the economic and social structures in which students operate, even in the rich western world, suggest that new mixtures of traditional and distance learning will begin to have more appeal. The way potential students perceive that leaders and policy makers rate these options, in both proclamation and practice, will also play a major part in how they are taken up. In the UK, the proposed national 'e-university' (e-U) is based on the premise that it will support existing UK universities and other partners in the development and delivery of online programs and services.[1] Such big, top-down planning often falters at the operational level because implementation throws up all those messy human factors that need to be addressed with the same resolution that fuelled the initial policy enthusiasm. The government backed e-U prospectus, for example, claims that most distance education can be provided purely by electronic means, and that peer group interaction can be accommodated entirely via chat rooms and bulletin boards, a claim that may need some revision before the show gets on the road. The high cost of Internet use in the UK is also a hindrance that needs addressing. If broadband access is made available on the kind of pricing structure that currently operates in the UK, then take-up will be slow and all the promised fast streaming of information will be enjoyed by only a minority for a long time to come. Academics excited by the innovative presentation of graphic materials that could so enhance net learning will become frustrated and again blame lack of national support for achieving supposed national objectives.

Traditional universities, though sometimes battered, have shown themselves to be very resilient at handling the economic and social changes of the past fifty years. Their 'legacy system' may be creaking, but they have opened their doors to more and more students – and the more nimble of the universities have learnt to follow the myriad funding changes they have been subject to in order to maximize their share of a regularly diminishing cake. I expect them to be equally invigorated by potential online competitors, both by embracing ICT to accommodate distant students themselves and in using it to better serve their on-campus customers. As in the commercial world, a mixture of 'bricks and clicks' may prove a mixture fertile in both richness and reach. Those traditional universities that can use their brand value, independently or in consort with others with similar brand power, may find in the Web a golden opportunity to extend their reputation and influence, particularly in recruiting qualified overseas students who are unable to travel to them.

For example, London University is building on its 150 years of distance-learning experience by adding a virtual campus to its External

Programme to offer online student services, information and course materials that will eventually provide Web-enhanced learning to its entire portfolio of over eighty undergraduate and postgraduate qualifications. Oxford University is exploring the possibility of offering an Open Oxford first year program online to students regardless of entry qualifications. Successful candidates would be offered residential places and scholarships for subsequent years. Such an innovation could do more for extending the net of access to an elite university than a cartload of central directives and quotas. Cambridge University is discussing with the OU its 'Open Cambridge' project, which includes a bid by both institutions to the UK's e-university. Nettuno, a national consortium of thirty-eight universities in Italy, has found that the Internet has reinvented TV as an effective educational medium because it adds the interactive component that all TV-based material cries out for. Perhaps the most striking development so far has been the decision by the Massachusetts Institute of Technology to make all its electronic course material available for free.[2]

This clear indication that disseminating content on its own is only a part of the story may give impetus to the 'open source' movement for courseware that Sir John Daniel, late of the OU, and others are calling for:

> Good distance-learning providers believe that the value they offer to students lies not primarily in their courseware but in the academic support they provide, the formative and summative assessments through which they help students learn, and the awards through which they certify student achievement. If their belief is grounded, then making courseware freely available should not erode the financial base of these institutions. What it will do is increase the quality and quantity of electronic courseware as materials are refined, versioned and adapted to academics around the world and made freely available in these new formats.
>
> (Daniel, 2001: VIII)

There are also clearly opportunities for both for-profit and not-for-profit entities to market online programs in continuing professional development in a variety of areas. Both individuals cut off from the possibility of institutional attendance and nations facing particular skill shortages desperately need high-quality distance-learning options in subjects such as business, finance, computing and nursing. The embryonic nature of current discussions, negotiations and alliances within the arena of Web-based learning means that any reporting of current examples must be seen as experiments that may or may not produce anything like the outcomes that are currently envisaged. It is clear that many permutations will come and go before the most successful formulas emerge. What cannot be disputed is that Web-based learning, either in a supporting or a primary role, is here to stay. Student take-up of such programs will ultimately depend on proof of their fitness for purpose and how they compare with what could be obtained by other options at a similar cost.

Advocating an open mind on the riches that Web technology may be able to offer students does not mean uncritical acceptance, and much has been written over the past few years that suggests that a new realism has replaced the initial missionary zeal and excitement. Awe and intoxication are no substitute for the critical faculties we would apply to any other suggestions regarding changes to our mode of delivery. We have already seen a number of false dawns, particularly in the over-optimistic predictions about the economics of Web-based production and delivery. Within the melting pot of the current debates about what constitutes the defining moments of an higher education experience, the values attributed to the old mixture of 'fixed' and 'fluid' moments will come under more scrutiny than ever before. The motives for this scrutiny will be mixed, but in defending the value of an old order, we must be frank in accepting some of its failures and flexible enough to appreciate some of the advantages that students can reap from the new.

Academics, though rarely in the driving seat, are good at adapting to changes in educational policy. They will remember that:

> Charles I on reading a declaration of his treason squirted down a fibre optic cable from Cromwell's headquarters somewhere in England during 1649 still gets to hear that he is going to lose his head! The defining moment has nothing to do with the technology that brings him the message.
>
> (Haywood, 1999: 44).

Notes

1   The e-university has been allocated £62 million (about $90 million) of UK government funds between 2001 and 2003. A business model for it was published by the Higher Education Funding Council for England in October 2000 (see www.hefce.ac.uk/Pubs/HEFCE/2000/00_43.htm).

2   See www.londonexternal.ac.uk/news/Launches.html for details of London University's plans for its Virtual Campus. A note on Oxford and Cambridge Universities' tentative explorations with the OU and the UK's proposed e-university can be found in THES (2001). Details of Italy's

Nettuno model for mixing satellite television broadcasts and the Internet can be found at nettuno.stm.it/english/display2.html (English version). Key statements concerning the MIT OpenCourseware (OCW) project, including information on the $11m funding of the project by the Mellon, Hewlett Foundations, can be found at web.mit.edu/ocw/

3   Making the case online
Harvard Business School multimedia

Sylvia Sensiper

The Web, computer-based applications and other new media have provided educators with unique new modes in which to present curriculum materials. These demand different ways of thinking about structuring information and ideas as part of a process of re-thinking how students learn. In this chapter, Sensiper explains how Harvard Business School's approach to case studies as a method of teaching has been adapted to the Web since 1995, including the introduction of video, simulations and links to other online resources. She gives examples of how the move to online cases has enhanced the presentation of cases, explores the implications for the ways in which students approach them, and highlights key lessons from Harvard's experience.

Harvard Business School case studies

The Harvard Business School (HBS) began developing cases in the 1920s with the idea of providing students with 'experiential learning'. Each case presents a real-life business situation. It provides enough detailed information for students to be able to imagine themselves in the role of one of the primary managers described in the case and resolve issues encountered by this chief decision maker. Case writers are taught to present the business dilemma in a literary 'story' form, with a 'case protagonist' facing a potentially difficult issue.

Until computers made it possible to put text online, teaching cases had been written documents structured as narratives, created through industry research, field studies at a company location, examination of pertinent documents, and interviews on-site and over the telephone.

Cases are usually twelve to fifteen pages in length. Accompanying exhibits aimed at informing students' understanding of the issues could include financial statements, organization charts, advertisements, articles and product specs. MBA students prepare approximately three cases a day, with each case meant to take about two to three hours to prepare. The cases are also used with HBS executive education programs and in other institutions and organizations worldwide. Class discussions center on a detailed analysis of the case, with students ready to present a solution and point to evidence in the case that supports their analysis as the most well thought out and logical. Students may also be called upon to role-play one of the 'characters' in the case and to debate with another student some of the salient issues.

Moving into an online environment

In the *Computer as Medium*, Andersen et al. (1993) argue that the kind of intelligence necessary for programming does not necessarily bring forth the most engaging products. They claim what is needed instead is an environment that "removes programming from the clutches of logical-mathematical intelligence and hands it over to musical and spatial intelligence." At the Harvard Business School, we faced the challenge of re-creating cases in an online environment by a process that included not only the logical-mathematical intelligence associated with programming and research, but also the spatial and artistic intelligences associated with videography and graphics, and the organizational intelligences associated with producing and editing.

The HBS cases are unique, but there are similarities with producing other educational experiences online. David Siegel, a prominent Web designer, has proposed an evolving model of Web development that increasingly uses the new media in ways that take advantage of its properties (see, for example: www.dsiegel.com/tips/). He divides Web sites into three generations. In the first, the tendency is simply to repurpose existing material: many early Web sites were pages of text hyperlinked to other text pages, so that you could interactively pursue a topic given the links from page to page. In the second generation, Web sites moved towards an inclusion of graphics and video, but with no clear sense of an integrated experience of the site as a whole. This might be called 'thin multimedia'. Third generation sites take advantage of computer interactivity and utilize other elements unique to the Web and to computers in general. In particular, they have a flow in which the different media – visual, auditory, text – interact and enhance each other. This three-stage model is important because it reminds us that multimedia is valuable to the extent that it works towards a coherent purpose. Second generation sites can often distract more than they focus.

HBS started to adapt a number of traditional text cases to an online environment in 1995. This involved the introduction of video segments, including interviews with managers and footage of factory floors, as well as simulations and hypertext links to other Internet resources. During the next five years of experimentation, a number of models were tested. The new case format eventually settled into a structure that uses the individual elements of the Web – interactivity, graphics, text, and video – to create dynamic teaching tools. A corresponding evolution occurred with the production process. The traditional text case was written by a faculty member alone or in collaboration with a research associate, but the creation of an online case currently requires a collaborative production that involves faculty, producers, videographers, graphic artists and software developers.

Valuable lessons learned from moving text-based HBS case studies online

Allow a discovery mode of learning/searching and freedom to learn non-sequentially

People do not read on the Web in the way they read books or newspapers – they search and surf for information and expect to be able to drill down, up and across. In order to both encourage and accommodate this way of learning, many online cases have not followed the narrative of a traditional text case and the literary model of identification with a protagonist. Instead, online cases use a more active discovery mode in which the student takes on the role of a consultant. For example, in a recent case about Knowledge Management, students were asked to consider questions about how managers might deal with the tacit knowledge associated with design-type skills in three different companies. After students watched and listened to managers talk about this issue, their assignment was to create five to ten general principles of managing tacit knowledge.

Setting up the HBS Web cases in this way helps motivate students to explore the site to which they have random access, and gather the information they need to make a managerial decision. This method models the decision-making process they will follow in real time. In many recent cases, students are also asked to submit information or make a decision through an interactive poll which allows the faculty member to have that information prior to planning the class. These polls help professors identify different learning strategies among students, each of which might have its own value. This also allows every student to make a contribution to the broader knowledge base of the class – in a large class, often only a small portion of the students will speak.

Present material that engages visual literacy

All of us know how easy it is to see when a person being interviewed on TV is hiding something, is happy or is extremely confident and honest. But most of us are not explicitly aware of how much these impressions are conveyed by factors such as camera angle, focal length and shots of hands versus face, as well as the inter-cutting of additional video sequences of activities and actions. This kind of visual knowledge is what is often missing in video interviews, and the unintended effects – because there are always effects – can be quite random and unwanted.

Early online cases repurposed text, but also repurposed video interviews – the video interviews did not make use of a visual grammar to go beyond an audio interview. Students could see and hear protagonists/managers, adding the capability to see the person and hear intonation, hesitation, and facial expression. But our video-saturated culture means these videos are experienced with eyes accustomed to TV talk-shows, news programs and documentaries. Videos shot without attention to how an audience – students in this case – will receive it, can often be experienced as slow, as well as indicating that there is nothing visually specific to present.

Using video was of paramount importance, for example, in presenting a managerial issue concerned with relationship marketing that focused on motorcycle-manufacturer Harley Davidson. While research interviews existed of riders talking about their experiences of the company's products, the project really came alive with footage shot during the annual 'posse ride', a cross-country trip that occurred in the summer of 1999. Harley Davidson prides itself on understanding its market by 'getting close to the customer' and building a community of riders through various events. These 'brandfests' create bonds not only between the riders and the product, but between the riders and the company and, most importantly, between riders themselves. The video segments shot on the posse ride told a story about six participants as they traveled across middle America from South Padre Island, Texas to the Canadian Border. Interviews with the riders were intercut with sequences of the riders on their motorcycles, at group events and in intimate interactions with other riders and their bikes – all part of the experiences that create and sustain this subculture community. The video segments allowed students to 'get close to the customer' themselves and experience the ride 'virtually', in order to answer the managerial questions posed.

Incorporate the tacit understandings gained through video, graphics and simulations

As teachers and business leaders well know, learning is only partly cognitive, the greater part of learning consists of tacit knowing – knowing how to do something as well as knowing when to apply the knowledge that we have. In fact, Michael Polanyi's (1962) work on the tacit dimension of knowledge has shown that "we can know more than we can tell and [that] the tacit dimension of all knowledge, while rich and complex, is not easy to convey to others." It is not easy to explain in words how many manufacturing processes work, nor is it easy to capture an entrepreneur's passion for his new technology. A student may not understand the craft dimension of a particular industry or a cross-cultural barrier unless the distinction is clear. In the realm of making business decisions, all these cues are necessary and rich media can be more powerful than words.

Take the case of Volant Ski. For this small high-end company manufacturing steel-tipped skis, students were given a visually complete online explanation of the manufacturing process. Without viewing the step-by-step process, students would have little understanding of its labor-intensive nature which involves a great deal of personal handwork. In addition to the manufacturing vignettes, the case included interviews with essential members of the management team, a simulated sale and the testing process of new skis.

Create multimedia in partnership and be prepared to move beyond traditional teaching and curriculum development

Modern culture has come to rely increasingly on visual images to convey meaning. Yet, according to Sturken and Cartwright (2001): "our colleges and universities traditionally have devoted relatively little attention to visual media ... [and] higher learning remains primarily a text- and symbol-based curriculum." Overcoming this bias to develop compelling online curriculum requires a dual understanding of the phrase 'visual literacy'. It can be used not only to describe an ability to read and interpret images, but can also be used to talk about the ability to *employ* the language of video, graphics and film to create meaningful teaching tools.

In initial multimedia experiments at HBS, faculty members created online cases just as they would a text case: by researching and developing the case themselves or in collaboration with a research associate. Once the case was written, a software developer worked to put the case on the Web. As the process became more complex, with the addition of graphics, pictures, interactive exercises and video, the need for a more skill-intensive and co-ordinated process became necessary. The position of multimedia producer was created to be a liaison between the faculty and the newly formed multimedia department. The department, staffed with software developers, graphic artists, and video editors, worked to develop a user-friendly format and created systematic processes for developing cases.

While academic research and writing are primarily solitary activities, teaching in a multimedia age requires us to attend to a variety of factors that we do not encounter in the use of a traditional curriculum in the context of a seminar or classroom. Working with sound, visuals and interactivity necessitates a collaboration with experts who are conversant in various media and languages, and an understanding that students often have a great deal of sophisticated knowledge about visual media. At the Harvard Business School, it was the faculty's ideas for teaching on the Web that drove the process of innovation, but it was necessary to collaborate with other experts who could both facilitate and execute these ideas. Thinking and teaching in multiple media requires that we learn to work across, and with, different intelligences.

4 Targeting working professionals

The case of a Master of Arts in Gerontology

Edward Schneider, Maria Henke and Carl Renold

An example of the many new online degree courses that have emerged since the Web gained acceptance is provided in this chapter. The authors describe a Masters program in gerontology at the University of Southern California which they have helped to develop. They explain how this program has been designed to use Web capabilities to meet the needs of professionals working with the seniors. The main obstacles for students, faculty and administration created by the novelty of the ICT-based capabilities employed are also highlighted.

The growing demand for education in gerontology

Gerontology is one of the fastest growing academic disciplines (Peterson, Wendt and Douglass, 1994). The increasing demand for gerontological education is particularly strong among professionals who have an educational background in an area not specific to aging (e.g. occupational therapy, social work, and long-term care administration). Such students are typically trained to work with families, children or the general public – but often find themselves struggling to meet the needs of a rapidly-expanding elderly population once they enter the workforce.

An indication of the burgeoning interest in gerontology is shown by the escalation in the number of US colleges and universities offering credit courses in the subject. In 1957, there were fifty-seven such programs (Masunaga, Peterson and Seymour, 1998). By the early 1990s, the number had risen to 1,639 campuses (Peterson, Douglass, Seymour and Wendt, 1997). Despite this growth in academic programs and on-campus students, few professionals working with older Americans have ever had any formal training in gerontology. In addition, new research findings in related areas, such as sociology, psychology, health care, social work, public policy and pharmaceuticals, can dramatically affect the lives of older persons. In order to better meet the needs of the elderly, professionals must therefore gain an understanding of how developments in these diverse areas impact their particular area of expertise.

The Web-based Master of Arts in Gerontology at USC

The Ethel Percy Andrus Gerontology Center at the Leonard Davis School of Gerontology, University of Southern California (USC) is the nation's oldest and largest private educational center devoted entirely to gerontology. However, many students, especially those tied to specific geographic regions due to family and professional commitments, cannot attend traditional classes on the USC campus. To help overcome this problem, in the autumn of 1998 the Center's online division introduced an interactive Master of Arts in Gerontology (MAG). One of its main priorities is to help busy professionals involved in the care of the elderly to acquire the education and training they need in order to keep pace with rapid changes in the multi-disciplinary field of gerontology. The program's online capability offers students the convenience of using the Internet to attend class from their own computers, on their own schedules.

The MAG program consists of a total of twenty-eight graduate units, based on seven four-unit courses. It started in 1998 with an introductory graduate course (Gerontology 500), called *Perspectives on Aging: An Introduction to Gerontology*. A new course was offered each subsequent semester, with the entire seven courses first becoming available in Fall, 2001. Several additional courses will be created in order to allow students some choice in elective credit. Initially, a new cohort of students enters the program each semester, by enrolling in the introductory course; the following semester, all cohorts are combined and take the next available course, until the cycle of seven courses is completed. Students may choose to enroll in any of the courses after the introductory course is completed.

As it is online, MAG can be updated frequently to reflect the most recent findings in the various pertinent fields of study. In addition, it can be easily linked to many large databases available on the Web to help keep students current, and to provide them with the research skills needed to prosper in today's economy.

How the MAG program operates

The program is entirely Web-based, requiring students to attend 'class' on a password-protected Web site. No special software-based 'course-ware' is required to access the program, so students can access their courses from their home, office or while they are traveling – twenty-four hours a day, seven days a week.

The fifteen weeks of the course are conducted asynchronously in one-week blocks of time. For example, if the first assignment is given on a Wednesday at 1:00 p.m., then it must be completed by the next Tuesday at 1:00 p.m. (co-ordinated according to Pacific Standard Time). Students may log on to the site at any time they choose during the duration of the week. They are encouraged to do this early in the week, and as often as possible, in order to develop a dialogue with their classmates and instructor.

Online students are an integral part of the Andrus community, interacting with classmates and faculty in one-on-one and group discussions. Professors and staff are available throughout the program to discuss the lecture topics and class work, and to assist with any technical problems that may arise. Students are given their own computer account, which provides access to USC information services and library resources. For example, students may access the USC Gerontology Library's 'LibraryWorks' online services to borrow books, request journal articles and utilize the 'Ask the Librarian' reference service.

Efforts are made to make available to online students special lectures and presentations from distinguished academics visiting the USC campus. Online students are also informed of all televised USC sporting events and other extra-curricular activities. In addition, students are strongly encouraged to attend the annual meetings of the Gerontological Society of America and the American Society on Aging. There, students have the opportunity to meet each other, Andrus faculty, staff and alumni, as well as traditional students from campus.

MAG online courses provide a variety of learning experiences within the structure of each fifteen-week Web-based course. Students are invited to participate in vigorous online discussions with class-mates and instructors about issues affecting the elderly. Not only are students encouraged to interact with, and respond to, one another and their instructor; they are also given ample opportunity to interact with, and respond to, the course. Weekly innovative electronic exercises have been designed especially for each course, in order to reinforce and better explain concepts. For example, in addition to reading a lecture about cataracts, students have the opportunity to look through an interactive 'Vision Simulator' to see what the world looks like to someone with the disease. They are able to click on several aids to view how vision impairments can be corrected or minimized.

Each week of a course consists of the following components: required readings from a text, as well as supplemental readings from the university's electronic reserve or from a printed course reader; a lecture written by the course instructor, or by a guest lecturer who is also a leading expert in a specific area of gerontology; interactive exercises that further enhance understanding of the subject matter; an essay assignment that is sent via e-mail to the instructor; and, finally, a discussion in a cyber-classroom. The 'lectures' are supplemented by links to other related Web-based materials, animated graphics, short video clips, useful facts – 'factoids' – and definitions of new concepts and terms.

As students read through the lecture, they encounter various interactive exercises, charts, graphs, or figures that will pop up when clicked. Students are also able to click on selected terms that will take them to a glossary. These activities are designed to further explain and illustrate the lecture's major concepts. At the end of each week's lesson, students are required to compose a three to five page essay that integrates the week's material. During the established course duration, students are expected to keep pace with assignments and deliver them on schedule to the instructor for review and analysis. In order to keep up with the course, instructors recommend that students schedule a specific time each week to read the required text and supplemental materials, 'attend' the lecture, view the interactive exercises, participate in the cyber-classroom and complete the essay assignment. This should be at a time convenient for the student, and when they will least likely be distracted.

Challenges posed by introducing an innovative online approach

When the MAG program was first introduced, students, faculty and administration had to deal with a number of obstacles associated with its development and delivery. These stemmed from the novelty of the program's utilization of new technologies. The MAG was implemented within a university structure that had no previous experience with students who were unable to come to campus. While the University administration was supportive of the new program, there were no formal policies in place to implement the program effectively at its launch. All student services had to be performed at the departmental level.

One significant problem was that many potential students were reluctant to enroll in a program offered via the Internet. Many expressed anxiety over their ability to access and navigate the courses effectively; several had never accessed the Internet, and two had not found it necessary to own a computer until enrolling in this program. This problem was overcome by providing technical assistance over the telephone. Each student entering the program was assured that the courses were designed to be simple to use and that technological barriers would be easy to overcome. Technical support was offered to students by faculty and staff during normal hours of operation. In all but a few cases, students rapidly adapted to their online classroom.

The MAG is designed to be accessible to the widest possible audience; therefore, instructional design is facilitated by easy-to-use and readily-available software. Program administrators became acutely aware of the gap in technological expertise between university personnel and the average end-user. So, it was necessary to sensitize technical support staff to the needs of students without any previous computer experience.

Faculty also require training in order to help them teach online and in an asynchronous manner. In addition, faculty require release time from their regular duties to prepare their fifteen-week courses and be trained to teach in the new format. It has been the experience of the Andrus faculty that online courses require more preparation than their traditional on-campus courses. As teaching online requires as much time as traditional courses, online courses must be scheduled into the existing faculty workload.

Future developments

In order to continue the growth of the MAG program, several strategies need to be implemented in the future:

- continuation of efforts to develop personal relationships between faculty and online students;
- greater recognition of the need for faculty training;
- increased support from the wider campus community including formalized policies to ease the registration process and access to student services;

- more course offerings with other units on campus, so that students can take advantage of dual degrees and minors, a concentration in a complementary field through a set of prescribed courses;
- increased technical support staff in order to keep pace with growing enrollment.

The Andrus online MAG program has made tremendous strides since it was launched. By the Fall of 2001, enrollment had surpassed original projections by nearly a third. If this rate continues, revenue is likely to surpass the on-campus program by 2005 (student numbers have already surpassed campus-based enrollment). USC's 2002 Commencement ceremony was attended by 11 graduates from the MAG program.

5   Students' difficulties in a Web-based distance education course

An ethnographic study

Noriko Hara and Rob Kling

Hype and promotion are often essential to encourage individual and institutional change, but the reality of distance education and distributed learning is not problem-free and will require as much attention as has been given to traditional classroom instructional technique and training. This chapter explores this reality through a study that offers an in-depth qualitative analysis of the distress felt by students in a graduate-level online course at a major US university. Hara and Kling describe their study and its findings, which aim to help enhance understanding of instructional design issues, communication practices and the preparation needed by instructors and students for effective Internet-enabled distance learning.

Internet-enabled distance education

Cutting-edge digital communications and learning technologies enable universities to implement distance education to reach more diverse populations and to provide more available learning environments twenty-four hours a day, seven days a week. Internet-enabled courses that rely primarily on asynchronous, text-based communication media are a rapidly-growing means of providing such courses (National Center for Education Statistics, 1998)[1]. Here, we describe a detailed study of one such course, particularly the students' feelings of distress.

There are at least five major kinds of literatures about Internet-enabled distance education, covering:

* specialized research (such as the *Journal of Asynchronous Learning Networks* and the *American Journal of Distance Education*);

- practitioners (e.g. the *Chronicle of Higher Education*);
- instructional materials for specific courses;
- popular accounts of such courses;
- marketing descriptions.

Most of these diverse sources emphasize the likely value of Internet-enabled distance education institutions for reaching new students, and generating new revenues. The prospective students are attracted to convenience and, possibly, enriched educational experiences.

There is some debate about the actual costs and profits of distance education (Green, 1997). Among academic practitioners, there has also been considerable concern about whether universities or their staff own the instructional materials they develop for these courses (Noble, 1998). Some research studies have also examined the difficulties faced by instructors in developing and teaching such courses (Rahm and Reed, 1998). However, it is hard to find studies that give the students' perspectives, other than through course evaluation forms and concise characterizations of students' comments and experiences (Wegerif, 1998; Rossman, 1999). The majority of practitioner and popular articles tend to emphasize the virtues and minimize the difficulties of routinely providing high quality and effective Internet-enabled distance education courses (e.g. Barnard, 1997; Yakimovicz and Murphy, 1995). This promotional bias has been characteristic of similar literatures about computerization (Kling, 1994). Further, many characterizations of this form of education deftly intertwine themes of needed educational reforms to improve accessibility and a larger cultural narrative about "the death of distance" (Iacono and Kling, 2001).

It is anticipated that the demand for distance education would increase in the future. As a result, many first-time online instructors and students could face similar issues addressed in this chapter.

Background to the study of students' experiences of an online course

In 1997, we undertook an ethnographic case study of student experiences in a specific online course. The first author (Hara) conducted interviews and observations on the course[2], and collected course-specific documentary data. We chose to study this particular course only because of the availability of in-depth data made possible by the instructor's permission to allow observation of the online class and interviews with the students, thus allowing more observational and ethnography data than was previously reported.

Our original research question was: "How do the students in this course manage their feelings of isolation in a virtual classroom in order to create the sense of a community of learning?" However, during the study we learned that student isolation was not a major problem, although some prior studies have cited its importance in distance education (e.g. Besser and Donahue, 1996; Rahm and Reed, 1998). The recurrent experiences of other types of distress, such as frustration, anxiety and confusion, seemed to be pervasive. Possibly because of the small class size, the students supported each other and developed a sufficient sense of community.

A few studies of online courses have mentioned students' frustration with technical problems or anxiety about communication norms (Dede, 1996; Feenberg, 1987), but emphasized the value of the student learning. We felt that the substantial distresses about such aspects reported in our study were not incidental, and could actually impede learning (Hara and Kling, 1999). So, we shifted our focus to examine the conditions that led these students to be distressed, and to some of the consequences. We also reviewed the literature of Internet-enabled distance education, but found only one study reporting on such phenomena (Wegerif, 1998).

The practitioner literature includes some high-quality advice for the instructors of face-to-face lecture classes (e.g. McKeachie, 1999). However, we could not find materials of similar quality about online courses which could help to avoid the difficulties we observed. Handbooks to enhance face-to-face teaching often anchor their tips in specific research, and flesh them out with contextualized examples. In contrast, articles with tips to improve online teaching are rarely explicit about the basis for the recommendations and often do not provide examples of ways that students and instructors can utilize the typically generalized advice (such as "emphasize interactivity"). The huge discrepancy in the quality, quantity and accessibility of the materials for face-to-face versus online courses leads us to suspect that the difficulties experienced in our study might also be experienced by students in other Web-based courses.

This small-scale case study therefore raises interesting and important issues that merit serious engagement well beyond this class or this university. The key issue is to understand how people work with their innovations in practice, without censoring what is problematic. This chapter may help stimulate a better understanding of instructional design issues, instructor preparation, student selection practices and communicative practices that should be widely encouraged.

The course we studied

We studied B3002[3], a graduate educational technology course at a major university in the USA. In the course, students learn how to use information technologies in their areas of expertise. It was taught through a Web site developed the previous summer by graduate students working with close faculty supervision. The site contained links to reading materials, activities, discussion questions, additional readings, the course syllabus and assignment instructions. After students entered their user names and passwords, they would see the menu screen. This page used the metaphor of a traditional classroom, so that the student could be situated in a familiar environment.

In 1997, B3002 enrolled eight students studying for a Masters degree; six of them completed the course. Four students had only minimal experience with computers, but one was enthusiastic about technology and spent thirty to forty hours a week on this course at the beginning of the semester. One student was very familiar with computers, as well as knowing about course content through friends who had taken B3002 during the prior summer. The sixth student trained teachers in integrating computers into a curriculum, but lived far from the university and thus did not have direct access to university facilities. This was the only student who had taken a distance education course prior to B3002. The instructor was a PhD candidate. She was also an experienced educator, although this was her first experience teaching in higher education and by distance education. She had taken B3002 in the summer of 1996, audited B3002 again over the previous summer and participated in the B3002 Web site design team. This site was used in a traditional class version of B3002 during the previous summer, but was not substantially altered for the online version of B3002. Instead, the instructor sent weekly e-mails to inform students about the differences in some activities.

The inquiry used three methodologies:

- *observation* of relevant activities, such as classroom discussions and during students' interactions with the course Web site, when they were asked to "think aloud" while using a computer;
- *interviews* of about one hour with students immediately after they had finished online tasks, as well as informal conversations with some students and the instructor;
- *document review*, including the course syllabus and reading assignments.

Comparison of the information collected from various sources helped to verify the data. This was done to check that different data collected from a given informant supported each other, and that different informants tended to report similar issues. Informed consent was obtained before each of our observations and interviews, and interview transcripts and interpretation were validated by participants. Pseudonyms are used in order to protect the informants' identities.

Student distresses in an online course

The students did not report that all of their course activities were distressing. However, the following examples illustrate the distressing events that stood out for them.

A virtual field trip

The following observations were made at a special event in the middle of the semester which provided an opportunity for the students to visit the virtual online SchMOOze University[4]. When people join SchMOOze University electronically, they see text-based screens. People can also use simple commands, such as "go to east", to explore different virtual buildings to meet others from all over the world. Prior to this event, the instructor had used e-mail to send out instruction and a map for the SchMOOze University.

All students and the instructor were supposed to gather at a virtual meeting room at 8:30 p.m., so that the instructor could see who was online. I was observing one student, Kathy. She started the field trip at her home by typing *@knock MMM* (instructor's name), but the computer replied:

> > I don't know

Kathy said, "It doesn't understand. How stupid it is. Let's try with a different name." Then she typed *@knock MMM* two or three more times, but continued to receive the same response. She murmured, "I don't know what I am supposed to do. Maybe I am already in." Several messages then appeared on her computer screen, where conversation proceeded very quickly, making it very difficult to follow. A student complained:

> > Sheryl: Please slow down.

However, the conversation never slowed. When Kathy saw the message:

> MMM: everybody seems familiar with commands.

Kathy typed: *I practiced this afternoon.* When she typed, Kathy seemed very careful about spelling and capitalization.

> Sheryl: I like the action of calling rows.

Kathy remarked, "I think what she means is 'calling role.' Sometimes it's confusing, half of the students are non-native speakers." Kathy then saw the message:

> Julie: Julie is here

She tried to respond to it. While she was typing, she commented, "By the time I type in my response, the conversation is gone." She typed: *Welcome*, intending this comment for Julie, but at this time several people who were not in the class joined the discussion.

The first thirty minutes went by very quickly while Kathy tried to identify who was there and what to do. Kathy explained, "This is the first time we talked together." She complained, "What are we supposed to do?" and glanced at her watch. It was almost 9 p.m. and, according to the instructor's guideline, students were supposed to leave the original meeting room, go to different buildings at SchMOOze University and look for possible student activities. Therefore, Kathy typed: *Are we supposed to move around now?*

> MMM: choose building

When she saw the instructor's message, she murmured: "I'm going to be out, go to lobby, and go to Mall." However, she couldn't find anybody to talk to at the virtual Mall, so she maneuvered back to the original meeting room. She saw on the screen that there were still students from the B3002 class continuing discussions. She said, "Now, I'm back to the discussion" and typed: *Guess I need to stay put.*

> MMM: go to the building

Kathy said, "I feel like nobody is answering my question," and complained, "I've already been around the campus and…"

While she was deciding what to do next, the online discussion at the meeting room was continuing. When she saw a message referring to Ann, she typed: *Who's Ann?* The situation was chaotic in the room because different simultaneous conversations were overlapping. Before identifying Ann, Kathy said, "Maybe I'll explore the campus now." She suggested to her classmates that they go to a virtual bar, by typing *How about the bar?* She then saw everyone's agreement, as well as a message saying:

> \> Knock, knock

Kathy suspected that somebody had knocked at her door. She responded by typing: *Enter*, but received no answer. She muttered, "What am I supposed to do? I'm confused," and looked at the instructor's guide. Kathy assumed Julie was sending a message that knocks at her door because she saw Julie's message asking her a question, and thus she tried to find where Julie was. Kathy then moved to where Julie was and Julie sent a message to her:

> \> Julie: I don't want to leave you at the bar alone.

Kathy laughed when she read the message. Julie tried to instruct her how to respond to a knock in this text-based environment, but Kathy was still struggling. Kathy looked at her watch and said, "This is exactly an hour." She told me, "If I have one complaint about this class, it is that time goes so quickly. I can be hooked up with a computer for a whole day and then realize that I haven't had a dinner or I haven't prepared my lesson plans."

Kathy had tried to be well prepared for this special event, including visiting the SchMOOze site earlier in the day – although no one had then responded to her attempts at conversation. Nevertheless, she had experienced many difficulties during the field trip. She was overwhelmed by her first experience of the fast pace of communication and felt frustrated at not being able to figure out why she could not operate her intended commands. There was no one to ask for help, so she had to attempt to resolve the difficulties by herself.

Another student, Amy, was also frustrated by the problem she had with operational commands at SchMOOze University. At a computer lab a few days after this event, Amy commented that she had "got lost" at SchMOOze University when she planned to meet with the classmates. She added:

I talked to other people from different places at SchMOOze University, but not my classmates. I was so frustrated because everyone else could do it, but why not me? Not only for the SchMOOze University activity, but I put in lots of time for this course overall, but I couldn't see the results. Like I paid a hundred dollars, but I only got ten dollars back. I probably spend a hundred minutes, but I can get ten dollars worth.

Julie also had a distressing experience with this virtual trip. The slow connection from her computer meant her responses were significantly delayed. On the day after the virtual field trip, another student also reflected on the trip in a personal e-mail to the instructor:

I thought your [the instructor's] preparation for our visit to SchMOOze U was excellent. ... I did not enjoy our class excursion there however because the technology did not live up to expectations. I also felt more encumbered by knowing people there. I was more cognizant of hurt feelings and other people's frustration, and it narrowed my exploration.

There were, however, some positive comments about the virtual field trip. John seemed to be excited about the new technology he was experiencing, and was generally enthusiastic about the SchMOOze University activity, despite encountering some negative aspects:

I'd loved the MOO session. I felt like doing that, we're really sort of like a community. I was totally laughing, at my computer, laughing. It's so weird to laugh at the computer. But I was laughing because I really felt somebody's there talking. And I met a person that was kind of cold to me and asked me weird questions, and they never really answered my questions. That hurt, you know? So it's real feelings that were involved.

Working alone at night

It is common for students in many online courses to work alone, often at home in the evenings or weekends. However, it is hard for students who work under these conditions to resolve potentially frustrating problems that can typically be discussed and resolved more readily in a face-to-face class meeting. The dynamics of this issue is illustrated by the experiences of one student, John, whom I met unexpectedly when he was working alone after midnight in a campus computer lab.

The week's topic was "feedback and time." John was working on an assignment to evaluate a set of lesson plans that used information technologies in education. He was to use the Internet to find these plans, which had been developed by various unknown instructors located by the B3002 Web design team. John started talking:

J: I am frustrated because I am here too long (*laugh*).
I[5]: How long have you been here?
J: Ohhhhh, I…probably nine o'clock, I guess.
I: Four hours?
J: Yeah. So, my eyes are tired. Of course, a part of the problem is not totally the class's fault. Part of the problem is finding things really interesting. They don't completely relate to the class. I mean, we are looking for things, lesson plans that we have to evaluate, right? And there are all kinds of great lesson plans. I am looking for ideas for my classes and I just get stuck. Then by the time I'm at the place where I really need to be doing my work, I'm totally frustrated because I really want to go home. I don't want to be here anymore…
I: Too much information?
J: Perhaps. I mean these links on the B3002 Web site have all the lesson plans that we can give to a class. I think this one (*pointing to a link*), just tons and tons of activities, but most of the stuff on these, I don't like.

John went on to explain that he was frustrated and distressed with the poor quality of many of the lesson plans he had found for his assignment. He reported significant distress during this interview. He still had not received specifications for the assignments from the instructor and was confused about her expectations.

When I left the computer lab, John returned to his assignment and declared, "I will finish this work anyway. It'll probably take an hour and it may not be a good work. … But just do it." It was almost 1:20 a.m.

Interactive communication tool: e-mail

The students and instructor relied upon e-mail as a primary means of communication. In fact, the instructor required that students post e-mail to the class discussion forum "at least five times during the course" and "to check the list daily." The students and the instructor generated quite intensive online discussions through e-mail, and all of the students posted far more than five one-to-two page-long messages. On the surface, this indicates a lively class. However, we found that there were some underlying problems with the reliance on e-mail.

First, some students did not read other people's postings before writing their own e-mail messages. Second, some students were unable to make time to read and post e-mail during short intensive discussion periods; some reported being overwhelmed by the volume of e-mail. For example, the student who posted the fewest number of messages to the online class discussion sent an e-mail with the subject line: "Ah ... I cannot catch up with all of you." Some of the student difficulties were a by-product of using e-mail differently from the "standard view", in which students read e-mail online and reply immediately from their computers.

My observations of Amy, who did not have a computer printer at home, revealed a more complex way of working. She logged in from a campus computer lab and copied all of her e-mail messages into a word-processing file. "After that, I delete the messages because it's too much e-mail." At the lab, she printed out all the e-mail messages and readings for B3002 and then read them at home. She replied to messages on another day, when she returned to the campus computer lab.

Another student, Eric, also commented about the overwhelming e-mail messages:

> I don't like, I have to say, turning on the computer and finding that I have eleven messages on my e-mail. It's a pain. I mean to answer that many things, just talking in conversation would be so much easier, rather than replying and doing all the stuff you have to do. So, that is just time-consuming, but it is a part of at a distance. I think if you are doing that, you have to be aware that you're gonna be spending more time with computer problems, not getting online, software freaking out, crashing, whatever it's gonna happen, gonna take you a lot longer, waiting in a line at a lab. There are so many things that make it kind of difficult to do.

It appeared that students in B3002 were competing with each other, or felt obligated to produce a notable number of thoughtful and detailed e-mail messages. The category "e-mail messages" includes short conversational notes and more elaborate multi-screen memos; these are mixed with the student's other more general e-mail flow, such as messages from other students, friends and administrative announcements. The instructor also commented that at the beginning of the semester she was spending all day reading and responding to e-mail messages. Later in the semester, she was able to reduce her workload, but still spent a large amount of time on this course.

Other research also indicates that it can be very demanding for students and instructors to read all their messages when they are sent asynchronously at different times (Hiltz, 1998; Wegerif, 1998; Hara, Bonk and Angeli, 2000).

Understanding student perspectives

Complexities of working alone

A valued advantage of asynchronous distance education is its ability to allow students to work at different times and in different locations. However, students in our study reported some confusion and anxiety because of the absence of physical cues in communication interactions, as B3002 had no video support. For instance, when John was working on a B3002 activity in a computer lab, he pointed to an e-mail message from the instructor and said:

> I agree with her, but I am not sure if I should send a message saying, "I agree." That's the problem with this e-mail. If this is the classroom, you can just nod your head to show your agreement. I am not always sure that if I am contributing enough or not. Other people, like Julie and Kathy, are really active. I feel a sense of competitiveness. So, my survival skill is not to respond. In fact, I haven't gotten any feedback about my contribution. I cannot tell from the e-mail. You can tell from the classroom what the professor thinks about you from the body language and the way they talk. So, I am not feeling that I'm getting enough assessment.

Eric also indicated his frustration with not getting enough feedback, while Sheryl expressed her frustration with the lack of immediate assistance from the instructor, as well as the difficulty of finding information on the Internet. When working on a B3002 assignment, Sheryl typed the keyword instructions for evaluating "electronic learning" at the Yahoo Education site. The computer responded:

> There is no Web site to match your inquiry.

Sheryl looked unhappy. It is likely that she had used too specific a phrase rather than a careful selection of keywords. She next went to the AltaVista search engine because one of her friends had told her that "AltaVista is much better." AltaVista helped her to locate one Web site, but that didn't help her. Sheryl did another search with the keywords *educational assessment*, which produced too many matching pages. She tried to narrow down her inquiry by adding *assessments* and *education*. When this seemed to produce a more reasonable list of the sites for her topic, she printed out two pages for her assignment. While she was assessing the Web sites, she also read the e-mail instruction from the teacher again to make sure she was on the right track (she carried a three-inch-thick folder with all the e-mail messages for this course). Sheryl next went to the Web site referred to in the e-mail instruction, but she did not find relevant readings there. So she went to yet another search engine, InfoSeek. After three different keyword searches, she found a promising reference. However, when she tried the links on that page she could not reach the sites she was looking for. Sheryl compared this experience to what she had heard about the B3002 class that had been taught over the summer: "They had more resources. They saw a teacher in person, so they might have had the same problem, but not as much frustration as this."

Commentary on working alone

In contrast to John's positive comments on the virtual field trip, he seemed to be unsure about the communication conventions appropriate for participating in the online class. Eric had indicated the same problem. Some of their anxieties and communicative confusions were caused by the lack of feedback from the instructor because they couldn't see her physically. That is the byproduct of having limited social cues, such as gestures and facial expressions (Harasim, 1987; McIsaac and Gunawardena, 1996; Feenberg, 1987).

Sheryl expressed frustration at her poor background in understanding effective Web searching and a lack of immediate help. One gap in the 1997 version of B3002 may be the (tacit) assumption that graduate students in this program all had good online search skills. (The face-to-face version of B3002 included interns who could consult with students at their PCs when they had technical problems.)

The lack of prompt feedback from the instructor was certainly a major source of anxiety and frustration for students because they were concerned about their performance. According to McIsaac and Gunawardena (1996), "the concept of interaction [including feedback] is fundamental to the effectiveness of distance education programs as well as traditional ones" (ibid: 407). Bonk and Cummings (1998) also suggest the significance of feedback in Web courses. In B3002, the instructor did apologize later in the semester for not providing "enough and prompt feedback."

Technological problems

During the interviews, some students reported frustration with technological problems and the absence of personnel to provide technical support. Unlike the other students, the following informant was taking the course from a distant site. She indicated three areas of frustration:

> First of all, inappropriate prerequisite statement. For example, there is nothing to say that you should know HTML, but our first assignment was creating a Web site. Fortunately, I knew it. I'd explored learning how to do HTML by myself. If I didn't know, I just cannot imagine how to get through. Secondly, this course is very time specific. The course I took before, I could go in anytime and finish anytime. However, this course is very specific in terms of time. For example, I got into the class a week late and the instructor sent me e-mail saying that they had already started. As an old learner, I felt so intimidated. I felt pressure to catch up. Third, accessibility to technology. This is related to the prerequisite. There is nothing that says we should have access to a Web server. However, when we developed the Web site as an assignment, we had to have the server access. Since I work for a school, one of the technical people helped me to connect to the Web server. If I didn't have these resources here, I would have dropped this course.

Some students expressed their anxieties and frustrations with the course in their e-mail messages. For example, on a Friday evening a student wrote the following to the instructor: *I have spent one hour trying to follow your directions. I am getting an error message. The first time I tried to download it as a zip file, the error says, cannot access this file. I am getting extremely frustrated.*
On Saturday afternoon she wrote another e-mail message regarding the same issue:

> This computer is very frustrating. I would imagine it is like sitting in a class and only understanding some of what was said, then asked to answer a question. I have felt it ... *panic ... isolation ...*

frustration ... anger. This has been a very good lesson. I will keep trying.

About thirty minutes after this message, the student sent an e-mail message saying that she had solved the problem.

The instructor's personal reflection notes expressing her problems and frustrations with not being able to solve the student's technical problems offered a different perspective, and helped us better understand the class dynamics. For example, the instructor wrote:

> I may need to understand more about how network and ISPs [Internet Service Providers] work. This to me is a hardware issue that I really did not want to touch and that I don't know how much help I could give to people. But, Julie and the previous two real distance students (who dropped out after several frustrated experiences) keep pushing me to this knowledge domain.

Because of their e-mail interactions, the instructor knew that students had difficulty dealing with technological problems and felt frustrated. During the interview, she commented:

> even though we provided them with very good, we thought, very good job-aids, but still they had difficulties. Help themselves learn. They are not in that kind of mode yet. They still need help. I guess both them and us, we are not used to this kind of environment at all. If you are in a classroom, a teacher can lead them during the process, so whenever they have problems, we can just fix it, right on a spot. However, if you give them the job-aids, if there is anything wrong there, there is no way we know. There is no way we can fix it right away and make it smooth for them. So that's frustrating for them and also frustrating to *me* because sometimes you feel that you've done everything you could, but it just doesn't work out that way.

Commentary on the technological problems

The problems with technological hardware and support reported by students on the courses is reflected in several research studies (e.g. Burge, 1994; Wiesenberg and Hutton, 1995). However, these studies do not thoroughly investigate the issue, although the importance of computing support for professional work and even the public's use of the Internet has been well reported in other research (see Kling and Jewett, 1991; Kling, 2000).

Pedagogical issue – ambiguous instructions

Much of human communication is inherently ambiguous. But people can often adequately resolve key ambiguities when they are face to face. When the primary communication medium is written text, resolving ambiguities may be more difficult for many people, as Amy indicated in the following interview excerpt:

> Though I understand each sentence and word in the e-mail that the instructor sent us, I don't know how to use the instructions to compose the programming. Because in her instruction, sometimes I can follow steps 1 and 2, and then I can't follow from steps 2 to 3. So I go back to the beginning and start over. The instruction is all in text, no graphics because she sends it to us through e-mail. ... So, when I submit my assignment, I always put a note to her, "please let me know if I need to do more, or if I need to delete something" to make sure I do the things that I am supposed to do, because I don't know exactly what the instructor wants.

Amy identified two recurrent sources of communicative ambiguity. She had trouble adequately interpreting both the instructor's weekly e-mailed instructions, as well as the instructions on the B3002 Web site. For instance, one of the activity instructions on the Web site was:

1. Review the sample testware package that you have. What does it test? How do you think it facilitates learning? OR Visit one of these sites: [*List of URLs*]
2. Read at least two electronic portfolios (student works) in Student Project page [*URL*]. How would you give feedback to the students?

OR

3. To create a quiz on the Web, here are some tools you can use: [*List of URLs*]

The instructor's intent was to give the students flexibility. However, some students did not consider this flexibility to be an advantage, and they wanted more structure and clearer direction. Sheryl, for example, said:

I think the biggest problem [in this course] is the instruction of our assignments. I usually don't understand what she wants, either e-mail or from the Web site. Actually I shared the printouts with my friend. He is a doctoral student, and he looked at the instructions. He thought that our instructor was not a very good presenter because he also agreed that those instructions were so ambiguous that it's very confusing. There were no points at all. Sometimes, she takes all kinds of responses and she would say, "it's good you are creative," but sometimes I got her response saying this is not what I want. So I felt very frustrated because we were supposed to be creative and that's what I came up with, but she said that's not what she wanted.

Sheryl went on to relate her dissatisfaction with the amount of content provided by the course, particularly that of theoretical orientation to the material. Unlike the other students in the class, Sheryl had no prior background in the subject area. Given the course's lack of clear instructions, background information or even explicit definitions of terms, she found herself having to attempt to glean this information from the general class discussions, and felt that she had only gained a general sense of the material. Like Amy, Sheryl also gave up trying to clarify the instructor's expectations after asking her a few questions.

Kathy's frustration was that she was uncertain what the instructor expected because she could not see the instructor physically. She also gave an example in an e-mail message of how she misinterpreted the instructor's message:

You sit in a [traditional] classroom with somebody and you analyze who they are, and what they like. You cannot analyze these things online because you've never seen them. So, you are only guessing at what the teacher really wants. You don't know how to interpret what they say because you don't know their personality. Like one time, the teacher was joking and I took her seriously and it really hurt. She was saying that, I can't remember what it was now, but something about that nobody is working ... since none of you are working at this, maybe we should do such and such and I wrote her back, "what do you mean we are not working. I am spending 6 hours a day" and she wrote back and said, "it was only a joke". ... but I think if you are, like, very careful in what you write and communicate often with people, you can put them easily to get to know you.

The instructor knew that the instructions on the Web were too ambiguous, and attempted to clarify them. For the final project, she sent out an e-mail message saying "I think we need a set of very clear criteria so that you and I know exactly what you are expected to do and how your project will be 'judged'." However, this attempt did not succeed, as a few students posted questions about her "clear criteria."

Both the students and the instructor reported periodic distress with this course. Even so, during interviews the students complimented the instructor's overall performance. They appreciated her support. Some students even sympathized with her because she also had to resolve many technological problems. The distance education format amplified the difficulty of interpreting the student messages, as the instructor reported receiving periodic e-mail about ambiguous expectations for the course.

Commentary on ambiguous instructions

Three student concerns stand out. First, the asynchronous 'anywhere-anytime' format of B3002 often led to significant delays between the times that students raised questions and the times that the instructor could reasonably answer them. In face-to-face courses, in contrast, students can reduce major ambiguities by conversing with the instructor and each other during class meetings. Second, this course's Web site was originally developed for the same course offered in summer in a traditional classroom, so did not always fit the distance requirements of B3002. For example, students were instructed to form teams, although in the Web-based distance education course students had to work individually. Third, the Web site had been developed before the course had started, and some links to other Web sites were no longer accessible. Not all the students in B3002 were familiar with the technology used in the course and some were feeling rather overwhelmed. Therefore, the unclear instructions and expectations for B3002 probably amplified their anxiety.

Dealing with distresses

Amy stopped discussing problems with the instructor after one bad experience. She dealt with her distresses with B3002 by talking with a classmate of similar ethnicity in her own native language. Amy explained:

A: I am calling a friend every week, just to complain. She is a good listener, whenever I complained, she just listened and I felt better.

I: Did you complain to your instructor?

A: Once.

I: Why just once?

A: I complained once about the difficulty of searching on the Web, and she gave me the tips for searching as I told you before. After that, I didn't complain because I felt stupid. I should have spent more time on this, but I couldn't because I'm too busy. If I hadn't taken this many courses and also work, I could ... if you want to take this course, you *have to* spend time. I want to complain, but it's not the instructor's problem, or the class's fault. It's my problem. There is nothing she can do about it.

Despite his periodic frustrations, John expressed a different view in an informal conversation. He believed that his frustrations were a good learning experience because now he understood what his students might experience when he teaches similar courses in the future.

B3002's instructor did try to help her students resolve their difficulties. Later in the semester, she started to ask students for their suggestions to improve tutorials and teaching materials. She believed that at this point the students felt less frustrated. In her personal reflection notes she wrote:

> It was from the MOO week that I started asking them for improvement ideas, and it seems to me that this opened a new door for communication. ... All of the sudden they agreed that it is all right to be frustrated when following instructions that are with flaws, because flaws give opportunities to think and to gain real control.

Commentary on dealing with distresses

If students could deal effectively with their frustrations, B3002 might not be a negative experience. In fact, the students supported each other by sharing their frustrations with their friends or classmates. We suspect that without this mutual support, none of the students would have completed this course. Some students felt a community of learning with their classmates. The instructor also helped create a sense of community among the students. Bates (1994) claims that one of the major contributions of two-way technologies is allowing interactions among students as well as between students and instructors, and there was some active interaction among students in this course. Many researchers note the importance of virtual community to support students (e.g., Burge, 1994; McIsaac and Gunawardena, 1996). In this case study, however, it seemed that student distresses – confusion, anxiety and frustration – recurred throughout the term.

Conclusions drawn from the B3002 online course

Instructors' misperceptions of student distress

From the interviews and observations, we found two foci of student distress in B3002. The first was technological problems, with those students who did not have access to technical support being especially frustrated. The second involved course content and the instructor's practices in managing her communications with students. Students reported confusion, anxiety and frustration when they wanted prompt feedback from the instructor, and when they found ambiguous instructions on the Web and in e-mail messages. The instructor did not appreciate the duration of the student distress. She believed she had effectively eliminated their anxieties and frustrations during the term, noting during an interview:

> They [the students] thought that the problems they had were basically their own; other people did not have the same problem until we opened up the conversation and they realized that, oh, yeah, we were all in the same boat. Now, they have this peer support coming in. That [problem], I think, we took care of pretty well.

However, her students still expressed their frustrations and anxieties during observations and interviews late in the semester. Part of the reason for the instructor's misperception resulted from the student's reluctance to express all of their anxieties, frustrations and confusions to the instructor, probably because of the frequent power differential between students and instructors in university courses. We suspect that these difficulties were exacerbated by the weaker social cues of asynchronous text-based communication. After all, small elective graduate courses are often highly rated. There are two important reasons for this: instructors can better appreciate their students' experiences and preferences than in larger courses, and the smaller courses have greater latitude in flexible adaptation during the term.

The pains of innovation

We caution against emphasizing only the virtues of computer-mediated distance education, as is done in most articles written for practitioners (i.e., administrators and teachers) and lay people (e.g., potential students). In some of these upbeat studies, students may not have had opportunities to express their confusions and anxieties with Web-based distance education. At the end of the semester, students might make positive comments about the courses because of a relief in finishing a course and concern about hurting the instructor's feelings. For example, one B3002 student posted this "thank you" note during the final week:

> I do believe you all are the best classmates and instructor I have ever met. I can see your hard work, your enthusiasm and your patience learning along. I'd like to say that the most successful condition I've learned from this class is a warm and supportive class atmosphere.

If students give public evaluations like this in courses like B3002, the positive results of many studies – including such findings as students enjoying their experiences despite communication break-downs and technical problems – can be artifacts of the research methods. Unfortunately, only a few scholars (e.g., Bromley and Apple, 1998; Feenberg, 1999; Jaffee, 1998; Wegerif, 1998) examine important limitations and pervasive problems and their studies are found in the specialty research literature rather than integrated into the practitioners' literatures.

We found some discrepancies among the different data sources: observations, interviews and e-mail messages. Triangulating various kinds of data sources enabled us to see this distance education course from a different perspective. We recommend that future researchers use this kind of multi-source methodology to study distance education courses.

Understanding instructional work and communication in practice

It is time to examine seriously actual experiences for students in distance education courses, and to discuss critically the wide array of practices and experiences that undermine the outcome of distance education. It is easy to place the burden of student frustrations wholly upon the instructor's limitations. One might argue that this course was a unique case of an insufficiently experienced instructor poorly teaching an online course, which tells us nothing about online courses in general. We disagree. In this era when the number of online courses is growing rapidly, many instructors teaching them are likely to be leading their first online course. Yet, we have not found any widely publicized articles that encourage faculty who are starting to teach an online course to prepare in special ways.

We believe the students' ongoing concern about "prompt unambiguous feedback" is much more difficult to achieve in text-based asynchronous courses than in face-to-face conditions, for instance because of the way students worked on the course during late evenings and weekends. This issue could be even more significant in larger classes. What is needed is for students and instructors to learn how to manage their expectations about when they should be able to have reliable, fast communicative responses.

Part of the communicative complexity of constructing adequately unambiguous conversations via text-based media comes from trying to anticipate the level of detail and phrasing that will be sufficiently helpful to others. But, as our informants noted, they were also unsure what meta-communicative conventions would be appropriate in their online conversations. E-mail that represents the nodded heads of a face-to-face group could be valued by an instructor to confirm others' understanding. Or it could result in yet more e-mail glut. These kinds of practices need to be negotiated within each group. In B3002 and many other courses, both face-to-face and online, participants don't explicitly question and negotiate meta-communicative conventions, even when they are confused and frustrated. These discussions and negotiations require a higher level of social skills from all participants. And their enactment, such as creating a strong social presence in a written medium, also requires time and expressive capabilities. This is not well explained in the literatures of online instruction. Clearly, we need more student-centered studies of distance education designed to teach us how the appropriate use of technology and pedagogy could make distance education more beneficial for more students, with the best of such research translated into the practitioner literature.

There is, of course, broad public appeal for the hope of inexpensive and convenient education, especially for people who are working or who have extensive family commitments. Unfortunately, little of the practitioner literature and even less of the popular literature about distance education effectively identifies the complexities of working and communicating with "new media". It appears that few academic administrators, especially those that are a few levels away from the front lines of teaching, understand these complexities very well. With the increase of distance education courses, we may expect that the instructors and students in online courses would be aware of the types of problems found in this study. However, they are unlikely to learn much from the literature, unless we continue research on difficulties, as well as benefits in distance education courses.

One might argue that more advanced technologies in the future would reduce the problems in distance education courses. However, Kling (1994) and Ragsdale (1988) suggest that more socially realistic analyses are needed before accepting enthusiastic attitudes toward technology. Cuban (1986) also observes an unrelenting cycle of technology promotion and adoption in classrooms by reviewing the literature on the educational use of media since the 1920s. The cycle indicates a pattern of failure to effectively use technology in education. Thus, advanced technologies by themselves are unlikely to provide adequate solutions for problems in distance education.

Administrators who want to encourage their faculties to teach online courses coax instructors into viewing them as easy to take on, rather than as a complex instructional engagement that can require new materials and new behaviors. High quality education, both online and face-to-face, is neither cheap nor easy. We have not heard of administrators in traditional universities who encourage regular faculty to teach online courses also insisting that these instructors immerse themselves in the most sophisticated literatures about distance education and computer-mediated communication before they are allowed to teach online.

We understand that there are many high quality online courses taught today. However, a careful reading of the literatures suggests these courses are usually taught by highly dedicated and very experienced instructors. They are said to be much more labor-intensive for their instructors than comparable face-to-face courses. Analysts argue that some of these courses can be much better learning experiences than their in-place equivalents. But given these requirements of unusual instructional skill, experience and dedication, we would be surprised if these constitute a majority of today's online courses.

Even so, we see some signs that the "floor of professional practice" is improving at a few universities that offer numerous distance education courses. There are some new internal consulting groups and workshops for prospective instructors. In some cases these are mandatory; however, they are more commonly discretionary. We have not examined the ways that these support resources work in practice. However, if they help participants to understand the communicational complexities of asynchronous text-based communication, they may help to raise the level of instructional and student competencies for effectively teaching and learning with new media.

This chapter reports on one case study; explicitly theorizing the conditions under which such courses are organized and taught is well beyond our scope. That is an important next step. Part of the theoretical analysis would have to examine the socio-technical complexity of the communication and computational support for the courses, as well as faculty and student abilities to work with and through them (Star and Ruhleder, 1996; Kling, 2000; Kling and Courtright, in press). Another critical part would include the political economies of the participating universities, such as the ways academic administrators are being encouraged to embrace Internet-enabled distance education as a new source of revenue (Carnevale, 1999). Other elements would include an understanding of the conditions under which potential students take such courses and faculty teach them. Most seriously, the necessary theorizing would involve the conjunction of these conditions, social processes and practices: the various ecologies of games (Dutton and Guthrie, 1991; Dutton, 1995) in which administrators, students and instructors come together in making Internet-enabled distance education programs happen.

Notes

1   An earlier and more extended version of this chapter, including more material on the study's background and methodology, is available at: www.slis.indiana.edu/CSI/wp00–01.html More interview data are also reported in Hara and Kling (1999).
2   The first author is therefore referred to as "I" in the text relating to observational descriptions.
3   B3002 is a pseudonym.
4   SchMOOze University is a multi-user, text-based virtual university campus available worldwide via the Internet to enable people to meet online, have synchronous discussion and play games (Blankenship, 1993). It is designed as an 'English as a Second Language' learner and is a MOO (abbreviation for Multi-User Dungeon Object-Oriented).
5   In the interviews reported in this article, 'I' indicates the interviewer, while the informants are represented by their first initials.

Part II

Reconfiguring institutional arrangements

The production of higher education

6 A new game in town

Competitive higher education in American research universities

Lloyd Armstrong

Research universities are such complex and expensive organizations – carrying out multiple interrelated tasks and serving numerous constituencies – that the value structure they have evolved has created many impediments to rapid change and competitive pressures. This chapter examines the impact of the new types of for-profit and non-profit organizations that are beginning to provide competition in targeted segments of higher education, particularly through distance education and distributed learning. While Armstrong looks only at American research universities, his conclusions may be applicable elsewhere. The strategic perspective provided here by Armstrong emphasizes both the real competitive threats to the vitality of academe, and why he regards the ways universities respond, rather than the technology as such, as the key determinant of outcomes.

Growing competition in higher education: the implications for research universities

'Competition' in higher education in the USA has traditionally had rather genteel connotations. Universities compete with other similar institutions on the athletic field, and for faculty, students, donors and grants. While some of these competitions can be longstanding and quite passionate, they do not cause fundamental changes in the institutions involved. However, the sheltered status of institutions of higher education is changing. New types of for-profit and non-profit organizations are beginning to provide competition in targeted segments of higher education. Although rather minimal at the moment, this competition is likely to become more pernicious from the standpoint of traditional higher education than generally understood – and is gaining pace through the take-off of distance learning mediated by the Internet. Distance learning will also allow the institutions of higher education to access each others' constituencies in new ways, leading to new kinds of competition among traditional institutions. Intense competition, as known on the broader economic scene, is therefore coming to higher education.

It is important to recognize that competition can produce results that are both good and bad, both desirable and undesirable. Increased competition will provide more options for students, and students will respond by maximizing benefits to themselves as individuals. The sum of these individual decisions will not always lead to global changes that are positive. Simply saying that certain consequences of competition are negative will not stop them from occurring, however. Many of these negative consequences can be reduced by appropriate responses from higher education, but the face of higher education ultimately will be altered by this new competition in multiple ways.

These developments are applicable broadly across the many segments of higher education around the world. The impact of the new competition will not be uniform across the diverse face of traditional higher education, however. In the USA, many of the new competitive forces are aimed initially at students of the type currently served primarily by community colleges and by universities and colleges that are not generally classified as 'prestigious'. For those institutions, the challenges will be immediate and serious, but relatively direct and obvious. For the more prestigious colleges and universities, on the other hand, the impacts will not be obvious so rapidly, but are likely to be more subtle, more complicated and, in the end, perhaps more revolutionary.

This chapter focuses on the implications of this new competition on a small but highly influential component of higher education: the American research university. During most of the twentieth century, the face of American higher education was influenced in a major way by practices and values of the research universities. Faculty reward structures, disciplinary frameworks and belief in the value of research spread from the research universities into universities and colleges of all types. This spread was perhaps inevitable, since the research universities produce almost all of the future faculty in almost all of the components of higher education. It is contended by many that research universities will be relatively immune to the new competitive forces because of their prestige and great success in carrying out their multiple missions. I will argue to the contrary, that research universities have perhaps the most complex challenges to face in this new environment.

Institutions of higher education collectively value highly their stability, and their capacity to survive for long periods of time without revolutionary change. The value structure that has evolved for research universities is one that creates very high barriers to entry for new players, and numerous barriers to rapid change. These barriers are primarily related to cost, but there are also other types of obstacle. Paradoxically, many of the structures and practices that serve to provide stability in the current competitive climate will be those that put the research universities at greatest risk in the coming competitive era. Because of this critical paradox, it is important to begin by reviewing some of the organization and structure of research universities, and how they provide stability.

Stability in the research universities

American research universities have succeeded to a remarkable degree in integrating several functions that in many other countries are not considered necessarily to be organically linked. Broad and varied educational opportunities at both undergraduate and graduate levels, research, credentialing and a highly evolved social infrastructure are melded together into a distinctive offering. The research component itself plays a complex role, since it serves both the educational mission of the institutions and the needs of the broader society. This highly integrated structure is very expensive and involves considerable cost shifting and sharing between the components. Three elements of this structure serve to provide considerable protection against traditional forms of competition: quality and the cost of producing it; credentialing; and physically-imposed size limitations.

Quality of the educational experience and its cost

Because undergraduate education is typically the largest part of the educational component of universities, it plays a key role in the form the integration of functions takes. Following the highest aspirations of education, universities focus much of their rhetoric and efforts on providing an undergraduate education that will prepare the student for a lifetime of achievement and successful adaptation to change. That is, much of the focus is not on skill development for the first job, but on aspects of a liberal education – such as critical thinking, love of learning, curiosity, judgment, etc. – that prepare the student to be a lifelong learner. As valuable as these attributes are, they are very hard to measure. Consequently, in economic terms, an undergraduate university education becomes somewhat of a 'credence good', whose value is very difficult to quantify by analysis of data or even by experiencing it (Darby and Karnia, 1973). In such cases, various surrogates are used to value the product. Using a somewhat circular argument, the cost of the product is often one of those surrogates: the more it costs, the higher its quality must be. This phenomenon is well known in higher education. A university that increases its tuition by an amount that is large compared to the increases of its peers will almost always see a significant increase in student applications. The existence of this response has a great effect on the price and cost structures of universities, and acts against many efforts to hold down price.

Another surrogate for the quality of an undergraduate university education is the quality of the faculty. In the research university, it is the research productivity and visibility of the professors that primarily defines the quality of the university to the general public. The importance of using the people who actively create knowledge to teach students has been widely propounded by the research universities for decades, and is now widely accepted by the public. Thus, assembling a star research faculty is imperative for the university that wishes to ascend to, or remain in, the first ranks.

Research, however, is a very expensive enterprise. It requires very costly facilities: libraries for the humanists, laboratories for the scientists, computers and networks for everyone. It requires a large infrastructure of accountants, grants specialists, compliance officers and technicians. The direct external cash flow to cover the research function of the university comes primarily from grants and contracts from government, foundations and corporations. However, most of these grants and contracts will not cover the complete cost of the research, and implicitly or explicitly require the university to share costs. In addition, competition for the faculty who do the best research is quite intense, and they are relatively expensive to hire. Thus, the revenues attributable to the research component of the university are less than its costs. As a consequence, the research component of the university requires considerable internal subsidization.

PhD programs are a perfect example of the integration of the research and educational functions of a research university. However, educating a PhD student is among the most expensive forms of education ever invented. It requires an immense amount of faculty involvement and university infrastructure. The value system in place generally dictates that PhD students should not pay for this education and, indeed, should receive some support from the university to defray costs during their studies. Although some portion of the cost of educating some of the PhD students is covered by grants, most of the total cost must be covered by internal subsidization.

The social infrastructure of the contemporary university has become highly evolved, and this too has become a surrogate for quality of the undergraduate educational experience. For students who come to the university immediately after high school, the university is a place of great social growth. Students are exposed to new situations, conflicting ideas and people from widely different backgrounds and social classes. Universities have created a complex infrastructure to help channel these potentially disruptive experiences into productive outcomes. Residential colleges, social organizations, intercollegiate and intramural athletic teams, cultural events, student counselors and student unions are all components of these infrastructures. This, too, is a very expensive infrastructure. It is, however, of greatest importance for the traditional undergraduate, and of significantly lower importance for older, non-traditional undergraduates and for graduate and professional students.

The breadth of offerings is yet another surrogate for the quality of the undergraduate educational experience. This leads most universities to sustain numerous majors that attract very few students, yet require a significant investment in faculty and departmental infrastructure. Similarly, excellent academic physical plant classrooms, teaching laboratories and state of the art electronic infrastructure are yet more surrogates for quality. All of these components, taken with the relatively high cost of the excellent-quality faculty found in most research universities, mean that the undergraduate educational function itself must also be internally subsidized.

To create and sustain a research university that is of high quality, therefore, is a very costly enterprise. Student tuition and research funding do not cover these costs, and so a variety of other major sources of income are required. Among the most important are endowments, gifts and, for public institutions, taxpayer support. In addition, continuing education in its many forms is a very important source of revenue for many institutions, and commercialization of intellectual property is rapidly becoming more significant. Without these multiple sources of income, the research university would be unable to maintain its multiple interlocking activities.

The high cost of research universities presents a tremendous barrier to entry for any new entrants seeking to compete on the same basis, thus providing stability against new competition. In addition, most of the sources of revenue that support this cost also change only slowly, thus providing stability to the competition between existing research universities. For example, increasing total tuition revenue by having more students requires increasing the costly social infrastructure beforehand; similarly, to increase research significantly requires major investments in facilities and new faculty. Increasing donations typically requires years of cultivation of potential donors. Thus, the cost structure of research universities has provided a high barrier to entry by new institutions with a similar mission, and a brake on rapid change in competitive position among existing players.

Credentialing in higher education

The credentialing function of higher education has also created barriers to entry and thus provided stability. A component of credentialing resulting from accreditation has legal ramifications. Accreditation by a recognized regional accrediting agency or professional group is required in order to receive many types of federal funding, and for the licensing of graduates in many professional areas. Accreditation is also an important part of the credentialing power of institutions of higher education, for it provides external evidence that they are of sufficient quality that they can in turn attest to the quality of their graduates. However, accrediting standards have also been used to frustrate, or at least delay, new forms of competition. For example, the Western Association of Schools and Colleges refused to accredit a non-traditional California institution that was just starting up. As a result it moved to Phoenix, Arizona where it was accredited by the North Central Association of Colleges and Schools under the name of the University of Phoenix. The American Bar Association currently refuses to accredit Juris Doctor degree programs taken through distance learning and consequently law schools are being protected from competition from non-traditional sources.

An even more important component of the credentialing power of universities, however, is reputational. The degree or the certificate from a highly-ranked prestigious university is a statement that the holder met very high entrance standards and was able to pass the rigorous courses required by the program. This form of certification that the holder of the credential is among the best of her or his generation and has learned some useful skills is of great value to employers, which in turn makes it of great value to prospective students and their parents. As more very highly-qualified students want to go to the highly-ranked university in order to gain the desirable credential, this further increases the value of the credential. This non-linear system is an example of a winner-take-all situation (Frank and Cook, 1996). The reputation required to provide credentialing of value takes decades (or centuries) to build, however. This means that a new entrant to the university market holds a very weak credentialing power, and has a correspondingly weak attraction for the best students. This clearly discourages new entrants into the market.

Geographic limitations

One final but quite important stability-providing component must be mentioned. Traditional research universities exist primarily in one physical location, with perhaps a few professional schools (e.g. the medical or agricultural school) located at other sites. There are limitations to the number of students who can be enrolled in this single primary location while still maintaining the image of quality education. These considerations provide a physical limitation on the number of students who can be served by a single university, which reduces competition for good students between universities of comparable quality. There is not the physical capacity in a single university, or a small number of universities, for the winner to take all in practice – even though many characteristics of the competition (such as those discussed in the previous section) would otherwise favor this result.

The new competition

Within the shadow of these stability-providing barriers, American research universities have reached levels of excellence admired around the world. Research critical to the economic, social and political well being of the country is produced by academics with an international reputation. Graduates of these universities are disproportionately represented in positions of visibility and influence. However, new forms of competition are developing to circumvent the barriers that have thus far provided stability. In this section, I will describe several of these that are completely external to the research universities: for-profit colleges; non-traditional non-profit colleges such as the Open University (OU); and new alternative credentialing agents.

The direct impact of these organizations may as yet be minimal on traditional institutions, but I will argue that they have the characteristics of "disruptive technologies" (Christensen, 1997) – with the potential to grow to have major direct and indirect effects on research universities. A disruptive technology (or business model) is defined by Christensen as one that initially provides a product that is inferior to the mainstream product, but that brings a new and desirable set of values. The new product appeals initially to a set of 'fringe' customers who are offered more than they need, or are willing to pay for, by the existing mainstream product. Over time, improvements in the new technology (or the new business model) lead to significant increases in product quality. This improved quality, in conjunction with its other desirable values, then enables the new product to displace the mainstream product. Later in the chapter, I will attempt to show how distance learning will increase the disruptive potential of these organizations.

For-profit educational institutions

For-profit colleges with shares traded in the public market have been around for many years. Among the largest and best known of these are the University of Phoenix, the DeVry Institute and Argosy. Traditional higher education has generally given this sector little consideration, considering it to be a provider of lower level skills to a non-traditional set of students, primarily working adults. If these institutions have been viewed as providing competition, it has been with two-year colleges and the lower end of the four-year colleges, where there is some overlap in mission and student demographics.

While this view still has considerable reality, these colleges are now moving aggressively into some of the areas normally thought of as belonging to the traditional non-profit sector. Many are now regionally accredited and offer Bachelor degrees, with some offering Masters and Doctors degrees as well. Among the students enrolled in four-year undergraduate programs in for-profit universities at the end of the 1990s, more than 47 per cent were 'traditional' in the sense that they entered the programs directly from high school (Phipps, Harrison and Merisotis, 1999). Part of this trend reflects evolution in mission, part increased quality as the model is elaborated. Most important from the standpoint of the research universities, these colleges use strategies that are quite different from those employed by most of the non-profit sector, and correspondingly offer students a distinctly different value structure.

The most obvious difference in the approach followed by these for-profits is that they focus on only the educational component of the mission of higher education (Nicklin, 1995; Strosnider, 1997; Kartus, 2000). The expensive components of research and social infrastructure are almost non-existent, leading to a very different cost structure. Facilities are often rented rather than owned, and generally contain nothing other than faculty offices, teaching laboratories and class-rooms. Student facilities such as dormitories, athletic facilities and elaborate student unions are non-existent. Capital costs are corre-spondingly quite low in comparison to those of a traditional institution of higher education.

There are, however, other equally important differences. Con-venience for the student is a major emphasis. Most for-profits offer their classes in multiple accessible locations, at times appropriate for working students. They also emphasize an education that is career-focused, meeting the needs of employers. Advisory boards and focus groups of business people give constant input into an ongoing and rapid (by normal university standards) process of curriculum develop-ment. Many have introduced general education into their curricula in response to input from these groups (Kartus, 2000), thus moving their product more out of the 'trade school' model and into greater overlap with that of traditional higher education.

However, while the research university emphasizes at the under-graduate level learning that will be a basis for future intellectual growth, these for-profits primarily focus on preparation for the next job. In effect, they have embraced an alternative concept of lifelong learning: students are simply expected to return for additional courses as job opportunities evolve. A consequence of the close coupling between curriculum and job opportunities is that the graduates of these institutions have a very high probability of finding appropriate work in the area of their training (Merrill Lynch, 1999; Strosnider 1998; Kartus, 2000).

The curriculum in multi-campus, for-profit colleges is usually centrally controlled. This means their educational experience will be very similar from campus to campus, and from semester to semester. Course materials are prepared by experts in specific areas, and gener-ally taught by faculty who have had practical experience in the area. Significant financial resources are put into the development of new curricula. Evaluation of the faculty is quite rigorous, and focuses primarily on one dimension – teaching effectiveness. Most institutions spend heavily on skill training for faculty in order to build and main-tain that effectiveness in the presence of rapid curricular change. The predictability of a course's quality level and coverage in such a system is impossible in the research universities, with their traditions of academic freedom in teaching and their need to evaluate faculty on a multi-dimensional grid.

Multi-campus for-profit institutions are highly scalable. Their flexibility in student intake derives from the predictability of quality level, focus on near-term benefits to students (jobs in the area of study), and relatively low requirements for capital investment. Such institutions can expand enrollment in a region, or enter a new geographic market with relative ease. In addition, their emphasis on near-term educational benefits makes it easy to quantify the value of one of their degrees or certificates. Value surrogates are not required when value is defined by the quality of the first job after graduation. All these characteristics are very different to the situation in traditional research universities.

Although for-profits are not major players overall in the graduate arena, there are some areas where the for-profits already have a significant presence. For example, almost 10 per cent of the doctorates in clinical psychology in the USA are awarded by the Argosy Education Group (Kartus, 2000; Blumenstyk, 2000b). Many of the for-profits are quite active in the MBA arena. Only about 4 per cent of the Masters level business degrees were awarded by for-profit universities in 1997, but the percentage is growing. The University of Phoenix accounted for almost two-thirds of that number (Mangan, 1999).

These institutions appear to be on the first steps of a path in the business world that is described by Christensen (1997) as a disruptive technology. They have identified a set of potential customers who were over-served by the existing providers – in this case, working adults who found little value in the socialization and research aspects of traditional higher education. They then provided an educational product having values – student-centric and focused on job-related education – that appealed to this set of potential customers. From the perspective of the research university, these institutions provide an incomplete, inferior product. However, from the perspective of the students of the for-profit colleges, they offer an alternative value structure that nicely fills a real need. This is reflected in enrollment growth rates for the industry in the range of 10–20 per cent a year, and in the striking result that the University of Phoenix is now the largest private university in the USA in terms of enrollment. The quality of the approach has improved over time, as the model has been refined.

The business history of other similarly-defined situations would suggest that this continuing quality improvement, and the alternative benefits and values that this approach brings, will lead eventually to increased penetration into the markets of the traditional suppliers. That is, the for-profits increasingly will provide a viable option for all students to consider for some portion of their education. One should expect that an increasing number of students will consider this option in circumstances when they are uninterested in the social and research aspects of research universities, and weigh more heavily the quantifiable value measures and convenience of the for-profits. As I discuss below, the advent of Internet-mediated distance learning is likely to greatly increase the rate at which the for-profits enter into the traditional markets.

Even before they improve to a point that they can effectively enter the markets of the research universities, however, the for-profits can have an impact on the universities. They provide an increasingly visible alternative metric that the public can use in evaluating educational approaches. The for-profits have a very different business model from the research universities at almost every level, and a radically different model of valuing education. The more successful and visible they become, the more the public may question the integrated model of the research universities, with their associated high costs and traditional arguments for valuing education.

One area in which the for-profits are already directly challenging the research universities is continuing education, which provides one of the important revenue flows that enables research universities to support their expensive integrated education. Loss of continuing education revenues could therefore have a significant impact on many research universities. It is obvious that many of the for-profits compete directly with traditional university schools of continuing education in terms of clientele, subject matter and quality. That is, they provide recreational and skills enhancement courses and certificates to individual working adults.

However, several for-profits also compete with continuing professional education programs in schools such as business and engineering, by offering degree and certificate professional programs to employees of corporations. For example, according to the Apollo Group (1995), the University of Phoenix has an "educational partnership with AT&T to provide graduate and undergraduate degree and certificated learning programs to 200,000 AT&T employees worldwide." Jones International has similar contracts with Ball Corp. and AT&T Broadband Internet Services (Michaels and Smillie, 2000). DeVry lists on its Web site (www.devry.com), GTE, National Data, Nortel and Sprint as companies for which it has provided professional development programs in management, electronics and communications. Although many of these programs focus on lower-level professionals who traditionally would not have been of interest to university programs in continuing professional education, others are increasingly moving to higher-level professionals who once would have been the exclusive realm of universities. It is also increasingly common to hear of young graduates of the most prestigious universities turning to the for-profit sector for some just-in-time continuing education focused on job-related needs, rather than returning to a university for a traditional postgraduate degree. Thus, strong and meaningful competition in the continuing education area is already a reality, and will only increase with time.

A different non-profit competitor: the Open University

The OU in England provides an interesting alternative model that is in many ways intermediate between the for-profits and more traditional higher education (see also Palattella, 1998; Blumenstyk, 1999; Chapters Thirteen and Fifteen in this volume). It is a highly successful non-profit university that now enrolls one of the largest number of students in the world – over 200,000 in 2001. It has several hundred regional centers that serve as sites for tutoring and associated activities. Its curriculum is centrally designed, as are the multimedia course materials that are the core of the asynchronous instruction it provides. A relatively small core of rather traditional research staff – about 900 – create this curriculum, supported by numerous outside experts. Very significant resources – \$2.5–\$3.3 million per course (Palattella, 1998) – are committed to producing the highest quality educational programs.

While courses in the for-profits typically involve lectures given by adjunct faculty following scripts prepared centrally, the course material in the OU is presented entirely through the centrally-prepared multimedia materials that are accessible to the students asynchronously. This enables the OU to focus its interaction time on tutorial sessions. Groups of roughly twenty students are assigned to tutors who both grade centrally-defined assignments and provide tutorial sessions.

This combination of a small cadre of research faculty creating advanced curricula, significant resources dedicated to producing effective asynchronous courses and the intimacy of tutorials has made the OU a very effective institution. A recent study of seventy-seven universities by the Higher Education Funding Council for England ranked the OU tenth in the quality of teaching (Palattella, 1998). As reported on the OU Web site (www.open.ac.uk), objective measures of research performance collected by the UK government put the OU in the top third of all UK universities, indicating that the research faculty does indeed fit traditional definitions. While not yet a competitor for

Oxbridge or the other very top tier universities in the UK, the OU has clearly become competitive on both teaching and research levels with a number of highly regarded universities. In doing so, it has demonstrated the potential for an alternative approach to higher education to create a recognizably high quality product.

The OU has recently started the United States Open University. This new enterprise will modify some existing OU programs for an American clientele, and develop new programs specially designed for this market. It expects to pay particular attention to the executive education market. One should expect that this new entity will provide serious competition for many segments of American higher education in the coming years.

Institutions providing alternative credentialing

In the past, credentialing has been defined effectively through the awarding of a degree. Within the set of degree-granting institutions, those that are accredited have had by far the greatest credentialing power. New organs of credentialing are appearing, however, that focus on certifying that candidates possess a well-defined set of skills (Adelman, 2000; Irby, 1999). Because they focus on certifying specific skills, these certifications have considerable value for employers.

These credentialing agencies, which do not seek traditional accreditation, can be of many types. Among them are: vendor corporations, such as Microsoft and Cisco; industry organizations, for example, the International Information Systems Security Consortium and the Certified Financial Planners; and US government agencies, such as National Institutes of Health (NIH) and Department of Agriculture. At present, most of these agencies operate in the area of information technology, but the model has been, and probably will increasingly be, extended to other areas. These alternative credentialing agencies can work with all the forms of new competition, and thus provide strong competition in certain areas to the more traditional credentialing of the research university.

Distance learning: enabler and catalyst for competition

The institutions discussed above have the potential to increase competitive pressure on traditional higher education through more vigorous application of well-known approaches. Internet mediated distance learning, on the other hand, will bring a new and potentially explosive kind of competitive pressure to bear on traditional higher education.

As Cisco Systems' CEO John Chambers has commented (quoted by Friedman, 1999): "The next big killer application for the Internet is going to be education."

Through distance learning, the traditional institutions will compete with each other in a manner in which many previous size and geographic limitations on competition will disappear. For-profit entities will enter the competition both as partners of individual institutions and as direct providers, and alternative forms of credentialing will take on a new power. All areas of the teaching function of universities eventually may be impacted. Access to distance-learning courses is no longer restricted to a location, as are traditional university classes, or to a time, as are traditional classes or televised distance-learning courses. Instead, learning becomes global and asynchronous to provide maximum flexibility and opportunity for the student.

Traditional classroom lectures adopt a linear learning approach in which students follow the pace and path of the professor through the subject matter. The new distance learning allows non-linear learning approaches based on cognitive learning theories, permitting students to move at their own tempos within an organizational structure that responds to their comprehension of the material. Flexibility in responding to different learning styles is increased dramatically compared to the traditional lecture.

The current model being used to create non-linear approaches leads to a very different faculty role from that which has been found in universities. Traditional teaching is 'vertically integrated', in that one individual chooses the material to be covered in the course, then teaches the material and, finally, evaluates the learning of the students. Non-linear distance-learning courses more typically have one or more subject specialists who define the course material, experts in pedagogy who map that course material on to the non-linear medium in the most effective manner, and testing experts who devise the evaluation materials. The 'unbundling' of the faculty role in non-linear distance learning is similar to that already found in many of the for-profit universities discussed above.

This new distance learning has the potential to be highly scalable, that is, to be extended to larger and larger numbers of students without significantly changing the basic approach. This removes many of the limitations on size that have reduced competition between institutions of higher education. Most students will still not be able to go physically to one of the most prestigious colleges or universities, but they will be able to take courses and degree programs from them. The scalability also increases the potential for creating significant profit, thus making this a field of great interest to the for-profit world.

Because of all of these attributes, the new distance learning itself is likely to be both a sustaining and a disruptive technology. It will be used in a sustaining way (Christensen, 1997) by universities to better serve some of their existing constituencies such as alumni and students, but as a disruptive technology when accessing constituencies currently served by other universities. In addition, distance learning will be used by alternative providers as a disruptive technology to accelerate their penetration into the marketplace of the traditional higher education providers.

The alternative providers discussed in the previous section have already demonstrated that there is a large set of potential customers who feel over-served by the research universities with their bundled products. Distance learning extends significantly the convenience factor highly valued by those students, and removes geographic and space constraints that even a multi-site for-profit experiences. It is not surprising, then, to find that many of the for-profit colleges are moving heavily into the new distance learning. For example, the University of Phoenix set up a very successful tracking stock, UOP Online (online.uophx.edu), for its division of distance learning (Blumenstyk, 2000c). By 2001, UOP Online courses were showing an annual increase in degree enrollment of 86 per cent, reaching a total of 25,700 students (Trigg, 2001). The parent of the University of Phoenix, the Apollo group, joined with Hughes Network Systems to form another distance-learning company. DeVry recently won accreditation for online Bachelor programs in business and information technology (Blumenstyk, 2000a).

Other established corporations in the education field – such as Kaplan, Thomson and Sylvan – also moved into distance learning. Kaplan purchased Quest Education Corporation (www.questeducation.com) largely because of its presence in distance learning (Blumenstyk, 2000d), started an online law school, Concord (www.concordlawschool.com), and offers a wide variety of other online programs through the Kaplan Colleges (www.kaplancollege.com). Thomson joined with sixteen universities to set up an online university called Universitas 21 Global (Cherney, 2001). Sylvan played a major role in creating Caliber Learning Network to provide online courses to businesses. In addition, many new for-profit distance-learning corporations appeared, such as UNext (www.unext.com), notHarvard (now Powered) (www.powered.com), Hungry Minds (www.hungryminds.com), Pensare and University Access (now Quisic) (www.quisic.com).

Not all of these experiences have been happy ones, and the failures have demonstrated that many in this new field are still struggling to find a business model that works (Chandrasekaran, 2001). For example, Caliber and Pensare have taken bankruptcy protection, and many of the remaining original wave of companies have changed their business plans several times. Failures such as these should be expected in a rapidly developing field that seeks to provide a new product using a new medium.

Even in the successful university and for-profit efforts, distance learning is not yet of the quality that it is a significant competitor to the classroom experience offered by the research universities. However, the for-profit colleges are showing that there is a very considerable market for Internet-mediated distance learning among their students, even at the current levels of quality; many universities are also experimenting with distance learning for targeted groups within their traditional student bodies. In addition, many developing countries where traditional capital-intensive educational infrastructure is lacking are experimenting with distance learning, often with funding and encouragement from the World Bank (Carnevale, 2000b; Bollag, 2001). If the evolution of other new disruptive technologies is a guide, it is likely that distance learning will be improved and elaborated within these growing secondary markets, until it becomes competitive with traditional forms of classroom teaching as a learning experience.

The nature of the threat from the new competitors

All of these new forms of competition significantly increase options for students at all levels – certificate, undergraduate, graduate and professional levels. They focus on a single aspect of the complex role of the American research university education as reflected in the teaching function. These competitors can make inroads into the current student base, to the extent that those current university students who are primarily interested in this teaching function are over-served by the additional services offered to them via a bundled price. They will compete by offering new benefits such as convenience, flexibility, ability to take courses from a more highly ranked institution, focus on job-related skills and a lower cost structure. By focusing on a single component of the bundled structure of the research university, all of these modes of competition manage to bypass the barriers that have provided stability in the past. To the extent that they can funnel off some portion of the teaching revenues of the research university, they make the bundled whole unstable.

The situation is potentially similar to what is occurring in medical schools, whose missions have traditionally bundled together teaching of medical and PhD students with research and the provision of health care. The revolution in health care has introduced fierce competition into that part of the mission, and many for-profits have moved into markets once held by the faculty practices and university hospitals. Not surprisingly, the Health Maintenance Organization (HMO), the dominant mode by which the for-profits have moved into this arena, is identified as a disruptive technology by Christensen (1997). The HMO seeks to severely contain health care costs by hiring or contracting with groups of medical professionals to provide specified and carefully monitored health services to subscribers for a predetermined annual fee. The resulting decreasing cash flows into faculty medical practice have produced fewer revenues that can be transferred to the other functions of the schools, and have put great pressure on many faculty to increase their time devoted to the practice mission. Many faculty must now spend so much time on their practices that they can no longer devote sufficient time to their teaching and research functions. As a consequence, the clinician-scientist may be a disappearing model. At present, the pressures are so intense that it is not clear how the traditional vision of a medical school can be maintained.

For the university as a whole, the tuition (teaching) revenues play a dominant budgetary role similar to that of clinical revenues for a medical school. Once those revenues come under attack, the entire integrated system risks collapse. As the teaching function is partially stripped away from the university of matriculation and moved to alternative providers, pressures will be transmitted to the other components of the functional bundle. Students who spend less time at the university will contribute fewer dollars to the fixed costs of the social infrastructure. Some marginal costs will disappear, but the fixed costs will be hard to decrease in a timely fashion. The football team costs the same no matter how many students watch the game; dormitories are difficult to convert into other uses when the student body shrinks. The cost of expensive research faculty, previously carried roughly equally by the research and teaching functions, will be moved further on to the research function.

Should this happen, in all but the very best endowed institutions the faculty who are in areas where research grants are plentiful will be forced to move more of their time and salary to the 'soft' money that such grants provide. Research in areas where grant support is very scarce is likely to decline. It is also likely that, as the teaching and research functions separate, the research activities of the faculty will play a decreasing role as a surrogate for quality in the pricing of education. As students take more courses from alternative providers, they will take a smaller fraction of their courses from research-active faculty, thus weakening the perceived relationship between teaching quality and research. The result will be that the salaries received by relatively highly-paid research faculty for their teaching activities will appear to the public to be too high.

The general public's attention to the price/value relationship will be increased by continuing growth of the for-profits with their very clear, one-dimensional value equation – immediate placement in appropriate jobs. Universities should therefore expect to see growing interest in the success of their graduates in their first jobs. Although not an inappropriate concern, this will put pressure on the universities to readjust the balance between long- and short-term goals of their education.

The effective legal credentialing monopoly of traditional higher education has already been broken by the for-profits that have achieved accreditation, and the alternative credentialers that have created valuable certification without accreditation. Further serious inroads into the credentialing monopoly of universities will probably occur as more for-profits are drawn into this area, and as yet unimagined business plans are unveiled.

Over the somewhat longer term, the possibility of truly revolutionary change exists. Higher education in the USA is a $240 billion per year market (Merrill Lynch, 1999), and the world higher education market is estimated to be about $400 billion annually. The entire market is very highly fragmented, with no single provider having any significant portion of the market. In many dimensions, the market is similar to those which existed in health care and banking not so long ago – markets that now have consolidated into only a relatively few major players. This new distance learning, because it is scalable, greatly increases opportunities for significant consolidation in the education market.

Truly effective distance-learning courses will be expensive to produce, and it will be necessary to spread initial costs over as broad a student base as possible. However, scalability provides opportunities for large profits once the initial costs are covered, if a sufficiently large student base can be reached. In addition, as English becomes increasingly the language of commerce and technology, distance-learning courses in English will increasingly find a worldwide market (Bollag, 2000), thus increasing the possibility of consolidation on a global scale. American for-profit educational corporations are already moving to establish themselves in this new world market (Blumenstyk,

2000; Lively and Blumenstyk, 1999). If the educational market moves significantly towards worldwide consolidation, universities will have to devise rather radical strategies to compete.

By 2001, most of these threats were not serious for the research university. Distance learning was not yet of a quality that can compete with the classroom experience in most cases. The for-profit colleges could not attract many students who would be considered prime candidates for matriculation at a research university. Corporations were still looking to the major business schools for their upper level professional education, not to the for-profits. However, evidence on every front indicates distance learning is improving in quality; the for-profit colleges are moving into greater curricular and demographic overlap with traditional institutions; and corporations are hiring the for-profits to do much of their in-house training. Thus, it is likely that these new modes of competition will become much more intense in the future. Distance learning, in particular, is moving very rapidly, and the competition between universities in this arena is likely to increase dramatically in the near term. Thus far, these new forms of competition seem to be following quite closely the evolution predicted for a disruptive technology.

Responding to the new competition

Universities will not be impacted uniformly by this new competitive environment. At both the undergraduate and the graduate and professional levels, universities with lower reputations for traditional quality will be affected first, but the impact will rise over time to more highly-ranked universities. Within individual universities, all academic areas will not be impacted equally, due to variations in parameters such as student demographics (e.g. age, academic achievement), importance of facilities (lab versus lecture courses) and the relative economic value of a name-brand degree (e.g. lower for education than for biology). Similarly, responses will vary by field, as universities prioritize within the framework of their own particular situations. In order to compete successfully in this new environment, universities will have to react in many areas. I will discuss four of these areas: mission focus, excellence, organizational change, and distance learning.

The significance of mission focus

The nature of its educational mission will need to be well understood and implemented by individual institutions, and the mission's value clearly articulated to the public. A central tenet of such a mission for the bundled research university has been that education and research are inseparable components of an organic whole, and that students gain a uniquely valuable education from this system. Therefore, a key initial response to the new competitive situation must be an increased focus on ensuring that this mission of the research universities does provide real and unique value to the student. At the undergraduate level, the best way to preserve the viability and desirability of the research university's bundled-function mission is to make sure those functions are truly synergistic.

At present, most undergraduate students at research universities do not participate directly in research. The courses that students take are often very similar to those taught at colleges where the faculty is not seriously involved in research. A large number of the courses in many universities are, in fact, taught not by research faculty, but by adjuncts or graduate students. These self-imposed decouplings of research and teaching functions actually serve well the interests of external competitors that seek to capture some portion of the teaching function of the research universities.

Some corrective actions for this problem are straightforward but not necessarily easy to implement. Significantly increased participation of undergraduates in research, for example, is more a matter of choice and policy than resources. Teaching undergraduate courses in innovative ways that weave recent research into the course material is difficult only in that it requires more time and creativity than a course that parallels a widely used textbook. Both actions add greatly to the value of the research university undergraduate experience, however, and should be a part of the response of every university.

Other actions needed in this realm are more complicated to achieve since they run into existing competitive strategies. For some universities, getting research faculty into the classroom more often is clearly required if the necessary teaching/research synergies are to be built and maintained. Unfortunately, teaching relief – especially at the undergraduate level – has become a bargaining chip commonly used by many universities in attracting the best researchers. While this is a strategy that is very counter-productive over the long term, it provides a short-term advantage that makes it irresistible to many universities.

Even in the absence of this special treatment of star faculty, the number of courses taught per year by the average faculty member in a research university has shrunk over the past thirty years, in order to enable the faculty to increase their research productivity. Thus, there is real conflict in the balancing of the research and teaching roles of faculty, with both gains and losses to the overall mission of the university to be found in any adjustment of the balance. Persuasive arguments can be made that the balance has swung too far to the research side in many universities to sustain long-term stability. However, rebalancing can cause significant internal dissension, as well as external competitive difficulties. Nevertheless, tighter coupling of the research and teaching functions is almost certain to be necessary in order to preserve the viability of the traditional model of the research university.

In a similar vein, the social structures of the university must be well integrated with the teaching and research functions, such that these structures contribute significantly to the education of the student. Residential colleges in which resident faculty help bring intellectual excitement to the living experience, student organizations that encourage exploration of a profession or development of leadership skills, student research fairs and similar integrating activities are by now commonplace on most of our campuses. As time goes on, they will become even more important in demonstrating the viability of this model. The days are past when student affairs can be considered to be separate from academic affairs, and creative new ways must be developed for increasing the integration.

Looking to the future, universities must better define the prospective student body that is encompassed within their teaching missions. For many research universities today, the core educational mission really applies implicitly to students who are able to spend full time on campus. Continuing education of non-resident, part-time students is done primarily to make money rather than as part of the core mission. As opportunities arise to provide high-quality education through distance learning, universities must decide whether or not their missions encourage them to embrace the opportunity to extend educational opportunity to a much broader set of students. Whether distance learning is used to further core mission, to make money, or to defend against encroachment by alternative providers will be important in determining how the individual institutions respond to this new technology.

The competitive need for an increased focus on excellence

Increased competition in higher education will have the same effect as competition in the corporate world: excellence will be essential for institutional survival. Many of the practices that persist in the still relatively sheltered world of academe must change if institutions are to compete effectively. Both faculty and administrators must focus on the creation and maintenance of institutional excellence as their highest priority in this new environment.

Because of the strong tradition of shared governance in American universities, faculty must play a key role in creating and maintaining institutional excellence. This means that faculty must strive to achieve individual excellence in their own research and teaching activities, at the same time as playing a major role in creating broader group excellence. The minimal levels of institutional accountability generally admitted by tenure mean that faculty encouragement and faculty pressure become critical in creating high levels of group excellence. In many institutions, however, most faculty have accepted – or at least tolerated – colleagues who do not seek to perform with excellence in the core missions of the institution. The notion of lifetime employment that is implicit in tenure leads to a stability of community which has benefits, but also major drawbacks. Among them is that criticism of fellow faculty for not performing at high levels is typically muted, as a price for maintaining collegiality in this stable world.

The critical concept of 'academic freedom' is often misused as the rationale for allowing peers to ignore these critical core missions of the institution while following their own interests (academic or otherwise). In order to create the necessary levels of excellence, faculty must take the lead in demanding it of themselves, as well as of their colleagues. Tenure, if it is to survive in this increasingly competitive world, must be used to protect the academic freedom of those who are actively seeking and achieving excellence, and not to protect those who have found comfort in mediocrity. Without this understanding, universities will be pushed to a much more clearly corporate mode, in which administrators enforce the growth of excellence through unilateral decisions concerning individual achievement.

Administrators must also focus on creating conditions that allow academic excellence to grow. For example, the for-profit universities and the OU spend very significant sums every year to create new courses. Traditional universities seldom expect to spend more on the creation of a new course than a one-course release time for a faculty member. As we move into an era when multimedia teaching becomes the norm, universities will have to devote more of their resources to creating high-quality, innovative courses. Similarly, the for-profits spend heavily to assure that faculty keep their teaching skills up to date, while little of this occurs in universities. More will have to be invested in programs to develop and expand teaching skills, and institutional expectations must be created that faculty will avail themselves of these programs regularly. Facilities are increasingly important for excellence in both teaching and research, and universities that lag in this area will find that they are not able to achieve their aspirations for quality. Administrators, working with faculty, must make the hard prioritization decisions necessary to focus the resources of the institution on the building of excellence.

Greater attention will have to be paid in universities to developing methods of helping faculty remain at their most productive levels throughout their careers. The combination of tenure and lack of fixed retirement age make this a high priority if necessary institutional excellence is to be achieved. Industry generally invests enormous sums to constantly upgrade the skills of its employees, in order to maintain a competitive edge. Universities will have to behave in a similar fashion. The effectiveness of sabbaticals in this regard needs to be re-evaluated in the light of changing family situations, such as two-earner families. Perhaps there are more effective ways to encourage faculty to broaden their interests and experiences. Internal resources will need to be made available to stimulate new directions of research and creative activity. Fuller recognition that individual faculty members at different points in their careers may want to emphasize different aspects of their university activities can lead to a changing profile against which excellence can be measured. This will enable faculty to better focus their efforts on activities that most interest them, and are of most benefit to their institutions.

As teaching takes on more varied forms with the development of distance learning and distributed learning, faculty roles will become more diverse. Some will become content providers for multimedia material, while others will act as facilitators for those multimedia presentations in the classroom. Some may become experts in mapping content onto the new media in a pedagogically powerful way. Yet others will continue to provide more traditional classroom teaching. New standards for evaluating teaching excellence will have to be created in order to properly weigh these various contributions, and to determine appropriate teaching loads.

An even greater emphasis on institutional excellence than exists now will also have the effect of increasing the importance of having on the faculty individuals of great national and international visibility. Greater emphasis on student satisfaction will require that those individuals of most value are also excellent in one or more of the appropriate modes of teaching. This increased focus on a relatively few individuals will certainly increase their market value and, correspondingly, put downward pressure on the salaries of faculty who do not fall into this favored class. In other words, there will be an exacerbation of the winner-take-all (Frank and Cook, 1996) climate in higher education.

Organizational change leading to greater efficiencies

As pressures develop on one or more of the revenue streams that support the integrated research university, it will be necessary to begin to rationalize both the administrative and academic cost structures of the institutions. In doing so, it is necessary to note the difficulty associated with using price (or expenditures, in a balanced budget) as a surrogate for quality in higher education. For example, in higher education rankings published by *US News and World Report*, high expenditures per student is explicitly defined as a measure of quality. Numerous accrediting agencies carefully monitor expenditures per student, and issue dire warnings if the school is seen to be decreasing the expenditure per student. Thus, resistance to significant changes to cost-structure within the academy will be strong – until the competition has made significant inroads into traditional markets and can no longer be ignored.

Nevertheless, universities will have to become much more efficient in their internal provision of services. Typical university administrative rivalries (e.g. between academic and administrative computing) that limit performance and create inefficiencies will no longer be acceptable. Increasingly intelligent use of technology to handle business matters inexpensively and rapidly will be necessary, as will purchasing and construction practices that more closely parallel those found in industry. For many institutions, a more corporate-like clear delineation of administrative and fiscal authority will need to be put into place to enable effective response to rapid change and greater accountability. In addition, most universities will have to recognize that they cannot cover all academic and research areas, and will have to begin to focus their resources on activities that are most important for strategic reasons. In some cases, this will mean closing programs completely, and in others it will involve closing some parts, such as graduate studies. This raises both external and internal issues.

Higher education has numerous important and powerful external constituencies. Alumni, professional groups, governmental entities, donors – all feel a sense of ownership of the institutions of higher education. These important constituencies will often put immense pressure on universities to prevent closing or modifying academic programs. Graduates fear that their hard-won diploma will lose value

if the program from which they graduated disappears, and professional groups often feel their profession will be demeaned by the
closing of a program that trains people for that calling. Because all
universities depend on good relationships with government, donors
and alumni for resources, they cannot easily withstand major public
disapproval – no matter how misplaced.

It will be necessary for universities to develop strategies that enable
them to convince their many external constituencies of the need to
sharpen focus in this way. It will also be important that universities be
able to close out programs in a cost-efficient way. Tenure rules in many
institutions require that faculty in closed programs be found a new
home in another program. Not only does this limit the savings that can
be gained by closing the program, but it usually means that faculty
find themselves moved into positions for which they are only
marginally qualified. These are constraints on resources and quality
that will place those institutions at a serious disadvantage in a more
competitive environment.

Faculty governance will also need to be reorganized in many universities. For universities to respond appropriately to the changing
competitive scene, the faculty must participate actively in determining
the responses. Unfortunately, most faculty governance does not work
effectively in meeting the challenges of rapid change. Many faculty, for
all of their understanding of how much effort is required to become an
expert in an academic discipline, tend to think of themselves as experts
in all areas outside of their disciplines, whether or not they have actually given that area any thought and study. Much of faculty
governance then becomes spirited debate among the uninformed,
where political agendas tend to carry much more weight than desire to
find meaningful solutions to real problems. The difficulties become
even more serious when the important new issues are partially within
the academic experience and partially without. In this more competitive environment, faculty must devise governing mechanisms that
provide more rapid and better informed input if they wish to be heard
as a group. Otherwise, administrations will be forced to seek critical
faculty input from special committees or from individuals.

The transformational potential of distance and distributed learning

Distance learning will begin to make inroads into the undergraduate
experience, both as a pre-college component and as an external supplement to what is offered at the student's university. Most universities

will find it advantageous to create distance-learning programs that represent their particular strengths and approaches. In this way, they can extend themselves beyond their geographic limitations and gain new students and new revenues that can support the core activities. In doing so, they can also hope to more than make up the losses suffered when their own students take courses from competing purveyors of distance learning. As noted above, however, each university will need to understand where distance learning fits within its own educational mission.

Once students have experienced effective and innovative distance-learning courses, they will be difficult to satisfy with traditional lecture courses. Consequently, innovations in on-campus education will have to occur at a more rapid rate than they have in the past. In particular, the teaching methods developed in distance learning will need to be adapted to on-campus teaching. This form of 'distance learning' – distributed learning – will change the way in which many courses are organized and taught, with corresponding redefinition of faculty teaching roles. For example, something more like the OU model might be appropriate for these courses, in which the basic subject matter is presented in a distributed-learning mode, and classroom time is spent in a tutorial mode. For these courses, the vertical integration of the teaching function could cease to be the norm as different faculty assume different roles in the process. With the flexibility of asyn-chronous methods, courses mediated by distributed learning will not need to fit into neat semester-long packages, and the classroom will be only one of the many locations where learning takes place.

Universities will have to find a way to accommodate increasing student demands to be allowed to take distance-learning courses from competing institutions without harming their own credentialing authority. A possible solution would be to allow the students to choose among a restricted set of authorized distance-learning courses that have been found by the faculty to be of appropriate quality. This situa-tion is similar to that which has traditionally happened with transfer credits, although the pressure to accept more distance-learning credits than are typically accepted as transfers will be high. Alternatively, students could be allowed to choose among certain competing distance-learning courses as the distributed learning component of the Open University type of course described above, thus incorporating the outside distance-learning courses into the course structure in a natural way. Accommodations to this new pressure will, of course, have both financial and academic implications that will need to be carefully considered by each university.

At the graduate and professional level, the changes are likely to be even more dramatic. Here, the bundling of research and teaching is obviously important. However, as remarked above, the primary social structures of the university at this level are generally of much lower importance, and these students are adults who are forgoing significant income in attending school full time. Consequently, many graduate and professional programs will find it advantageous to use distance learning extensively in order to provide the flexibility that will attract the best students. Brown and Duguid (1996, 2000) have argued that one of the primary roles of graduate and professional programs is to provide a socialization into disciplinary communities, a process that requires a mentoring experience. Although there is considerable variation from field to field, it is obvious that major components of most graduate and professional training do require intense mentoring experiences. Consequently, graduate and professional programs that are strategically balanced mixtures of distance learning and place-specific, person-to-person interaction are likely to be most effective in attracting the best students. Creative use of such programs would also enable universities to increase significantly the number of students who could be educated effectively in chosen programs. This could provide important financial and reputational benefits.

In order to compete effectively in the arena of non-degree continuing education, universities will have to pay close attention to the needs of the market, and the innovations of the competition. Anecdotal information regarding recent graduates of prestigious institutions indicates that many are choosing to get any necessary additional education from non-traditional suppliers (e.g. online courses certified by alternative credentialers) for reasons of convenience and responsiveness to specific job needs. The continuing education market of the future will be considerably more varied, demanding and unforgiving than the market of the recent past.

Most universities will find it necessary to partner with other universities, and with a variety of for-profit corporations in building their distance-learning programs. Effective distance-learning programs will be expensive to produce, and it will be counter-productive for all if every university produces the same set of programs. Thus, finding the right partners will be critical, and there is clearly a benefit to those universities that move to ally themselves with high-quality partners who bring complementary strengths. For-profit corporations will be important potential partners, because they can provide capital and types of expertise not typically found in universities, such as marketing and production skills. All of these partnerships will put great pressure on administrative structures and traditions of shared governance because they will require careful attention to interests outside the university, and to faster decision times than those which usually occur in academic settings.

Universities and their faculties will have to come to grips with at least two distance-learning issues that, from certain perspectives, seem to be relics of the pre-competitive era. Ownership of – or share of profit from – distance-learning courses is a major issue on many campuses today. In the competing for-profit sector, all ownership of, and proceeds from intellectual property go to the corporation, not the creator. However, this has not kept that sector from creating valuable intellectual property at a remarkable rate. The for-profits can then put almost all profits from courses back into the creation of new courses. Universities, on the other hand, are being asked to liberally share profits from a course with faculty involved in its creation, thus limiting the institutional resources available to create the next course. In a competitive world, this is a formula for falling behind.

Similarly, many faculty are now arguing for the right to contract individually to create distance-learning courses for corporate entities. These same corporate entities may then enter into direct competition with the faculty member's university, using the faculty member's course. In a system that is not strongly competitive, such activity on the part of faculty is not particularly damaging to the university. However, in the competitive world that we are entering, it is contrary to the long-term interests of both faculty members and their universities.

Faculty members will also increasingly have to recognize that their individual actions can actually damage the long-term viability of their university in a competitive era. Attention to the long-term health of the university that provides the job and the tenure will have to become a more important characteristic of the faculty–university relationship in a more competitive world.

Conclusion: how to respond effectively to increased competition in higher education

It is critical that those in higher education consider changes that increased and varied competition might bring. The system of higher education in the USA is competitive round the world, drawing students from many nations. It is incredibly diverse, serving a tremendously broad spectrum of student needs and aspirations. It encompasses institutions that have achieved a remarkable synthesis of the dual missions of research and education. Overall, the current system serves America well, although certainly not perfectly.

However, competition often maximizes a narrow, rather than a global, good. Thus, increased competition has the potential to have a negative effect on the overall strength of the American system of higher education. Only by understanding more clearly our core missions, and by understanding the ways in which increased competition might affect those missions, will it be possible to respond in such a way as to preserve and increase the strength of our university system.

7 Jones International University™

A pioneering virtual university

Pamela S. Pease

Launched in 1993, Jones International University became the first fully accredited 'University of the Web' in the USA. Here, Pamela Pease – its President – provides a brief overview of the University's aims, achievements and future ambitions. She focuses particularly on the University's innovative features, such as having geographically-distributed staff and students and its Web-cast 'cybergraduation' ceremony, as well as summarizing its post-accreditation experience.

A virtual model for higher education: the mission shapes the university

Jones International University (JIU) is a viable and operational virtual university, which illustrates the important role of private, for-profit entrepreneurship in higher education. As a new for-profit university with no legacy as a branded 'bricks-and-mortar' institution, JIU was developed from inception in 1993 to be fully online. Its academic offerings and organizational structure were shaped by JIU's founding mission. This included four distinctive goals that were operationalized in 1995 when the university began offering courses, certificates and degrees:

1 to serve adult learners worldwide as a global university;
2 to provide accessible and affordable programs – overcoming barriers of time, distance and cost;
3 to develop and deliver rich content and learning to adult learners across the world via the Internet and Web; and
4 to demonstrate a new model for higher education.

A global 'virtual' campus allows anyone, anywhere to participate in JIU, as exemplified by the enrollment of students from one hundred countries. With over 50 per cent of adults representing the demand for academic courses and programs in higher education across the US, online learning serves to provide convenient access and an alternative to traditional programs. The adoption of an asynchronous, Web-based campus provides flexible and convenient access by faculty and students alike.

JIU's administrative headquarters are located in Englewood, Colorado in the USA. The organizational structure is entrepreneurial and dynamic to encourage change and to increase the response time for meeting the educational needs of its customers – working adults. The new model introduced by JIU ensures a cost-effective and a lean infrastructure 'on-the-ground' by leveraging online resources across the world. There is no residency requirement, as JIU's campus is entirely located on a Web-based portal. Thousands of students and over 400 faculty actively participate in teaching and learning. Students graduating from the degree programs are conferred degrees in a live 'Web-cast' at the JIU Cybergraduation (graduation.jonesinternational. edu). A visit to JIU's campus Web site (www.jonesinternational.edu) illustrates its current and leading-edge developments.

Receiving accreditation status for a virtual university was a critical milestone in higher education. On 5 March 1999, JIU achieved inter-national visibility as the first 100 per cent online university in the USA to be granted regional accreditation from the Higher Learning Commission of the North Central Association (NCA), which accredits colleges, universities and other degree-granting institutions of higher education in the USA (www.ncahigherlearningcommission.org). This provides evidence that a new virtual model for higher education can meet the rigors of accreditation, and hold the same status earned by more traditional universities. It is a feat that took more than five years and millions of dollars to achieve.

The NCA's decision to grant accreditation was unanimous. Among US institutions, this is the same type of accreditation that all tradi-tional universities aspire to and seek validation from. For JIU, accreditation provides key validation of quality and an accelerated market acceptance by the higher education community and potential students. Because of the importance of accreditation to JIU's evolu-tion, its growth may be categorized as either pre-accreditation or post-accreditation. The pre-accreditation or foundation phase for JIU represents the period from its inception in 1993 to accreditation in

March 1999. Post-accreditation is focused on sustainability and growth of the University that commenced in 1999.

Pre-accreditation: the foundation of a virtual university

JIU is distinctive in that its mission and organizational structure are designed to demonstrate a new model for higher education. Between 1993 and when it was launched in 1995, the University was committed to extensive market research and development of innovative approaches to instructional design for an effective online university. The research results indicated clearly that adult learners were interested in alternatives to traditional modes of education. Potential adult learners identified the following three top factors cited by adults for selecting virtual learning:

- flexibility and convenience to overcome time and distance challenges;
- high-quality but relevant education; and
- value for their money.

For JIU, it became clear in 1993 that a virtual campus, using the asynchronous attributes of the Internet and Web, would meet the needs of adult learners. The 'anytime and anywhere' aspects of online learning provides a venue for a flexible and convenient learning environment. Issues of affordability for students contributed to the implementation of a largely virtual organizational model, where capital expense is earmarked for content and course development, rather than for bricks-and-mortar buildings. In addition, JIU demonstrates that interactivity and community building can be successfully accomplished using Web-based student and faculty forums.

The hallmark of JIU is its commitment to developing high-quality content and facilitating learning. The development of academic content optimizes the attributes of the Internet and Web. JIU has achieved this by implementing a multi-tiered faculty structure that indicates a changing role for faculty in some models of online learning. JIU's multi-tiered faculty consists of:

- an academic advisory board for each degree program;
- content experts who develop courses;
- teaching faculty who implement the courses and facilitate learning; and
- a chair for each degree program drawn from the full-time faculty.

Content Experts are the course developers and have renowned expertise in the subject matter of the course. Freed by the Web from the need for physical presence to develop a course, the Content Experts are selected from prestigious universities across the world; these have included Columbia University, Oxford University, London School of Economics and Stanford University. They work on a contract-for-hire basis, and rarely implement the actual teaching of the course. It is a Teaching Faculty member who actually implements the online course and facilitates discussion with students. All development is conducted in a team consisting of a Content Expert, instructional designers and Web architects. Courses are modular, with clearly defined performance outcomes and with assessment strategies that blend theory and practice. JIU does not replicate face-to-face instruction but, rather, develops each course to optimize the use of the Web and its multimedia features.

Post-accreditation: growth and sustainability

A new organizational perspective grew with the advent of accreditation. JIU realized it has the ingredients to be successful. This has led to increasing student revenues by aggressively expanding its marketing and, when necessary, its staff and faculty. To accomplish this, millions of dollars are earmarked for marketing and public relations. There is an on-going effort to brand the University and recruit students.

The expansion of the degree programs from two in 1999 to twenty in 2001 – and more than forty by 2003 – assists in broadening the appeal of its academic offerings to a more diverse student population. By 2001, seven of its degree programs in business had been localized to Spanish. This makes it possible for students to take courses in English or Spanish.

The foundation of the pre-accreditation phase for JIU has resulted in a dynamic organization poised for rapid growth. Jones International University continues to be recognized for its attention to quality, rapid speed to market of its products and competence in serving students in over 100 countries. In April 2001, for example, JIU was selected through a competitive process by the United Nations Development Program (UNDP) to establish a Virtual Development Academy. This project is similar to establishing a virtual 'corporate' university. JIU has developed a Web portal, content and faculty for this high-profile project. There are other customized and innovative projects including delivering content through hand-held Personal Digital Assistants (PDAs), such as the PALM Pilot.

Since 1999, the success of JIU grows with each year. Student enroll-ment, the broadening of the academic offerings and the strengthening of its staff have contributed to the maturation of the organization. Admissions have grown ten-fold and enrollment by 300 per cent during this period. At this rate, the strategic business plan to recognize a return-on-investment and serve students across the globe soon becomes reality.

8 The Open University of Catalonia

A European virtual university initiative

Emma Kiselyova

The Open University of Catalonia was one of the pioneers in the provision of higher education based on a virtual campus. In this chapter, Kiselyova provides an analysis and overview of its innovative model of education in the digital age. She highlights its aim of enhancing the human capital of society and identifies the University's main challenges in scaling up to offer higher education to a wide cross-section of society.

Pioneering Internet-based education at the Open University of Catalonia

The Universitat Oberta de Catalunya (UOC) was initiated in 1993 with a very clear vision: to open up the possibility of higher education at a cost all Catalans could afford, by offering distance learning that maximizes the use of ICTs. This base was also seen as a springboard to win and maintain a competitive edge in an increasingly challenging global educational environment. To achieve this, the University had to innovate, because it was started at a time when there were few examples of online education success and no organizational models to follow. Table 8.1 summarizes UOC's track record since it accepted its first students in 1995.

A private virtual university with a public mission

The initial proposal to build a new type of university was directly addressed to Dr Gabriel Ferrate, who was then the Chancellor of the prestigious Universitat Politecnica de Catalunya in Barcelona (UPC), because he has a reputation for creativity, aligned with strong leadership, political influence and great personal charisma. Dr Ferrate has

Table 8.1   Universitat Oberta de Catalunya: history and organizational background

- Initiated in 1993 by the Catalan government as part of a national strategy to strengthen the political and cultural autonomy of Catalonia, boost economic and technological development of the region and reassert the importance of the Catalan language.[1]
- Co-financed by the Catalan government to create a private university with a public mission: to offer higher education supported by highly interactive learning and teaching techniques.
- Opened in 1995 with a pilot project of 200 students on two degree courses.
- In 2001, over 20,000 students were enrolled in fourteen degree courses (thirteen nationally accredited).
- Most programs are university-level degrees; others (about 5,000 enrollments) are university extension courses at postgraduate and Masters levels, summer university, programs designed for corporate customers and the Virtual School of Governance.
- All course materials are designed at UOC by eighty full-time professors. In addition, 800 consultants and tutors work on contractual part-time basis.
- Two teaching divisions, each with its own financial policy: the Catalan division is subsidized by regional government to offer low-cost education for residents of Catalonia; the Iberoamerican[2] division for the rest of the students, who pay three times as much.
- Sixteen support centers, mainly regional but also including four national and three international centers.
- The Virtual Campus platform designed by UOC is the main space for study and communication. This runs on an ISDN-based[3] computer network covering the whole of Catalonia.
- The Internet Interdisciplinary Institute (IN3), EduLab and other departments conduct numerous research projects on the information society and e-learning.
- Interdisciplinary PhD program on the Information Society started in 2000 by IN3 as a new initiative to foster in-depth research and teaching on ICTs. It requires two years of virtual seminars followed by a PhD dissertation based on empirical research. Participating faculty includes scholars from leading universities around the world.
- UOC has won a number of international awards for excellence as a digital initiative in distance education.[4]

said that he was given seed money, a free hand and "no limits" on his imagination.[5] So, he decided to build a virtual university from scratch without using UPC as a base; it was not based on "evolution but a rapture". He became Rector of UOC when it opened; his charismatic leadership role has been of crucial importance in its subsequent success. This kind of human factor is often insufficiently recognized in an era of technological triumphs.

In the search for a legal formula that would allow flexible dynamic operation and freedom for pedagogical and technological experiments and decision-making, the model chosen was of a private university with a public mission. This was achieved by making the university part of the private Foundation UOC (FUOC) which was established in 1994 with strong participation from the Catalan government in the Board of Trustees, its Standing Committee and in the Council of the FUOC. This ensured full accountability for UOC's appropriate use of public funds.

UOC's modus operandi

UOC was projected as a school for high-quality tertiary education that doesn't just use the Web, but is Web-centered, i.e. with its own virtual campus as a delivery platform for online teaching/learning. Initially, students studied only in the Catalan language, and since the year 2000 in Spanish as well. In order to secure high standards of teaching, it was necessary for UOC to recruit quality academic staff to work for it full time, and consultants and tutors who are employed at UOC on a part-time basis. This part-time group of faculty, specialists and professors come from other universities, which are paid an overhead fee for permitting their professors to teach at UOC. New staff go through an induction program at UOC: for one year they are coached by the senior faculty, attend interviews and methodological seminars. A 'Methodological Resources Assistant' program developed at UOC provides staff with guidelines and tools for creating effective software-based courseware.

The Virtual Campus platform (see Table 8.1) allows interactive, mainly asynchronous, communications between students and teachers, and between students and students. In addition, it allows students access to UOC's information resources – such as databases, bulletin boards and libraries – and administrative and third-party services, including the Internet, WWW and external databases. Web-based materials designed at UOC are increasing in number and quality, including facilities for easy distribution and updating of content.

The pedagogical model

UOC's pedagogical model is student-centered and aimed at overcoming space and time barriers. This requires a shift from the traditional teaching paradigm to a new approach to learning, based on the idea that the success of the educational process is ensured not by the skills and work of the professors and tutors in delivering information, but by the ability of the student to acquire this information, analyze it, digest it and transform it into knowledge suitable for continuous updating and assessment.[6]

The three 'pillars' of UOC's pedagogical model are: teaching materials, tutorial action and continuous evaluation. Teaching materials are in multimedia and paper form and/or Web-based, according to which is more appropriate and efficient for specific content. They are designed to guide students through the subject and to facilitate their process of learning, rather that to serve just as a source of information (Duart and Sangra, 2000).

Tutorial action implies a three-tier faculty body involved in the teaching process:

tutors, who are simultaneously a guide for the student, envoy of the university and personal coach;
consultants, who are specialists in particular subjects and motivate and support students in their study and continuous evaluation; and
professors, who do not participate in direct teaching/learning, but who develop the course program, ensure the quality and state-of-the-art of teaching materials and co-ordinate the work of consultants and tutors.

In Web-based learning, continuing evaluation is essential. The success of the process often depends on how well students understand evaluation criteria, the importance of following these guidelines and of maintaining a proper rhythm of study in order to reach objectives. UOC's students can choose between continuous or final forms of evaluation, both of which require the final exam to take place face-to-face (in 'presence form'). Although continuous evaluation is more demanding, over 80 per cent of students opt for it .[7]

Other elements of this pedagogical model are UOC's sixteen support centers and a 'virtual library' giving access to general information through the electronic library and catalogues of UOC and other universities' libraries. UOC's model also includes a human communication space for its students, faculty and staff. This is meant for both virtual and face-to-face social relationships and activities – thus completing the idea of building a 'real' campus life without bricks and mortar (Ross, 2001).

UOC's organizational model

FUOC was set up in 1994 to make this challenging project credible and popular among the broad public, politicians, university rectors and the media. Its overall aim is to promote the use of ICT in higher education in Catalonia, to control quality and to optimize the use of public funds. With time, its function and role have grown, and a number of strategic alliances with leading Catalan and Spanish institutions have been established. A specific problem for UOC is knowledge transfer during its continuing restructuring process, in a context where new units are younger, more dynamic and sometimes 'smarter' than the old ones.[8] It is a new challenge for UOC's management to make the necessary changes within its branched-out structure of a virtual university, to take account of shorter feedback cycles and to ensure the cross-fertilization of ideas brought in by new elements of the system.

Since 1997, the University's business model has taken the form of the UOC Group. Its aim is to widen the scope of core activities of UOC and to enhance its functional strength, opening the University's way to unprecedented growth – both in number of the student enrollments and business-oriented activities. These developments were followed by continuing changes of management mode, which first strove to build up horizontal organizational structures. In the early 2000s, there has been a move toward organizing functions as a flexible and dynamic network that can adjust its structure and management to meet the specific needs of new projects.[9]

Big challenges and smaller problems

The main challenge for UOC is to achieve excellence as a knowledge-building university. The Internet Interdisciplinary Institute (IN3) is the main element in this process, requiring long-term investment and clearly-defined priorities in order to secure a huge leap forward in building a global virtual university of high quality. It was established in 2000, with its key objectives including the co-ordination of numerous ongoing UOC research projects and encouraging a shift from market-oriented to academic research. To reinforce this effort, several high-level scientists joined the IN3 research team in 2001.

Another major challenge for UOC is growth. It has the highest rate of growth in the Spanish university system, at a time when all traditional universities in the country are undergoing contraction due to a falling birth rate. UOC's governing council is therefore discussing vital growth issues, such as: Is growth too fast? Is it sustainable? What can be easily out-sourced? Growth may be an important indicator of success, but scaling up also often comes into conflict with the goal of educational and academic excellence.

One more strategic decision taken recently is to 'go global' by opening up more to Iberoamerica and to the world. For example, UOC is running the research project 'Metacampus', which involves several European universities and is financed by the European Commission's ICTs Program. It aims to create a protocol that will make possible the interoperability of educational intranets, with a single user account and customizable appearance. This attempt to interconnect campuses throughout the world started in March 2001 with a pilot project with Latin America. Several campuses in Iberoamerica that had started their online programs by 2001 using UOC's platform will be integrated into the Metacampus project.

Conclusions

One of first discoveries at UOC was that quality education online is not as cheap as expected. Optimization of the costs of Web-based learning compared with the cost of learning in traditional universities requires further study, as does the optimal size of a university and its pace of growth. In its first phase of development, the University established the brand name and gained valuable experience, a creative team and a substantial implementation capacity. Early in the twenty-first century, UOC began preparing a new phase: scaling up in qualitative and quantitative dimensions at the same time. This may or may not be possible, but it is a very challenging goal and resource-intensive ambition. The strategy chosen by UOC to try to achieve this will ultimately determine its capacity to be a driving engine for the Catalan autonomous community to advance in a competitive environment and economy of the information age.

Notes

1   The Catalan region won its political and cultural autonomy in 1979, when it was 'transferred' to Catalan governance, after a persistent and momentous struggle for independence from the national Spanish center. Today, Catalans identify themselves as "an autonomous European community located in the northwestern coast of the Mediterranean sea" (www.uoc.es). See also Stanford Study (2001).

2   'Iberoamerican' is a Spanish concept that covers Spain, Portugal and Latin America.
3   Integrated Services Digital Network.
4   The awards received by UOC were: 1997, The EU Bangemann Challenge Prize for the best European Initiative in Distance Education; 2000, World Information Technologies and Services Alliance (WITSA) as the "World Best Digital Opportunity"; 2001, *Computer World*'s "Best Project in Education Area"; 2001, International Council for Distance Education (ICDE) Excellence Prize as "the best virtual university".
5   Author interview with Dr Ferrate, 17 September 2001.
6   Nowadays this concept is becoming widely known; in 1993 in Spain, it sounded so futuristic and so out-of-context that the voting body of Spanish universities' rectors approved the UOC project simply because they were not aware how subversive it was potentially or "just because they did not believe that it could be done" (author interview with Dr Ferrate, 17 September 2001).
7   Interview with Josep Maria Duarte, academic director of Iberoamerican Division, 18 October 2001.
8   Interview with Dr Ferrate, 25 September 2001.
9   The management model of UOC *per se* may be a branded product for the distance and distributed education market. UOC strategists see the provision of such a product – for designing and making transferable an effective educational model online, including platform, content and project management as components – as a challenge to fill in a "strategic window on the global market" (interview with Carles Esquerré, member of the Strategic Committee of UOC, 26 September 2001).

9   Distance learning through highly-interactive tutorials[1]

Alfred Bork

New technologies can support a variety of educational and learning approaches. In this chapter, Alfred Bork makes the case for an alternative to the provision of conventional online Web-based content to students. His vision foresees efficient and effective computer-based distance learning which uses multi-media material to enable highly-interactive tutorial approaches to learning. Professor Bork's aim is based on a grand vision – to address major problems facing global access to educational resources, by enabling everyone in the world to be successfully educated, anywhere and at any time. His guidelines are gleaned from practical experience over several decades in the development of computer-based tutorial systems at the University of California, Irvine.

Visions of learning: goals for the future

Before looking at an example of a new global-wide learning paradigm enabled by computer-based systems, I would like to outline the future goals I believe we should be addressing. Ivan Illich (1971) stated the key challenge:

> Our present educational institutions are at the service of the teacher's goals. The relational structures we need are those which will enable each man to define himself by learning and by contributing to the learning of others.

As all individuals are unique, such learning experiences would be optimized to the needs of each student, exploring individual problems and offering tailored help to find solutions. Students will move at individualized paces through the adaptive learning units. The ultimate aim should be to ensure that everyone on earth can learn, lifelong, everywhere, at any time and in any subject area (Bloom, 1973, 1981, 1984; Bloom, Madaus and Hastings, 1981).

Everyone should learn well, through learning that emphasizes higher cognitive skills, problem solving, creativity and intuition. Learning should foster love of learning. We want creative happy individuals who can live and co-operate peacefully with others. The cost of learning should be affordable to all – for individuals, regions and the world. We need a global learning society that sees learning as a key activity at all ages. However, the dream of global educational opportunity for everyone on earth is likely to be:

> impossible if education is visualized as it always has existed in recent centuries: a school-room with a teacher and students ... an impossible model for world education at the beginning of a new millennium ...
>
> We need a completely new plan and vision for worldwide access to education at all levels, if the next century is to see a quantum leap in educational opportunities everywhere ... Obviously, this is a great challenge and no easy task.
>
> (Hesburgh, 1994)

This chapter envisages a practical way of meeting that challenge.

A tutorial-based learning paradigm

Most learning in human history has viewed the process as one of acquiring information. Typically, information is 'transferred' to the student in a class or other learning situations, or in reading a book or seeing a video. If the information is not transferred, or is not what is needed, little can be done.

A better paradigm for the future is *tutorial learning*, in which a highly-interactive dialog, a learning conversation, takes place between a skilled tutor and a student, or a very small group of students. There are many historical examples, beginning perhaps with Socrates. The student may work in a laboratory or solve problems, in addition to interacting with the tutor. Such a personalized tutorial interaction has been impossible for large numbers, because of expense and the small number of skilled tutors. But highly-interactive technology makes tutorial learning possible for all, if appropriate computer-based learning units are developed and made widely available[2].

New learning topics of global relevance can be introduced using this approach. For example, all materials can be directed toward encouraging everyone to live happily with other people, increasing problem solving, enhancing intuition building and encouraging creativity and love of learning. Learning should consider major world problems, such as population, violence and water availability.

Features of the new system

Current technology, both hardware and software, is fully adequate to support computer-based tutorial learning. Units work with or without teachers and professors. The basis of the new system will be highly-interactive, adaptive tutorial computer-based learning modules, used through distance learning or in formal institutions. The emphasis is on lifelong learning, from early childhood to old age, not just schools, universities and training programs within companies. Almost all students will succeed in these learning units.

The interactions will resemble a conversational dialog between a student and a human tutor, with the time between interactions no longer than twenty seconds. The computer-based learning programs will ask questions and respond to free-form student input, in the Socratic tradition. *All* interactions in both directions will be in the students' native languages, our most powerful learning tool. Multiple choice and pointing will very seldom be used, as they are weak forms of interaction that do not allow for full individualization of learning. Simulations may be part of the learning materials. The computer can also reply to student questions within a context.

The computer will frequently store information about the learner, such as problems and successes. These records will be used often within programs. For example, when a student returns after a break from using the system, the computer will know where to begin the new session. Information about learning styles will also be stored, helping the computer to work patiently with the student on each topic, until success is achieved.

Voice input, a natural mode of interaction for humans, will probably be used. New voice input systems from several companies are effective and inexpensive, and can be speaker independent in the highly-interactive learning environment (e.g., see Bork and Gunnarsdottir, 2001). Keyboards will be unnecessary, except for older users already addicted to the keyboard.

We will combine learning and assessment as one continuous process, with assessment determining what learning material follows. Therefore, tests will be invisible to the students, so not feared by learners. Success for all is our aim, while maintaining a positive attitude toward learning for all students.

At each point, the learning units will determine what should happen next for the student, as with Vygotsky's (1962, 1978) idea of the *zone of proximal development*. This is possible in highly-interactive, computer-based learning because of frequent high quality two-way student–computer interaction and long-term storage of student records. However, as discussed in the next section, designers of the learning units are responsible for these factors, not some computer 'magic'.

Production of tutorial learning units

The key to this new approach is the system for developing the learning modules. Most systems for generating learning software do not give major priority to highly-interactive tutorial units. So when my colleagues and I started to pursue this goal over thirty years ago at the University of California, Irvine, we began to develop a system for this activity. In subsequent years, Bernard Levrat and Bertrand Ibrahim of the University of Geneva joined us in this development, leading us to refer to this system as the Irvine–Geneva system (Bork, Ibrahim, Levrat, Milne and Yoshi, 1992). A major emphasis is on analyzing free-form student native language input. We do not use tactics from artificial intelligence, although they may eventually prove useful for this purpose. The designers make all the decisions.

We consider four stages in the development process, each requiring about equal costs:

Project management: An excellent idea can fail if the overall project is not well managed. We have learned much about how to manage this process (Bork and Gunnarsdottir, 2001), but it is not particularly unique to tutorial system and I would like to focus attention on three other stages for the purpose of this collection.

Design: This is the most important activity if we are to generate high quality tutorial units, effective for all students. All the details must be described at this time. The key people in design are very good teachers in the learning area, who should work in groups of about four. They identify student problems likely at each point of the interaction. They decide how to find these problems and determine what help is necessary for the individual student. This is essential for the tutorial approach which insists on mastery for all. In design sessions, the teachers formulate the questions asked to the students, and make all decisions about analyzing student input. Their experiences with students are pooled with those of others in the design group. Teachers' decisions are recorded in a script, initially on paper but now increasingly online. The script also describes needed multimedia.

Implementation: The script is the input to this process. Our script editor can write some of the program, from the stored design, but human coding will also be required. Specialists in the area create media mentioned in the design. Beta testing concludes implementation, to be sure that the program evaluated in the next stage is in a stable condition.

Formative and summative evaluation: Improving the learning units, and comparing their effectiveness with other ways of learning, is an important final stage. Typical students are evaluated using the material, which often reveals problems with the initial design that must be corrected. There can be multiple stages of evaluation and improvement. Much of the data needed for evaluation is stored online as it is generated as students use the programs.

Distance learning

Some use of the materials might be in existing institutions, but for learning to be available for everyone on earth, including the very poor, distance learning in informal environments is essential. These might include village centers, shopping areas, libraries and special areas for this purpose. In countries where there are facilities in homes, such as personal computers, they could be used for this purpose.

The term 'distance learning' has a variety of usages, but not all consistent with this vision. In the United States, for example, distance learning often means about 25 or 30 students at a location different from the teacher or professor. This is too one-way and reaches too few students for our vision. Information transfer is the paradigm. Because an instructor is still involved, it limits the number of students possible.

Another view of distance learning is to produce a video of a lecture, at several levels of video expertise. Stanford University and the University of Southern California have done this since 1972, starting with engineering courses for companies in the area, as has the Chinese TV University – perhaps the largest university in the world (den.usc. edu). The learning paradigm they adopted was again information transfer. Even when e-mail, chat rooms, and Web sites are added, the learning situation is not fundamentally different. Often only small numbers of students are possible.

Distance learning based on highly-interactive tutorials using computer-based learning modules can reach very large numbers of people. Since most students will not be in formal institutions, and will be without teachers, learning units *must* be intrinsically motivating and react to the individual needs of each student. Distribution will probably eventually be by satellite. Standard computers will be used initially. Later, inexpensive learning appliances can be developed.

Costs

Although development cost for this learning material will be high, the critical cost – an hour of student learning time – will be low. As with the United Kingdom's Open University (see Chapters Thirteen and Fifteen in this collection) very large numbers of students will use the interactive learning materials. So the cost per student, including development, delivery and other factors, will be much less than for current systems. We will seek the cheapest distribution method for each situation. Initially, CD-ROM and the Internet are likely modes.

The learning units will eventually be available in many languages, adapted to each culture. This will further increase the size of the market, and so reduce the cost for each student. The marketing of the units in developed countries could support the distribution to poor areas.

Next steps

We need more work to make this vision a reality. The following steps are suggested:

1   Little computer-based tutorial material is available. We need major experiments to attain an empirical basis for future development. We must develop many extensive units at all levels of learning and conduct professional evaluations with many students. International experiments will be desirable, with a very wide range of students including those of low economic status and living in very poor conditions.

2   If these experiments are successful, we need to plan and carry out the major activity of creating the large amount of learning material needed. An international management group will be needed to guide this activity. Major start-up funding will be needed, but

eventually the activity can be self-supporting, even profitable. We expect the cost for each student hour of learning to decline, as we learn more about this activity.

3   Using the new materials we need to conduct extensive research on learning, with many students. We have much to learn about the learning process, both in formal and informal environments. Professional researchers should plan and carry out this activity, with computers gathering much of the data as very large numbers of students use the units. Eventually, theories of learning with strong predictive value could be developed.

4   New organizational structures will be required. These organizations should be based on the new learning paradigm – tutorial learning – and must be capable of supporting very large numbers of students. We should consider how to keep useful features of current organizations.

5   We need continuing development, including evaluation, of new curriculum material. This includes replacing already-developed modules with new learning units. As we learn more about learning, we should be able to produce superior learning material. This will be a major on-going activity.

If we take these steps, we can look forward to an exciting future for learning!

Notes

1   The author of this chapter dedicates it to Bertrand Ibrahim, 1954–2001, who played a central role in developing the Irvine–Geneva system for tutorial computer-based distance learning described here.

2   More details of the capabilities and development procedure for such a system, as outlined in the remainder of this chapter, are provided in a book (Bork and Gunnarsdottir, 2001) and a number of papers (e.g. Bork, 1999, 2000a, 2000b, 2001).

10 Promoting scholarship through design

Tamara Sumner

This chapter provides insights into how new media can transform scholarly practice and the educational activities of teachers and researchers outside the classroom. Sumner focuses on a case study of a Web-based journal to show how this kind of technical innovation could change the social and institutional processes involved with the review and publication of refereed academic journals. She draws on this case, together with established cognitive and social theories, to derive design requirements and a theoretical framework which, she argues, could make a qualitative difference for the better in supporting scholarly tasks and communities.

Opportunities to transform scholarship

Digital documents and online communications have the potential to transform the way in which students, scientists and scholars work, learn and publish – in effect, to transform 'scholarship'. This is particularly salient in the area of ICT-based scholarly archives: collections of resources often managed by scholars for other scholars, such as e-journals, digital libraries or collections of materials supporting resource-based learning. These digital resource archives offer new opportunities, including the potential for new document interfaces to support discourse and knowledge-building in scholarly communities. Yet, these new media resources also require new literacies and new skills from both their producers and consumers. Balancing these activities in one document interface is the challenge for scholars working in the new medium.

Scholarship is a challenging concept, involving both cognitive skills and social enculturation. At the individual level, it implies recognizing the problematic nature of knowledge (Bloomer, 1998) and being skilled in information seeking and evaluation (MacDonald and Mason, 1999). At the social level, it implies belonging to a disciplinary community, being literate in their practices and literature, and contributing to the growth of knowledge in that community (Kuhn, 1996). The central thesis of the research presented here is that we can both support and promote these dual aspects of scholarship through effective design of scholarly archives.

Supporting scholarship: some preliminary design requirements

Scholarship is shaped through an individual's ongoing interactions with a community and that community's intellectual products. Being a scholar in a particular field means having familiarity with the discipline's literature, awareness of who other practitioners are and what they are working on and facility with accepted practices and criteria for judging research quality. Scholarly publishing has always played a mediating role in scholarship – by providing for the dissemination of the community's intellectual products and by setting up participation structures around which the community judges quality, such as peer reviewing mechanisms (Zuckerman and Merton, 1971; Cicchetti, 1991). In the following analysis, I review cognitive and social theories to draw out preliminary requirements for how the practice of scholarship might be better supported in future archive design. The purpose is not to present a definitive and exhaustive list, but rather to show how a scholar-centered design approach could contribute to archive design.

Interacting with a community

Being a scholar has become increasingly complex over the past fifty years (Bush, 1945; Odlyzko, 1995). The number of scholarly publications – both articles and journal offerings – is increasing at an exponential rate, driven by growth in the overall number of researchers (Odlyzko, 1995). It is increasingly difficult to keep up with both the literature in a field and with 'who's who' among other practitioners. This contributes to fragmentation, of both the sense of community and the research results, making it difficult for new research to build on existing work. According to Fish (1980), the stable interpretation of documents is not a function of the inherent qualities of documents per se, but a function of participating in a stable community centered on the production and consumption of these shared texts.

Shared texts have always played an important role in community formation and maintenance. It is not uncommon to hear colleagues refer to entities like the 'iCS community' (referring to the people that read and write for a particular journal). The juxtaposition of articles helps to define what is common knowledge and this shared knowledge contributes to the sense of belonging to an 'imagined community' (Anderson, 1983). Brown and Duguid (1996a) contrast two models of document use: documents as 'darts' – a paper-based transport mechanism carrying pre-formed ideas through space and time; and documents as a means of making and maintaining social groups. In the latter view, documents serve as a medium for negotiation within communities, as members struggle to reach a shared interpretation. These negotiations take on different discourse forms, including discussions, debates, annotations and even live events, such as presentations. In contrast, current publishing practices reinforce the idea of documents as 'darts'. Alternatively, archive designers could strive to support a broader 'social view' of documents, where shared texts and different discourse about the texts are integrated.

Cognitive psychologists and social theorists define 'communities of practice' as participation in a shared activity system organized around the things that members do, or the artifacts they make (Brown, Collins and Duguid, 1989; Lave and Wenger, 1991). Thus, it is not surprising that scholars conceive of communities such as the 'iCS community', given the importance of the production and consumption of texts in scholarly work. Lave (1991) uses the concept of 'legitimate peripheral participation' to describe the process by which newcomers learn the community's culture of practice and move towards full participation over time. Her analysis suggests that providing newcomers with holistic views of practice, access to the full range of activities and opportunity to talk within a practice are important aspects of legitimate peripheral participation.

In this light, current scholarly publications resemble gated communities more than communities of practice. Reviewing practices are hidden and conducted in isolation, all discourse is mediated by editors and only fairly established members of the community are able to participate. This is problematic because it inhibits participation by new scholars and it inhibits students from learning how to be scholars, since access and participation to practice are denied to them. This suggests that at least some archives could be designed to make reviewing practices and criteria more visible, and to provide opportunities for wider participation.

Facilitating interactions with the community's knowledge products

When interacting with a scholarly archive, or any repository, users engage in a cognitive cycle where they must first locate resources, comprehend the resources' content and decide whether the resource is relevant to their task at hand (Fischer and Stevens, 1991; Sumner and Dawe, 2001). Locating resources is notoriously difficult; searching by keywords is brittle and people rarely use the same keywords to describe resources (Furnas, Landauer et al., 1987). In the areas of Web information systems and digital libraries, much work has been focused on improving resource location, either through improved searching and browsing (Rao, Hearst et al., 1995; Schatz, Mischo et al., 1999) or social filtering (Resnick and Varian, 1997). Location tools are cognitive artifacts and well-designed tools help users to locate relevant resources and to gradually learn about the structure of the information space (Norman, 1993).

Scholarly archives are typically organized to reflect the publication process – by journal, volume and issue number. This organization reflects the publishers' view of the archive, rather than the users' tasks. For instance scholarship is partly a historical science: scholars often need to trace the 'intellectual lineage' of a particular document. What research does this document build on? What developments have taken place since this document's publication? Following bibliographic references is the traditional way to begin this process and there are tools for making bibliographic links active in digital archives in certain disciplines (Giles, Bollacker and Lawrence, 1998). However, following references will get you only part way there: a project's description is typically spread across multiple publications, and references won't help you find future work.

A diligent scholar, armed with a search engine and knowledge about the structure of the community, will be able to uncover quite a bit of past and future history. This is hard work, for which newcomers will not possess the necessary community knowledge, and students are unlikely to have the perseverance, knowledge or detective skills. Empirical studies of students engaged in resource-based learning have shown that they rely on keywords found in their assignment or other course material, and often settle for sub-optimal search results

(MacDonald and Mason, 1999). Archive designers could develop both task- and community-based methods to support resource location. These methods should be designed to help newcomers learn about the structure of the community, and how to engage in activities such as tracing intellectual lineage.

Comprehending and judging resource relevance are forms of human interpretation, which is always performed with respect to a person's background knowledge (Heidegger, 1962). For scholars interacting with texts, part of this background knowledge is the relationship of this text to other texts in the discipline – the web of intertextual references (Bolter, 1991). Newcomers to the discipline, such as students, will not share this rich intertextual background knowledge. One of the unique aspects of hypertext is the ability to make some of these intertextual relations explicit, which can support and influence the reader's interpretative process (Bolter, 1991; Goldman-Segall, 1995; Veltman, 1997). The architectural form of intertextual links provided in an archive is never neutral; it reflects the implicit or explicit goals and policies of the archive manager.

Studies of political Web sites show how these sites use intertextual links to control the 'spin' or interpretation of their party's platform document by carefully surrounding their manifestos with favorable poll results, media stories and other supportive materials (Yates and Perrone, 1998). In our previous work, we began to explore how surrounding academic documents with related secondary resources – such as survey data, video clips of use, demonstrations, positive and negative commentary – might support the scholarly interpretation involved in judging aspects such as the quality of results and the appropriateness of methods (Sumner, Yates, Buckingham Shum and Perrone, 1998). Archive designers could consider the interpretative processes important to their archive constituencies, in order to provide intertextual references to support these processes.

Approach: the contextually-enriched document framework

Given the current rapid pace of innovation, there is a disconnection between research community needs and the traditional practices of scholarly publishing. Simple dissemination is no longer an adequate model to ensure that science moves forward by building on the results of others. Rather, integrated approaches are needed that provide:

- opportunities for community-wide collaboration, negotiation and knowledge construction early in the document lifecycle; and

- mechanisms to publish a wider array of intellectual products for community-wide reuse.

For the past few years, we have been developing an integrated product-process framework for characterizing the communication and collaborative knowledge-construction processes that occur around digital documents in professional practice, and we have begun to explore how systems can be designed to better support the observed processes (Sumner, Domingue, et al., 1998). We call this admittedly preliminary theory the "contextually-enriched document framework." The motivations for this approach are rooted in empirical studies of the role of documents in scientific practice (Latour, 1990), business practice (Kidd, 1994; Boland and Tenkasi, 1995) and collaborative work (Bannon and Bødker, 1997).

In his studies of scientific literature and laboratories, Bruno Latour (1987) credits simple craftsmanship – the ability to read, write and argue using intellectual products such as texts, signs and diagrams – with explaining much of the divide between 'pre-scientific' and 'scientific' cultures. Traditional academic publishing contributed to scientific culture by creating "immutable mobiles"; i.e., published documents that traveled across space and time to disseminate new ideas. This publishing model is linear and one-way: it separates research (the process) from results (the product), and the producers of the research from the peer community. This model is largely anonymous, providing little opportunity for feedback from the larger community either before or after publication, and it assumes a stable environment where it is all right if communication delays between producers and consumers are measured in years (Marion and Hacking, 1998).

At the product level, our product-process framework suggests that document interfaces should enable practitioners to enrich documents progressively with important contextual information arising from social processes. This information can take on many forms, including discussions surrounding the document, shared vocabularies underlying the document, relationships to organizational or community structures and related intellectual products. It is important to capture this contextual information in such a way as to 'tightly couple' them with the base document. This 'enriching' approach appears to have three direct benefits:

The richer context supports improved human–human communication and interpretation, by keeping the context for interpreting a document coupled to the document itself.

The process of enriching is an incremental form of knowledge-building, encouraging practitioners to articulate their tacit understandings and incrementally refine them towards more explicit knowledge representations by reifying the context and its interconnections.

The richer context provides a form of social history, making the processes and the people that helped to shape the document more visible to newcomers. It also provides a richer machine-interpretable context that makes possible new forms of community and task-based resource location.

At the process level, the framework considers the new publishing practices required to support the enriched document lifecycle, including: the management skills, activities and tools needed for the extended lifecycle (similar to Terveen, Selfridge and Long, 1993); and participation and incentive structures that could enhance adoption and use. A key part of the framework is to characterize what proactive practices archive managers should engage in to facilitate use and assist practitioners in realizing the benefits of the new technology (Sumner, Buckingham Shum et al., 2000).

In the next section, I'll briefly present some findings from an ongoing e-journal project to illustrate both the framework and its potential for promoting scholarship through design. These ideas are also being explored through the design and development of other scholarly community-oriented archives – such as the Digital Library for Earth System Education (Marlino, Sumner et al., 2001) and the Unidata Meteorological Applications Discussion Area project (Hoffmann, Sumner and Wright, 2001).

Example: *The Journal of Interactive Media in Education* (JIME)

Reconceiving the journal review process

In 1996, Diana Laurillard, Simon Buckingham Shum and the author got together with the aim of founding a journal targeted at researchers and practitioners in educational technology (Buckingham Shum, Sumner and Laurillard, 1996). Besides offering a forum, we wanted to foster the development of an international community in this field and promote multidisciplinary debate on the theoretical and practical aspects of interactive media in education. With these goals in mind, we looked at our task from a design rather than a publishing perspective. We reconceived the reviewing process in terms of supporting 'design discussions taking place around an artifact' and launched *The Journal of Interactive Media in Education* (JIME, 1996: see www.jime.open.ac. uk for the online journal). The document-centered discourse interface shown in Figure 10.1 is used to support collaborative dialogue between reviewers, authors and readers during the peer review process (Sumner and Buckingham Shum, 1998).

Fostering multidisciplinary debate

In addition to making the review process visible, this collaborative dialogue approach appears to foster multidisciplinary debate. Figure 10.2 shows the outline of a thread with contributions from reviewers, the author, the editor and readers. The participants were engaging in collaborative knowledge construction across their disciplinary bound-aries as they discussed the meaning of 'strong versus weak multi-media'. One reviewer, a computer scientist, offers a definition based on 'immersion': virtual reality is strong multimedia and audio-graphics is weak. The author of the paper being reviewed, an economist, offers a definition based on 'affordable accessibility': strong multimedia systems are those that are widely accessible by the intended user group. A reader with a background in educational theory suggests, instead, that strong multimedia are those that best serve the pedagogical aims. This debate was published along with the final article, which was enriched to contain links to this part of the review debate (Soper, 1997).

Community-based retrieval is illustrated by the way readers use the fact that review comments are attributed to search for all articles reviewed by, say, 'Jane Smith'. You may be interested to read Jane's comments on other articles, or you may realize that Jane tends to review articles about leading-edge technologies in which you too are interested. This style of reviewing also appears to contribute towards widening participation in scholarly practices. We have received feed-back from some readers that indicate that visible and searchable review processes are useful for teaching purposes: they use JIME articles as objects-to-think-with when introducing peer reviewing practices into their classrooms.

In addition to publishing parts of the review debate, we also encourage authors to publish related secondary resources along with their articles, such as survey instruments, data, demonstrations and video or audio clips (e.g., see Repenning, Ioannidou and Ambach, 1998). The aim of including this information is to help readers to understand the work that is being presented, to judge for themselves

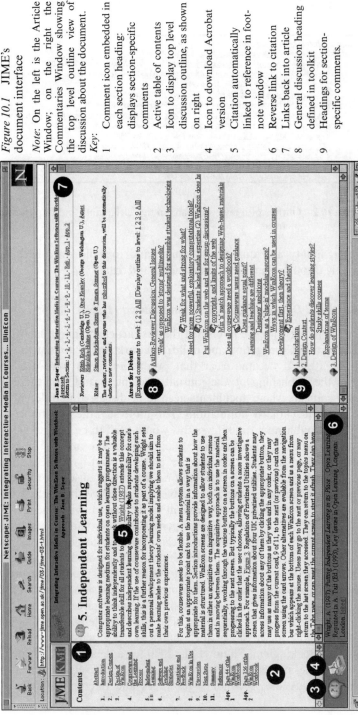

Figure 10.1 JIME's document interface

Note: On the left is the Article Window; on the right the Commentaries Window showing the top level outline view of discussion about the document.

Key:

1   Comment icon embedded in each section heading: displays section-specific comments

2   Active table of contents

3   Icon to display top level discussion outline, as shown on right

4   Icon to download Acrobat version

5   Citation automatically linked to reference in foot-note window

6   Reverse link to citation

7   Links back into article

8   General discussion heading defined in toolkit

9   Headings for section-specific comments.

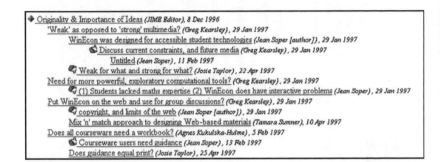

Figure 10.2   Outline of a review debate on the 'Originality and Importance of Ideas'

the credibility and quality of results, and to build on other's work directly through sharing of instruments and data.

The Digital Document Discourse Environment (D3E)

For the initial trial, we published the first article by hand, laboriously creating a rich navigation and link framework similar to that shown in Figure 10.1. It became clear that production tools were needed to make the publishing of the journal tractable – and that there were many contexts where documents need to be discussed in different ways by different scholarly populations. This motivated the requirements for a generic publishing toolkit. As this would need to be used to generate a variety of sites, it needed to be a tailorable environment. The project established to achieve this had the main research goal of gaining a better understanding of the factors that make discussions around media-rich Web documents desirable and effective. It resulted in the creation of the Digital Document Discourse Environment (D3E) Publisher's Toolkit, with tools for generating and managing a site and tools for supporting the document-centered discourse interface.

The article lifecycle of JIME (Figure 10.3) would not be feasible without such a toolkit to automate most of the production process. The entire process is structured to promote discussion between partici-pants, and to generate an initial discussion prior to the article becoming available to the public. The editor's role is to facilitate and moderate the discussion, and manage the discussion space (see Sumner, Buckingham Shum et al., 2000 for a detailed discussion). As the lifecycle proceeds, articles become progressively enriched with related discussions, secondary resources and intertextual references.

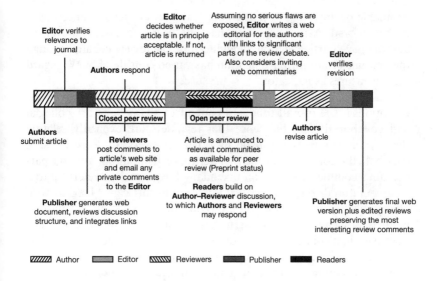

Figure 10.3   Lifecycle of an article under review in JIME

Figure 10.3 illustrates the key stages in the article lifecycle and the participants involved and their roles at each stage.

Successful aspects of JIME's archive design

Since the launch of JIME, we have been archiving all the review debates for both accepted and rejected articles. These archives contain the full debate, resulting from both the closed and open review periods and before the debate is edited for article publication. We are conducting a detailed quantitative and qualitative analysis of a two-year portion of these debate archives (eighteen articles in total) in order to assess the effectiveness of our archive design in promoting scholarly dialogues. I will use some of our preliminary findings to consider the effectiveness of our technical and social design activities.

Let's first consider participation in the overall process. During the review of these eighteen articles, 45 out of 46 reviewers (many reviewed more than one article) completed their reviews during the closed review period. While this is ostensibly their job and what they agreed to do, this level of reliable and timely reviewer participation is quite rare in any review process. When we initially proposed this model, a common critique was that it would prove difficult to find reviewers who were willing and able to conform to this rapid timetable.

This has not been the case. Also, we were concerned that authors may be unable or unwilling to participate in the review debate, since this is both new and extra work. This has not been the case, however, as authors have participated in all eighteen of the review debates, though the amount of author participation has varied considerably. We regard these measures as indicators of some success.

Examination of the review comments suggests that – with a few exceptions – the overall tone and content of the reviews are collegial and collaborative, in the sense that reviewers are explicitly relating their comments to those made by other reviewers. In some debates, over half the comments explicitly refer to, or build upon, another participant's comment. These can take many forms, such as referring to a commentator directly in the text of a comment; e.g., "I agree with Henry that ..." or "I think you are right but ..." Alternatively, participants refer to a comment using technical features of the medium. For example, they could select one of the predefined categories 'agree' or 'disagree', which causes 'thumbs up' or 'thumbs down' icons to appear with their comment, or they could physically include parts of a previous comment within a response.

Again, we regard these findings as indicators of some success, especially in light of prior research which attributes the high rejection rate in 'soft science' journals, especially multidisciplinary journals such as ours, to a lack of agreement about what constitutes 'good science' amongst reviewers (Zuckerman and Merton, 1971; Cicchetti, 1991). Indeed, in the best of cases, the debates reveal negotiations between participants about the meaning of important concepts, such as 'weak versus strong multimedia' or the definition of 'narrative'. As suggested by Kuhn (1996), when scientific communities do not share a common research paradigm such negotiations about fundamental concepts are the first step towards establishing a shared background. This style of collaborative negotiation and interpretation of key concepts is exactly the type of human–human communication and incremental knowledge-building the framework is intended to support.

Some JIME processes requiring improvement

While we are reassured that the overall process is basically working, preliminary analysis suggests that there is still plenty of room for improvement. One of our goals is to foster dialogue between multidisciplinary participants. While the participants are building on each other's comments, they are often *talking about* each other ("I agree with Henry that ...") rather than *talking with* each other ("I think you are right but ...")". Our preliminary findings suggest that negotiations such as those described above are most likely to occur when participants are talking *with* each other, rather than *about* each other. There are indications that the form of dialogue may be related to the asynchronous nature of the medium and the sparse days of active participation in the review process. During the closed review period, participants are typically active about 15 per cent of those days. With three or four reviewers and a month-long review period, this sparse rate of participation is probably to be expected. When participants are talking with each other, these comments tend to be clustered together in time (e.g., same day or successive days). When participants are talking about each other, there are often days or even weeks between comment postings.

This difference in behavior may be linked to the different reviewing strategies adopted by reviewers. Some reviewers come on line for one day and make all their comments at once, adding their own insights and responding to existing comments (a one-pass review method). Other reviewers adopt 'two-pass' methods: they come on line once and add their insights, then come on line another day and respond to the comments of others. A few reviewers come on line several times during the review period, adding new comments and responding to other ones as they are made. Clearly the opportunity for dialogue is limited when reviewers use the one-pass reviewing strategy.

As a next step, we are considering how to promote the use of two-pass and multi-pass types of reviewing strategies and how to reduce the sparse days of active participation. In one recent experiment, we took the approach of having twice as many reviewers in order to increase the activity level. This turned out to be 'too successful', in the sense that such a large number of comments were posted each day (sometimes around twenty to thirty) that the participants reported feeling overwhelmed by the volume and unable to keep up with the debate. This led them to resort to simply posting their own comments, without reading or responding to those made by others. Instead of more reviewers, we are now experimenting with shortening the review period to three weeks, and sometimes even two, in order to increase overlap in the active participation days.

Blurring the boundaries of authorship

Our evaluations to date have not been directed at assessing the value of the social history 'enriching' aspect of the contextually-enriched document framework. However, analyses of JIME's server logs indicate that readers do access parts of the debate during most visits to the journal's site. Another area of potential impact of enriching has to do with blurring the boundaries of authorship, as the document becomes a constellation of artifacts consisting of a central article and an integrated discussion, all authored by different participants. This form of multi-author enrichment could be negatively perceived by authors as a loss of control over the state of the final artifact. So far we have received no feedback from our authors that this is the case.

To reduce this concern, we try to make it very clear what the roles and responsibilities of each of the participants are in both the article itself and the front page of the journal. In addition to this explicit 'role signposting', each piece in the artifact constellation is attributed, so it is clear who authored what. The only issue with this model to date occurred with a reviewer who asked that his name be removed from the article's reviewer list on the front page of the journal, though his attributed comments should remain. His was the only 'dissenting' review, and he was afraid that being listed on the front page as a reviewer of the published article would constitute a positive endorsement. This has not occurred with other dissenting reviewers. However, since then we have sometimes chosen to highlight dissenting or opposing perspectives, where appropriate, by explicitly embedding pointers to counter-opinions in the articles themselves (e.g., see Repenning, Ioannidou and Ambach, 1998).

The strength of a holistic approach

It would be very difficult, perhaps impossible, to prove unambiguously that the contextually-enriched document framework led to JIME's success to date. For instance, our chances were surely helped by the general increase in 'comfort level' with the World Wide Web and computer-mediated communication technologies amongst participants over the past few years. However, our experiences with JIME and other cases suggests that the strength of the framework lies in its holistic approach to both technical and social design. While I believe our technical system has been thoughtfully designed and well conceived, it cannot be credited with 'causing' our success to date. This same technical system has been used in other application areas (including other e-journals) with widely varying degrees of success. Our own experiences suggest that having an explicit model of the desired participation structure – i.e., the JIME peer review model – and a battery of proactive intervention activities to reinforce and promote the new participation structure are extremely important components in the overall process (Sumner, Buckingham Shum et al., 2000).

Relationship to the state-of-the-art

The theoretical and empirical motivations for the research outlined in this chapter link with related state-of-the-art research in knowledge-building environments, document-annotation systems, digital libraries and online communities and collaboratories. These connections are outlined in the following subsections.

Knowledge-Building Environments

Knowledge-Building Environments (KBEs) are rooted in constructivist educational philosophy and support learners to articulate their own knowledge by providing scaffolding for particular conversational forms. Perhaps the best known KBE example is the Computer-Supported Intentional Learning Environment (CSILE), which enables students to create multimedia notes and link them together to create a shared collection. CSILE's creators cite as motivation for their design the desire to bring the knowledge-building activities found in scholarly reviewing into the classroom (Scardamelia and Bereiter, 1994). CoWeb, a collaborative Web authoring environment based on WikiWikiWeb, has a more 'free-for-all' philosophy: anyone can comment on, or add to, any other document. The emphasis is on providing an easy-to-use open authoring environment, relying on social conventions to provide norms for authoring practices (Guzdial, Rick and Kehoe, 2001).

The approach discussed in this chapter is certainly in the spirit of these efforts. However, there are two key differences. As pointed out by Guzdial and colleagues, these types of system emphasize creation, not production; the value lies in the process, and it is not clear what uses the final product will have. In the contextually-enriched document framework, the product is the centerpiece. The value lies in the enriching process, which in turn feeds back into and enhances the product. The other difference is the locality of use. KBEs tend to be classroom-based tools, whereas here we are considering community-wide tools. In effect, this research is concerned with integrating KBEs into scholarly archives.

Document-annotation systems

Document-annotation systems focus on providing the technical means for distributed users to comment upon a shared text, and they may not provide any scaffolding for conversational support. These systems come in two flavors. In systems like D3E or CoNote (Davis and Huttenlocher, 1995), the structure of the discussion space is determined at publication time. And in those like CU-Write (Scharff, 1998), users can stick comments – similar to electronic Post-It™ notes – anywhere in the document. The latter systems emphasize 'commenting' over engaging in dialog; with them, tracking the overall discussion may be difficult because they may not make available overviews of the entire commentary. D3E sits somewhere between a KBE and a document-annotation system.

Digital libraries

Much of the emphases in fundamental digital library research has focused on system-level issues, such as scalable system architectures (Phelps and Wilensky, 1996), interoperability mechanisms (Paepcke, Chang et al., 1998) and techniques for managing intellectual property rights and use charges (Stefik, 1996). As these libraries become opera-tional, many are realizing that digital libraries, like other information technologies, can be integrated into work practices more than physical libraries. Initial attempts along these lines have tried to articulate more user-centered information lifecycles, from retrieval to use (Borgman, 1996; Schiff, Van House and Butler, 1997). In this vein, the approach discussed here is focused on understanding, developing and supporting resource lifecycles based on task- and community-specific needs. It is concerned with how we might tailor digital libraries to better support the cognitive tasks and social interactions considered important within a specific community of practice (Sumner and Dawe, 2001).

Online communities and collaboratories

There have been numerous debates on whether online communities exist, whether they are more or less 'real' than physical communities and whether or not they are desirable (Rheingold, 1993; Doheny-Farina, 1996; Roberts, 1998). While some research (Kraut, Lundmark et al., 1998) may raise concerns about the social isolation effects of Internet access for average citizens, the effects appear to be more posi-tive for scholars (Hesse, Sproull, Kiesler and Walsh, 1993). Early studies on the impact of e-mail showed that it reduced feelings of isolation among faculty at smaller or poorer institutions, who were not surrounded with colleagues working in a similar area or blessed with large travel budgets. More recently, similar findings have shown that collaboratories can widen participation in atmospheric research by making remote instrumentation available and enabling new forms of collaboration across distance and time zones (Olson, Atkins et al.,

1998). To realize the potential benefits of the Internet, recent efforts have centered on using the Internet to create learning communities for primary and secondary teachers and students (Gordin, Gomez et al., 1996) or 'knowledge networks' supporting the professional development of educators (Schlager and Schank, 1997). While this research shares similar goals, its emphasis is on *integrating* knowledge networks and scholarly archives by examining how archive design can promote or inhibit collaborative knowledge building around shared texts.

Why design is the key to the future

Scholarly publishing and communications are undergoing rapid and far-reaching change. More journals are going online, more digital libraries are coming into existence and the Web is becoming increasingly embedded in the practice of scholarship. It remains to be seen if society can make the most of these changes: will these digital resources improve the practices of a privileged few scholars, or can they transform practices to encourage wider participation in scholarly endeavors? While the former would be beneficial, this work is focused on the latter ideal. The challenge is one of design. We need to reconceptualize archives as tools that can actively support inquiry and community-building, not as complex information repositories to be mastered. Then, we need to try to design them accordingly.

11 Infrastructure and institutional change in the networked university

Philip E. Agre

This chapter offers a critical perspective on the anticipated 'revolution' being fueled by the techno-economic forces that many people believe will bring massive structural changes to universities. Agre acknowledges that these forces are creating incentives for standardization and virtualization of approaches to higher education. Using an analysis of the relation between the forces of standardization and the 'places' in which university research and teaching is done, he argues that the future will be far from determined by these forces. His conclusions are particularly significant because they counter more conventional notions that the virtual university will inevitably lead to a more pluralistic and heterogeneous set of educational alternatives.

Universities and revolutions

The twentieth century taught us to be skeptical of revolutions. Proposals for revolutionary social change have invariably rested on superficial ideas about the world, and as a result they have changed both too much and too little, with tragic results. What, then, are we to make of the revolution that is supposedly being brought by networked information technology? After all, the case for an information revolution would seem straightforward. Information is everywhere, and every interface in the social world is defined in large measure by the ways in which people exchange information. Information technology liberates the content of these exchanges – the bits, in contemporary shorthand – from the physical media – the atoms – through which the exchanges have formerly taken place (e.g., Mitchell, 1995; Negroponte, 1995). This contrast between atoms and bits sounds like something out of pre-Socratic philosophy, with its attempts to reduce the universe to a small number of fundamental constituents. Yet perhaps it is the archaic character of the atoms-and-bits metaphysics that gives it such a hold over our myth-starved imaginations: it is the one secret, the one key that turns the lock. Separate the bits from the atoms, the story goes, and we will be freed from the encumbrances of the physical world.

The promise and danger of this story is that it offers a straightforward blueprint for the reinvention of every institution of social life. And in perhaps no other case are the revolutionary prescriptions so profound as they are for the university. After all, the university is in some sense about information, the life of the mind, for which the physical world is beside the point. Dissolve the campus, dissolve the classroom, dissolve the library, and the information-exchanges of teaching and research will transcend the artificial constraints of geography. Students will be matched with the best teachers, scholarly communities will achieve the cosmopolitan ideals of the Enlightenment in real time, and the rigidities of the bricks-and-mortar, pencil-and-paper, chalk-and-talk age will be discredited once and for all. That is the promise, and the vast millennialist traditions of the West make such a promise easy to say, easy to understand, and easy to want.

The question, of course, is whether it is true. Much of it can be granted. Networked information technology certainly provides the university with both the opportunity and the necessity of renegotiating its linkages with every other institution in society: with secondary education, industry, government, the media and the political system, among others. And the renegotiation of these linkages certainly holds the potential for pulling the university apart, as its many components become more closely connected with the great diversity of other social institutions with which they interact. All of this is possible. Before we can judge whether it is inevitable, and whether it is desirable, it will be necessary to consider some questions in greater depth such as: What, after all, is the university? How is it related to everything else in the world? And what is really at stake in the many attempts to reinvent the university for a networked world?

Incentives to standardization

I will take as my point of departure a single phenomenon: that ICTs amplify incentives to standardize the world (Rochlin, 1997: 212). These incentives need not be overwhelming, but they can be considerable.

When participants in a market, for example, can communicate data over long distances, it becomes useful to standardize the goods that are bought and sold. That way, goods that might be available for sale at widely dispersed locations can readily be compared for their properties and prices. In a sense, these kinds of standards are necessary for the very existence of a market; otherwise it would make no sense to refer to a given commodity – that is, a given standardized type of commodity – as having a price that emerges through the equilibrium of supply and demand. Likewise, ICTs reward organizations that standardize their processes: the very distinction between 'line' and 'staff' emerges when work done by staff – which is overwhelmingly information work – can be applied to the administration of large amounts of standardized line work. Finally, political systems can deliberate more rationally when prospective rules apply in a uniform way to a society that is standardized in the relevant respects. Technological societies have not been unanimous about the virtues of this kind of standardization – far from it. Yet, at the same time, the processes of standardization that ICTs encourage have been largely invisible to most ordinary people. After all, nothing is more esoteric or low-key than a standards organization, and hardly anyone is in a position to see the rising tide of standards as anything except an accumulation of small changes in their own local circumstances.

Of course, not everything can or should be standardized. The practical work of building an information infrastructure consists, in large part, of separating the things to be standardized from those that will remain diverse, and reconciling the tensions that inevitably arise at the border between the two (cf. Star and Ruhleder, 1996). Although these tensions will be part of any infrastructure project, they are especially acute in the case of the emerging generation of networked tools for supporting in fine detail the activities of research and teaching in higher education. One measure of these tensions is the conceptual complexity of the boundary between the network and the applications that the network supports. To say that the network's job is to move bits from point A to point B is simple enough, and research on that type of network can proceed without detailed knowledge of the uses to which it will be put.

Things become more complicated, however, when the network is supposed to offer services with specified quality or other such guarantees. Then it becomes necessary to survey prospective applications for the guarantees they require, and to reckon the utility of those applications against the difficulty of supporting them. More complicated still are those service layers, also standardized as part of a ubiquitous infrastructure, that embody some model of the interactions and relationships they are supposed to support, or of the worldly subject matters to which those interactions and relationships pertain. Examples include the services needed to build digital libraries or co-ordinate complex research collaborations. That kind of information infrastructure is easy to get wrong, given that nobody is likely to possess an adequate substantive model of the activities that the infrastructure is supposed to support. And an infrastructure that gets such things wrong can foreclose the possibilities that it was supposed to open up.

The places of education

For this reason, a style of research has begun to mature that works systematically back and forth between network architecture and the technology and sociology of network applications. This back-and-forth movement is a way of learning in its own right, and it deserves to be spelled out and systematized to the degree that it can be. I want to draw out and develop its consequences in a particular area: its role in the evolution of the places in which university research and teaching are done. By 'places' I mean more than geographic co-ordinates; I want to identify places in terms of the patterns of activity that happen within them, and the social and conceptual systems within which those activities are organized (Curry, 1996). A theater class, for example, is a place not simply on account of the room number, or even simply because of the architectural features that make it well-suited to theater work. Rather, a theater class is a place because of the social practices that routinely go on there: ways of talking, thinking, interacting, learning, changing, and so on. A physics lab is likewise a place for reasons beyond its equipment, and a mathematician's office is a place because of what mathematicians *do* with a chalkboard.

Viewed in this light, a university campus is an extraordinarily diverse assemblage of places – it is really a sort of meta-place that provides all of those places with a common administrative apparatus and physical plant. Now turn this picture on its side, and sort the university world in terms of the various types of places that it contains. Put all of the world's theater classes in one bin, all of the physics labs in another, and likewise the mathematicians' offices, registrars' offices, parking offices, scheduling offices, network administration offices, and so on. Networked information technology creates incentives, or more accurately it amplifies existing incentives, to do two things: first, to standardize all of the places in the university world in which the same activities occur; and, second, to interconnect those places so that eventually they merge, in some useful sense, into a single site of social practice. None of this will happen overnight, of course, and countervailing forces may prevent it from happening at all. But the effect is surely real, and it will be useful to draw out its consequences in the areas of research and teaching.

Colleges made visible

This process has moved further along in the area of research, and for a familiar reason: the institutions of research create powerful incentives for researchers to network themselves both professionally and technically with their peers in other universities and research organizations. These so-called "invisible colleges" (Crane, 1972; cf. Lievrouw, 1989) are in many ways more visible to the researchers than the physical campuses where they organize their places of work. The research world thus has a matrix structure: on one axis are the campuses and on the other are the research communities (Alpert, 1985). For all its efficiency, this system incorporates some tremendous tensions: the interconnections within the invisible colleges are subserved in large measure by an expensive infrastructure that must be paid for by the campus (Noam, 1995).

When the invisible colleges are loosely interconnected, the accounting is simple enough. However, the invisible colleges are now becoming more and more real. This reality can be measured crudely through the bandwidth of data connection between labs in a given field, but more importantly it can be measured in institutional terms. Physicists have for some time organized long-term experimental projects that include hundreds of researchers at scores of universities, but it is now possible to speak without irony of a 'center' that is located on several different campuses, for example the National Science Foundation-funded National Center for Geographic Information and Analysis at UC Santa Barbara, the University of Maine and the State University of New York at Buffalo. As this example illustrates, research funding policies have helped increase the strength of disciplines relative to the universities that house their members (Alpert 1985: 253).

On a technical level, research communities have begun to develop network services that encode their own distinctive methods, practices and concepts; and as broadband services become available this trend is accelerating. Some groups speak of these networked infrastructures as "collaboratories" (Finholt and Olson, 1997; Wulf, 1993), thereby recognizing, at least rhetorically, that the various places of research have been gathered into single functioning sites, and in some cases the interconnection is so detailed that globally distributed research groups must routinely negotiate the minutiae of their differing work schedules and interactional styles.

The scientific value of this development is not in serious doubt. The harder question is what it means for the university. It binds each community's participants more closely to one another while enabling each community to evolve ever more rapidly away from the others. The effect is surely real. But the dynamics of information technology are more complicated and more promising. Observe, first of all, that research communities themselves are not entirely discrete. They too have something of a matrix structure, whose axes are the subject matter being studied and the methods being employed to study it. Researchers who study the weather obviously have something in common, and they are accordingly grouped within the profession of meteorology. But researchers who engage in large-scale computer simulations also have something in common, regardless of what they are simulating; these researchers, too, have an incentive to be networked with one another.

Mathematical structures have long provided deep and unexpected points of contact for researchers from seemingly distant fields, as have the important theoretical writers in the humanities and social sciences, and now computational structures play this role as well. Information technology standards provide substantial economies of scope, and for this reason and others, computers now provide otherwise very different researchers with something to talk about. Each field can set out to develop its own infrastructure in its own independent direction, but in the long run the economics of standards, including the need for compatibility in a matrix-organized research world, will create incentives to abstract out one generalizable service layer after another. In many cases, such as teleconferencing, the generalizable functionality will seem obvious. But, even then, a great deal can turn on fine details, as well as on the ability to integrate one service with a whole environment of others (Star and Ruhleder, 1996). To the extent that a given field's collaboratory embodies that field's distinctive theoretical categories or epistemological commitments, painful negotiation may also be required to abstract a common platform.

Some dangers of standardization

An important lesson follows about the nature of standardization. In common language, standardization suggests the imposition of an arbitrary uniformity. But the concept is more complex. Standards can be a force for either uniformity or diversity, depending on how they are designed. If information, as Bateson (1972: 453) says, consists of the differences that make a difference, the key is to preserve information by standardizing everything that does not make a difference. The point seems obvious enough when stated in this abstract form, but its consequences are pervasive. Thousands of universities have arisen and evolved independently of one another. They experience many pressures toward isomorphism (Powell and DiMaggio, 1991), but their practices diverge in innumerable ways as well. The great opportunity here lies in the efficiencies that are to be gained by standardizing and networking all of the practices, in accounting systems for example, whose differences make no important difference to the local circumstances of a given campus.

The dangers are equally great. One is that we will standardize the wrong things, as can happen if particular standards achieve critical mass on a particular type of campus and then spread through economic pressures to campuses where they do not belong (Agre, 1999). This has already happened with the practice of giving letter grades,[1] and it could happen with the admissions process (impelled by economies of scale in Web-based submission of application forms), the academic calendar and the hours at which classes start and end (impelled by the spread of synchronous classes across campuses), the internal structure of individual majors (impelled by competition for students who assemble their own study programs from individual courses 'a la carte') and the introductory courses in many subjects (impelled by all of these factors and more). Indeed, in each case the pressures for standardization are well under way, for example in the tendency of a few introductory textbooks to dominate the market in many fields.

Implications for university teaching

These lessons also apply to the institutional problems of university teaching. By now everyone is familiar with a certain simple story: that classes will be conducted over the Internet; that students will pick and choose the classes that best suit them; that the resulting competition will improve the prevailing quality of instruction; and that the methods and resources employed in teaching will not be determined by ancient tradition but by the value that students place on the various course offerings as evidenced by their willingness to pay for them. For example, the long-standing question of the relative value of lectures and discussions will be definitively answered, and the answers may well surprise us, given the much greater opportunities for technology-supported economies of scale that lectures provide. Networked software can be interactive and finely modularized, can incorporate its own assessment mechanisms, and so on.

This picture has much to recommend it. But it is far too simple as it stands. For one thing, it passes over the many activities within the university that do require physical proximity, such as theater and dance, laboratory classes requiring access to expensive equipment, athletics and socializing. Consider also the questions of governance that it claims to address through the market mechanism. The market in courses will be a complicated place because the courses themselves will be complicated; institutions and standards will be needed to enable vendors to advertise the courses, exchange money, perform accreditation, record credentials and grades, exchange and store the many kinds of data, represent which courses provide prerequisites for which others and which can be assembled into large degree programs, clear copyrights, and so on. Each of these standards represents a possible point of leverage, whether for a software vendor, an accrediting organization, a regulatory agency or a university monopoly that might survive the same kind of shake-out that is producing monopolies in other areas of networked services. The revolutionary picture of a market in higher education, in other words, is quite capable of being true on the surface and false underneath.

The revolutionary picture also provides an inadequate account of the diversity of university education. On the surface, of course, that diversity would seem to be its whole point. Classes within the framework of a conventional university are constrained to uniform spaces and times, as well as uniform staffing arrangements, that the market picture would surely explode as each course sought its own economically optimal combination of arrangements. But universities fit together in more ways than the purely artificial. Teachers who also engage in research have incentives to remain up-to-date in their subject areas. Uniformity of courses enables students to combine different topics in a reasonably convenient way. And students must be able to follow trajectories through different kinds of courses, from freshman lecture courses – whose potential for considerable economies of scale is hardly in dispute – to advanced graduate education that is integrated with the institutions of research and ought to be much more so.

Perhaps, as the revolutionaries envision, competitors will come along that organize themselves to address one particular teaching model, so that the market becomes segmented by field, level of instruction or other factors. Will it still be possible to get a coherent education in that world? Will all of those markets behave as they ought to, or will some of them collapse into monopoly through their increased economies of scale?[2] Will the universities lose their vast abilities to cross-subsidize various fields and services (Noam, 1995), and will this necessarily be a good thing? In short, what do we really know about that world? We do not know much, I would suggest, because the simple market story does not incorporate any substantive understanding of what education really is, beyond the industrial distribution metaphor in phrases such as 'instructional delivery'. This is where more analysis is needed. Much could be accomplished, for example, by developing an analysis similar to that of the interconnected places of research activity (cf. Brown and Duguid, 1998).

Universities and the rest of the world

For education, however, another relationship between places is even more important: the relationship between the place in the university where teaching happens and the place in the world where the material being taught will be put into practice. This relationship varies, and it is a matter of conflict. The general idea is that effective teaching requires that the place of learning and the place of doing be homologous. Perhaps the two places cannot be identical, but the practiced patterns of activity, and not just the mental contents, must somehow carry over (Scribner and Cole, 1981). Let us consider how, and imagine the potential role of information technology.

The various styles of teaching can be analyzed in terms of their particular method of approximating this homology. In apprenticeship, as in advanced graduate education, the two places are the same, except for the role of the student's advisor. In an internship they are the same as well, ideally with some additional concurrent forms of supervision and instruction back in the places of the university. A teaching laboratory is a stylized and sanitized analog of the working laboratory, and the scientific and mathematical story problem is somewhat homologous to the narrative practices by which problems are framed in real scientific and technical work, even if a great deal is different about the social relations, the equipment and the information that is available. The liberal-arts classroom is held to be homologous with the public sphere, with its demands on one's spoken and written voice and, more abstractly, with the critical-thinking dimension of any real-world place. Students are often skeptical of these claimed homologies, and they often call for greater reality, relevance, usefulness and connection between the university's places and the places to which they aspire. It is a reasonable demand, even if opinions differ about its most essential features. The core of the students' complaint, of course, is that faculty learned the subject matter in graduate school, so that their undergraduate classrooms are more closely homologous to the places of graduate school than to the places where the students themselves are headed.

The great opportunity, then, is to use networked information technology to connect the places of university teaching with other places in the world. We can imagine many such connections. Classes can open video links to those other places, or they can be conducted remotely while the students literally occupy those places. Working professionals can visit classes and act as a jury on the students' projects. Many such experiments are being conducted.[3]

More fundamentally, the same kinds of field-specific technologies that allow research disciplines to coalesce into real-time online collaboratories could support the creation of hybrid sites of teaching and working, the details of which would depend on the particularities of the field: necessary equipment, forms of interaction, genres of documents written and read, the relationship between explicit and tacit learning, the role of embodied skills, the various forms of legitimate peripheral participation (Lave and Wenger, 1991) that both the classroom and workplace might afford, the relative role of verbal interaction and formal notation, the co-operative or solitary nature of the various activities, the degree of standardization of the subject matter itself, the degree of connection between teaching and research, and so on.

Informational substrate and professional skills

The great danger in moving towards these kinds of hybrid environments is that their many potential dimensions of diversity would be artificially homogenized by the uniform application, within a uniform technical and administrative framework, of a simplistic metaphor such as 'instructional delivery'. If 'instruction' is conceived as a homogenous data-stuff to be delivered to couch potatoes then the central pedagogical opportunity of the technology will be altogether missed. On the other hand, another danger is that teaching, like research, will be pulled in a hundred directions as technologies are developed that respond to the diverse inherent properties of the various subject matters, and that the university will be torn to pieces as a result.

To reconcile these tensions, we need to make visible two aspects of the university that are too often neglected. The first of these might be called the informational substrate of the university: the wide range of generally uncoordinated services that provide informational support of one kind or another to the university's teaching mission.[4] These include the library, instructional networking and computing, the telephone system, media services, the campus bookstore and course reader service and many paperwork-handling offices, such as those dealing with the course catalog and schedule. Academic staff pay little attention to these services because their relationship to teaching is uniform and changes slowly. With the rise of networked computing, however, and particularly with digital convergence, these services can support teaching in a greater variety of ways, so that teachers can adopt a wider range of pedagogical models. This will require coordinating the informational substrate organization in a way that enables its representatives to negotiate, class by class, what package of support they will provide, what pedagogical problems this support will actually solve and what it will take to staff and administer the result.[5] The key is that actual pedagogical problems be solved, and that instructors have a clear contract that guards against literature classes turning into computer classes, or physics classes from being disrupted by telecommunications breakdowns.

The second area of the university that needs to be made visible pertains to professional skills. Universities have not systematically taught the non-substantive, process-oriented skills that classes and employers both increasingly require: teamwork, consensus-building, professional networking, library searching, event organizing, online conferencing, basic Web site construction, brainstorming and innovation processes, study skills, citation skills, and so on. When these skills are taught at all, they are rarely made into required courses and are usually fragmented among a variety of marginalized units, such as the library and the career center. In order for faculty to conduct classes according to a greater diversity of technology-enabled methods that connect the places of learning and work, however, they will need clear contracts about the relevant professional skills that students will bring with them.

Once these two dimensions of the university are made visible, of course, it will be possible to ask how they should be organized. Once again economies can probably be achieved by merging some functions across campus boundaries and, once again, a leading principle will be to standardize only the differences between universities that make no difference. But which differences are these? In the current system, each campus can develop its own distinctive philosophy and culture. It is particularly important that we do not accidentally standardize these differences away by standardizing the details of the informational substrate and professional skills training where those distinctive approaches exist. We know little about these matters, for the simple reason that we have never been compelled to find out. Now that we *are* compelled to find out, we are probably going to discover that we have not been supporting our educational philosophies to anything like the degree that we would want, and the shock effect of new technology will be salutary if we decide to do something about this.

In the end, one of the most important outcomes of the process concerns the students' own personal and professional development. College has long been understood, in the USA anyway, as a place for students to discover themselves. Students do not automatically know who they are, and they find out who they are by moving back and forth between trying to explain it to themselves and others – a professional skill that should be taught from high school if not before – and joining in the activities of one professional community after another, through the relatively safe and convenient proxy places of the classroom. Students who have some idea of what they want to do with their lives will make better choices: they will know what they want from a given class, and the instructor can work backward from the students' life plans to what the course could usefully be. The newly reinvented university should be able to facilitate this kind of self-discovery, and should not undermine it by fragmenting itself in a hundred incompatible directions. Managing this tension will be a central challenge.

Governance in the networked university

Some conclusions follow about governance in the putatively new world of the networked university:

There is no simple thing called decentralization. Decentralization requires a framework of standards, and standards require a center. Centralization can thus happen by surprise, and decisions about such esoteric matters as desktop software can erupt into controversies about control over the future development of the places of teaching and learning.

It is crucial to design technology and governance at the same time. For example, the rise of multimedia courseware has led some university administrations to propose diluting instructors' traditional copyrights in their own teaching materials: if universities make substantial investments in multimedia courseware production, they figure, then universities should own the results (Scott, 1998). But these high costs may simply reflect an early, transitional phase. It would be disastrous to change copyright rules if multimedia courseware development tools are to become as routine and cheap as the desktop computers and library tools that faculty employ in designing their courses now. If any elements of multimedia production are *not* likely to become cheaper with time, then analysis should identify them early on, so that they are not institutionalized without adequate reflection.

Whatever endpoint we imagine for the networked university, the university community will experience major problems of both technology and governance in getting from here to there.   Some of the dangers derive from network effects (Shapiro and Varian, 1998): many potential innovations will be impractical until a critical mass of campuses are using them; and once a critical mass is achieved, the benefits of joining the club are likely to overwhelm any reasons to pioneer an alternative direction. As a result of this dynamic, the choices made by early adopters can be fateful for everyone else. The first universities and research communities to adopt new technologies and institutional forms will therefore have a great responsibility to everyone else. For example, if new technologies of research co-ordination are first developed by high-energy experimental physicists, then those technologies may be adapted to the unusual attributes of research in that field: very large projects with the attendant bureaucracy, high funding levels and the attendant politics, high levels of social cohesion, a deeply developed consensus about theoretical vocabulary and research assessment, and so on. Most fields do not fit this pattern, and yet network effects may cause technical and process standards from high-energy physics to spread to other fields, whether or not they are appropriate. The World Wide Web, originally developed at CERN provides a reassuring precedent, but the next standard to spread from the high-energy physics community may not generalize as well.

The future is not foretold.   Finally, I want to emphasize that my argument has been essentially normative. It has also been incomplete. The forces that encourage higher education to standardize its technologies and institutions interact with other forces that may push in other directions. Information technology is uniquely malleable, and it is easily shaped by the ideas and interests of whatever institutional coalition has the wherewithal to guide the development and implementation of new systems (Danziger, Dutton, Kling and Kraemer, 1982). The design space is thus political as well as technical. Serious conceptions of education might emerge from many quarters, and several constituencies – faculty senates and professional societies, for example – have at least the formal means of organizing around them. A predictive theory of the politics, however, would require more concepts than I have developed here.

Will we have a revolution in the university? I hope not. Revolutions are destructive. By caricaturing the old and idealizing the new, they falsely posit an absolute discontinuity between the past and the future. The last century saw enough of that, and even an elementary analysis has demonstrated that things are more complicated. In fact, information technology creates little that is new. It can amplify existing forces, it can increase efficiency by collapsing meaningless differences, it can decentralize some things and it can centralize others. It does not automatically dissolve power, and it does not eliminate the need for governance. Indeed, if issues of power and governance are neglected then it can lead to catastrophe. It is both a product and an instrument of human choice, and it leaves the burdens and dangers of choice squarely in human hands. If universities are to remain a foundation of a democratic society, then it will be necessary to make those choices wisely.

Notes

1 Letter grades in American universities have largely been standardized around a scale from 'A' for excellent to 'F' for failure, along with associated numerical values that permit grade point averages to be compared across students.
2 On economies of scale in higher education, see Goodlad (1983) and Maynard (1971).
3 See, for example, the project at Newcastle University to use online discussion groups to connect groups of medical students, including those doing their clinical rotations, to one another and to the university (Hammond, Quentin-Baxter, Drummond, Brown and Reg, 1997). See nle.ncl.ac.uk/nle/ (21 July 2001).
4 This notion is related to, but different from, Bates' (1999) concept of the "invisible substrate" of the field of information science, which consists in its reflexive, meta-level relationship to all of the other fields of study.
5 A more limited version of this proposal appears in Chapter Four of *The Follett Report* (Joint Funding Council's Libraries Review, 1993), which has

influenced the development of university information services in the UK. For a note on subsequent experience, see Rusbridge (1998). For the US experience with "integrated information centers", see the four papers from the University of Minnesota in Bonzi (1993).

Part III

Utilizing new ICTs and organizational forms in higher education

12 Competition and collaboration in online distance learning

Walter S. Baer

This part brings together a number of perspectives on emerging organizational forms designed to use ICTs in distance education and learning. It starts with a chapter by Baer which offers a systematic framework for discussing variations in approaches to distance education, based primarily on the balance struck between outsourced activities and those which remain the primary responsibility of colleges and universities. His robust analysis draws on evidence from the most important online-education initiatives under way in North America and beyond, in explaining why he believes it is critically important to understand how collaborations between for-profit firms and academic institutions develop, what forms they take and how they affect participants.

Introduction

Nearly every institution providing post-secondary education and training in the USA uses, or soon plans to use, the Internet for instruction. As an enabling technology, the Internet offers prospects for improving instructional quality, increasing access and potentially reducing costs – both for on-campus classes and distance learning (Baer, 1998). Some hail the Internet as a catalyst to transform faculty-centered instruction into student-centered learning. But others fear that Internet-based education will eliminate essential face-to-face interaction among students and instructors and turn higher education into commoditized packages of standardized courses and degree credits.[1]

Indeed, some critics talk about Internet instruction leading to the corporatization of colleges and universities into "digital diploma mills" (Noble, 1998). Part of their concern is driven by the recent success of for-profit, accredited, degree-granting institutions, such as the University of Phoenix, Capella University, Keller Graduate School of Management (a division of DeVry Institutes) and Jones International University. These for-profit institutions are investing heavily in Internet-based instruction and are attracting students to their online distance learning programs at a rapid rate. For example, as of May 31, 2001, University of Phoenix Online had more than 25,000 students enrolled in accredited degree programs in business, education, information technology, and nursing (Apollo Group Inc., 2001). Online enrollments increased 86 per cent over the prior year and constitute the fastest growing program at the University of Phoenix, which has become the largest accredited private university in the USA (de Alva, 1999–2000).

Blurring boundaries in post-secondary education

The major segments of US post-secondary education have been fairly distinct for over a century: education v. training; degree v. non-degree programs; full-time v. part-time students; on-campus v. distance-learning courses. Despite inroads by for-profit enterprises, such as the University of Phoenix, state and non-profit "private" academic institutions still dominate the higher education segment whose annual revenues exceed $230 billion. For-profit firms capture the bulk of the $75 billion training market. But information technology, and especially the Internet, is opening these segments to greater competition and smudging the lines drawn between them.

Certainly the distinction between learning for degree and non-degree purposes is becoming less clear. Degree-granting academic institutions see growing demands for, and attractive revenue streams from, continuing education and "lifelong learning"; at the same time, more and more students who complete certified professional training want their courses to count toward an accredited degree. Internet-based classes can serve these objectives in both the non-profit academic and for-profit sectors.

Information technology also helps blur the boundaries between on- and off-campus instruction for full-time and part-time students. Distance learning has traditionally served adult, part-time learners who can't or don't want to take classes on-campus because they hold full-time jobs, care for young children, remain homebound due to illness or disability – or just live too far away from the academic center. But with changing demographics and better technology, we find that:

- in 1999, 42 per cent of students enrolled in on-campus higher education were part-time (National Center for Educational Statistics, 2001);
- essentially all US students on campus have access to the Internet, and three-fifths of on-campus college classes use email and/or the Web (The Campus Computing Project, 2000);
- one fast-growing application for distance learning is for on-campus students who take classes for degree credit remotely from another institution, usually in subjects not taught on campus;
- many successful distance learning programs include on-campus and other face-to-face components, which provide a social context for individualized learning, help keep motivation levels high and raise course completion rates.

Distance learning uses all available media and technologies – print, broadcast, telephone and now Internet. The Internet has some real advantages over other media for distance learning, for example by offering more interactivity, greater flexibility in terms of both synchronous and asynchronous instruction, multimedia functionality and (at least potentially) lower costs. Of course, online distance learning must overcome major obstacles in aspects such as reach, current cost and the need for technical support. However, these problems are likely to be largely resolved in the early years of the twenty-first century. As a consequence, the Internet seems poised to become the preferred medium for distance learning, and in the process will supplant or subsume much past investment in videoconferencing and interactive television.

Still, the academic rollout of online distance learning has been proceeding rather slowly. Although the number of institutions offering Internet-based courses increases every month, the results so far have not been all that impressive.

Western Governors University (WGU), the most prominent "virtual university" to begin operation, has enrolled only a few hundred students in its first three years, despite the large investments of money and political capital expended to start it up (Carnevale, 2000a).

Many other virtual universities are little more than online catalogs of courses and programs offered by other institutions. A salient example is the California Virtual University, which then-governor Pete Wilson announced with considerable fanfare in 1997 as a rival to

WGU. Two years later, the state government quietly withdrew its financial backing, and by 2001 the University provided only a directory to other distance learning programs in the state.

Academic staff report that preparing online distance learning courses is very time-consuming and costly. Few colleges and universities have the support infrastructure in place for multimedia or Web-based instruction, and they provide little incentive for busy staff to take time from their research and classroom teaching to prepare online courses.

Many individual online courses have been plagued with problems, such as inadequate technical support, poorly thought-out structure and content, and student dissatisfaction with the interactive components (or lack of same) (Mendels 1999b). Such problems are not surprising, given the early stage of online learning development, but they can easily dissuade further efforts by faculty and students. Moreover, the general concept of Internet-based distance learning has come under fire in reports supported by the National Education Association (Phipps and Merisotis, 1999), the College Board (Gladieux and Swail, 1999) and the American Federation of Teachers (AFT, 2001), as well as from individual academic critics.

Meanwhile, for-profit firms appear to be making greater headway in using the Internet for training. Web-based training is the fastest growing component of the US training sector, and some recent consultant studies suggest that online training will grow from about $1 billion in 1999 to more than $11 billion by 2003 (Sambataro, 2000).[2] Information technology companies such as Microsoft, Oracle, Cisco, IBM and Hewlett-Packard do most of their training online. Other large and small firms sell online training to business, government and non-profit customers worldwide. For many of them, moving from online training to online higher education is a natural extension.

Models for academic/for-profit collaboration

Collaborations between academic institutions and for-profit firms take many forms. The simple taxonomy presented here distinguishes among them by the ways in which the partners divide responsibility for the key components of online distance learning:

- technology development and support;
- administrative services;
- promotion and marketing;

- content development;
- instruction;
- awarding credits;
- overall quality control.

Model 1: The firm as a traditional technology vendor

Table 12.1   Firm as traditional technology vendor

| | Responsibility | |
Function	*Academic partner*	*For-profit partner*
Technology		XX
Administrative services	x	XX
Promotion and marketing	S	S
Content development	XX	x
Instruction	XX	
Awarding credits	XX	
Overall quality control	XX	

Key:
XX primary responsibility
S shared responsibility
x secondary responsibility

In the conventional vendor model, an academic institution buys or leases hardware and software for providing online distance learning. For-profit firms – such as Blackboard.com, Cenquest, click2learn.com, convene.com, eCollege.com, VCampus Corporation, WebCT and IBM – have developed sophisticated technology platforms and authoring tools which they are aggressively marketing to colleges and universities. Their products usually include software for asynchronous and/or synchronous student interaction, as well as for registration, record keeping and other administrative applications. However, in this first model, the academic institution handles these functions, as it does for on-campus enrollments.

Academics, of course, often build and use their own platforms and tools, especially when the technology is at an early stage and commercial off-the-shelf (COTS) products are not readily available. Indeed, some of the commercial firms listed above sell technology systems that were initially developed by university faculty and staff. In other cases, universities continue to use the technology they have developed and may seek revenue themselves from exporting technology platforms and applications to other institutions. Over the longer term, however, home-grown technology systems will find it hard to compete with COTS products. Academics excel at R&D, but usually not at the technical support and marketing needed to maintain and grow successful commercial operations.

Model 2: The firm providing technology, administrative services and marketing

Table 12.2   Firm as provider of technology, administrative services and marketing

Function	Responsibility	
	Academic partner	*For-profit partner*
Technology		XX
Administrative services	x	XX
Promotion and marketing	S	S
Content development	XX	x
Instruction	XX	
Awarding credits	XX	
Overall quality control	XX	

Key:
XX primary responsibility
S shared responsibility
x secondary responsibility

The second collaborative model extends the for-profit firm's role beyond supplying technology to providing some administrative services and (often) marketing of online courses. Handling services such as registration, tuition collection and course record keeping is similar to the outsourcing that many colleges and universities are doing for on-campus administrative functions. Outsourcing for online courses is usually feasible because most of the technology vendors listed for Model 1 have included software applications for administrative functions in their overall systems, and the firms generally are eager to provide such services as well as technology. Vcampus, for example, provides most of the administrative functions for the distance learning degree programs offered by the University of Texas System, Northeastern University and Park University.

OnlineLearning.net has an exclusive arrangement to provide University of California Los Angeles (UCLA) Extension classes on the Internet. UCLA Extension hires the instructors who are responsible for course development and delivery, awards course credits and retains overall responsibility for quality control. OnlineLearning.net handles the technical and administrative aspects. Both the UCLA Extension catalog and OnlineLearning.net's Web site promote the online courses, which have expanded rapidly. Between 1996 and 2001, more than 20,000 students have enrolled in over 1,700 UCLA Extension online classes offered by OnlineLearning.net.[3]

Model 3: The firm and academic institution share content development

Table 12.3   Firm and academic institution share content development

	Responsibility	
Function	*Academic partner*	*For-profit partner*
Technology		XX
Administrative services	x	XX
Promotion and marketing	x	XX
Content development	S	S
Instruction	XX	x
Awarding credits	XX	x
Overall quality control	S	S

Key:
XX primary responsibility
S shared responsibility
x secondary responsibility

This model brings the for-profit firm into content development and instruction, in addition to providing technology, administrative services and marketing. That represents a major step involving important issues of instructional quality, cost and accountability.

Although first-generation online courses typically have relied on materials developed for the classroom or other media, using the Internet effectively usually demands course redesign to emphasize the Web's interactive, multimedia capabilities.[4] Many academic institutions find it difficult to provide the up-front investment and instructional support needed to develop high-quality courseware for online distance learning. One solution to this problem is to have a for-profit firm take on part or all of the initial financial risk in return for a larger share of future revenues from content distribution. From the firm's perspective, this provides incentives to market the courses widely and exploit economies of scale in distance learning. It also has the effect of separating responsibility for content development from that for subsequently using the content for instruction – which is, after all, the conventional textbook publishing model.[5]

As one example, Excelsior College (formerly Regents College) is an accredited, degree-granting institution founded by the New York State Board of Regents in 1971 to specialize in distance learning. It currently has about 17,000 degree students enrolled in thirty-two degree programs. In January 2000, Excelsior formed a joint venture with FT Knowledge, a division of UK-based Pearson plc, to develop and distribute business, management and information technology degree programs worldwide. According to the participants, the partnership blends "FT Knowledge's expertise in courseware development and international scope with Excelsior's outstanding assessment, advising and degree-granting strengths."[6] Since 1999, Excelsior College has also awarded degree-completion credits for certified information technology training courses developed and offered by industry. Students with an associate degree or equivalent, and employed in the information technology field, can obtain credits toward a Bachelors degree in Computer Information Systems by completing training programs that have been certified by Microsoft and the Computing Technology Association of America and approved by Excelsior College. Unlike the arrangement with FT Knowledge, this collaboration brings the for-profit sector directly into sharing responsibility for awarding credits, as well as for course development and overall quality control. However, Excelsior College retains the accreditation and responsibility to award degrees.

Babson College, known for its entrepreneurial management programs, is teaming with Cenquest to develop customized MBA curricula for Intel and other corporations. Babson Interactive, a for-profit subsidiary of Babson College formed in 2000, will take primary responsibility for developing the basic curricular material, which Cenquest will "adapt ... to include media rich online components to the Intel classes. ... Cenquest will also market the Babson onsite/online hybrid MBA program to other corporations."[7] Babson faculty will teach classes once a month at Intel corporate sites. The remaining instruction will be online and will include modules integrated with the students' ongoing work projects, as well as interaction via message boards, online discussion groups and instant messaging.

Some other recent partnerships have foundered due to the heavy seas encountered by Internet companies at the end of the 1990s. In 1999, Duke University's Fuqua School of Business signed an agreement with Pensare, Inc. to co-produce a new, accredited online MBA program targeted to corporations. The Fuqua School had previously pioneered in developing a Global Executive MBA that combined on-campus classes with Internet-based distance learning (Gubernick and Ebeling, 1997). Under the partnership agreement, Pensare would take over Duke's existing online delivery system and have exclusive distribution rights to the co-produced courses. Pensare's CEO commented: "We expect the Duke brand and business curriculum to resonate with major corporations on several levels ... This is the first time any private Internet company has licensed its complete curriculum from a university" (Woody, 1999). However, Pensare ran short of funding and declared bankruptcy in May 2001. Duke, which by then had established a for-profit subsidiary to offer degree and non-degree business programs to corporations, purchased Pensare's software and related assets. It hoped to license the combined e-learning system to other business schools (Anderson, 2001). [8]

Model 4: The firm providing all components, with some academic contributions

Table 12.4   Firm as provider of all components, with some academic contributions

	Responsibility	
Function	*Academic partner*	*For-profit partner*
Technology		XX
Administrative services		XX
Promotion and marketing		XX
Content development	S	S
Instruction	S	S
Awarding credits		XX
Overall quality control		XX

Key:
XX primary responsibility
S shared responsibility

A fourth collaborative model places the academic institution in a clearly supporting role of content developer and/or instructor for education and training programs run by the for-profit firm.[9] Colleges and universities have often collaborated in this manner under contract to "corporate universities" and other on-site corporate training programs, but not for corporate-run academic degree programs.

Prominent current illustrations of this model are the alliances UNext.com and its for-profit subsidiary, Cardean University (www.cardean.com), have made with top business schools at Columbia, Chicago, Stanford and Carnegie Mellon Universities, and the London School of Economics and Political Science (LSE). UNext.com was established in 1998 with seed capital from Michael Milken and Larry Ellison to become "the premier knowledge studio dedicated to creating and delivering educational products over the internet." (UNext.com, 1999).[10] Its initial offerings through Cardean University are "advanced business courses to companies around the globe," which Cardean will own, distribute and certify. Cardean is developing the curriculum and course content using senior faculty members from its academic affiliates, who are selected and compensated by their schools.[11] In return, the university reportedly receives a substantial up-front payment plus a share of the resulting profits. There have been reports (such as McGeehan, 1999) that Columbia, the first university to sign with UNext/Cardean, gets 5 per cent of profits, in cash or UNext.com stock, with a minimum payback of $20 million in the next five years.

Cardean's instructional model differs from those used in academic distance learning in its use of faculty, its cost and projected scale. Cardean expects to invest $1 million per course to develop an entirely new business curriculum, fine-tuned for Internet delivery to an audience of experienced executives and managers. Each course will be developed by senior faculty from the affiliated universities, working with instructional designers and other Cardean staff. Instruction will then be led by separate teaching faculty who are Cardean employees or adjuncts. IBM is under contract to develop a highly-interactive Internet-based platform for course delivery.

Unlike the arrangements in previous models, Cardean will market courses in its own name rather than under the names of its affiliated universities. For now, Cardean will provide individual courses and non-degree "course clusters" to its corporate customers. However, UNext.com and Cardean clearly intend to offer an accredited Cardean MBA and perhaps other degrees.

At an even more developmental stage is Universitas 21, a for-profit online university jointly owned by for-profit Thomson Learning and a consortium of sixteen universities in North America, Europe, East Asia, Australia and New Zealand (Cherney, 2001). Universitas intends to offer Masters degrees in business and information technology online, starting in 2003, primarily to students in Asia and Latin America. Thomson Learning will take responsibility for developing the courses, under the supervision of the academic consortium, and operating the online university.

Related models: Clearing houses and academic for-profit subsidiaries

Although not strictly collaborations between non-profit academic institutions and for-profit businesses, two other recent developments deserve attention here: *online clearing houses* for distance learning courses and *for-profit subsidiaries of academic institutions* that offer online distance learning.

Clearing houses: The growing number of online courses available from multiple sources has spawned Web sites that offer compilations and descriptions of such courses, as well as direct links to them. One such clearing house, Lifelonglearning.com, has been formed as a for-profit collaboration between Excelsior College and Peterson's Guides, a leading publisher of college guidebooks. Another, Collegelearning. com, is a for-profit firm with backing from the US Distance Learning Association that hopes to form revenue-generating alliances with many colleges and universities offering distance learning (Carr, 2000). Other clearing houses are organized by individual academic institutions, by state and regional educational consortia (such as the Southern Regional Education Board) or by firms that sell online distance learning technology (such as Blackboard.com and IBM). However, most clearing houses are new for-profit "dot.coms" – for example Hungry Minds University (now part of John Wiley & Sons), MindEdge and VirtualStudent.com – that expect to earn revenue from a combination of advertising, sponsorships and referral fees. Whether such "educational portals" will prove to be a viable and stable component of the online distance learning marketplace remains to be seen.

Academic for-profit subsidiaries: In October 1998, New York University (NYU) announced the formation of a for-profit subsidiary, NYUonline, to develop and market continuing education courses on the Internet. Unlike UCLA Extension's alliance with OnlineLearning.net, NYU chose to establish its own for-profit entity for online distance learning. A separate entity was needed, said Gerald Heeger, Dean of the School of Continuing and Professional Studies, because "[m]ounting distance-education courses is very expensive ... Being a for-profit gives us some options in terms of gaining capital support that a non-profit simply doesn't have" (Guernsey, 1998).

A few other colleges and universities have subsequently set up for-profit subsidiaries for online distance learning, including Babson

College, the Fuqua School of Business at Duke University, Columbia University, University of Maryland University College, University of Nebraska and National Technological University. Several others are in the planning stages.[12] Raising capital appears to be a principal motivation in each case, along with greater flexibility to operate in an increasingly competitive marketplace, including partnering with for-profit firms.

Fathom.com – the for-profit established by Columbia University in partnership with a dozen leading universities, libraries, museums and other scholarly institutions – intends to go beyond formal courses to offer access to museum collections, oral history archives and other forms of "authenticated knowledge." Although a good part of its site will be accessible for free, Fathom.com expects to bring in revenue from sponsorships and referrals, as well as fees for courses and certain other content.

Observations and issues

Diversity in higher education institutions means many collaborative models will be tried

Higher education in the USA is not really a single mass market but a series of markets, large and small, served by many diverse institutions. They include large public (i.e., state-funded) universities, colleges and two-year community colleges; elite private colleges and universities; other private non-profit colleges, some of which, like Park College, are highly specialized; for-profit trade schools and a few for-profit, accredited degree-granting institutions. They differ greatly in their overall missions, governance, programs and degrees offered and revenue and cost structures, as well as in the faculty and students they attract. Thus, it is no surprise to find that academic institutions differ in their approaches to online distance learning and their willingness to form alliances with for-profit firms.

Some colleges and universities prefer to go it alone. Others are trying a wide variety of collaborative approaches, including those described in the previous section. A few have concluded that expanding into online distance learning is not appropriate or necessary for them. For faculty in many academic institutions, collaboration with for-profit firms remains a highly contentious issue.

This is a healthy situation. Experimentation is highly appropriate at this early stage of online distance learning development. It is far too early to see, much less assess the results of current collaborative efforts.

Yet we can say with confidence that no single, one-size-fits-all model will fit the diverse set of academic institutions in the USA or around the world.

Collaborations will expand the markets for online distance learning

Bringing academic expertise in content and instruction together with corporate strengths in marketing and capital formation should accelerate the growth of online distance learning. The demise of some for-profit e-learning firms will slow, but not stop this trend. Indeed, the demand for "anytime, anywhere" access to quality instruction and learning resources seems ever-present and growing. Although some academic faculty and administrators express their concerns that distance learning will reduce student numbers and revenues for bricks-and-mortar campuses, their fears seem overstated. Instead, online distance learning is more likely to appeal to adults who are not presently enrolled in on-campus classes.

Expansion of distance learning may be analogous to the growth of air travel with the entry of low-cost, low-fare airlines. The major air carriers tried hard to keep them out of their lucrative big city markets. But rather than taking existing business away from the majors, the new discount airlines expanded into underserved areas and primarily brought in new customers who had previously flown very little. The principal effects of the new entrants have been to expand the overall market for air travel, create more market niches and force existing carriers to become more competitive. Collaborations and other new entrants into online distance learning seems likely to produce similar results in higher education.

For-profit instructional models separate content development from content delivery

The for-profit model unbundles the traditional faculty role of both course designer and teacher, and uses different professionals for the two functions. Content experts together with instructional designers create the courses, while separate teaching staff do the actual instruction and interact with students. This instructional model is used in online distance learning collaborations in which the for-profit firm plays a lead or strong role in content development, as well as by accredited for-profits such as Jones International University and the University of Phoenix. It seems well suited to distance learning and perhaps necessary for achieving financial success, in contrast to the high cost of online instruction observed at many universities.[13] However, role unbundling and its implications for student learning and academic careers has become a focus for academic staff objections to collaborating with for-profit firms.[14]

Many difficult issues remaining unresolved

Even without collaboration with for-profits, online distance learning presents colleges and universities with a host of old and new issues, including:

- standards for, and interoperability of, online courses and delivery systems;
- balancing investment in distance learning v. on-campus expansion;
- guidelines for effective online teaching and learning;
- intellectual property rights to online courses;
- individual and institutional conflicts of interest;
- maintaining academic quality control for online courses and degree programs.

For-profit collaborations may help with technical standards, interoperability and investment, but they make resolving other issues more complicated. Disputes between academic staff and administrators over who retains ownership of intellectual property rights to online courses may be exacerbated when a for-profit firm also becomes involved. And sticky conflict-of-interest issues can arise when a school partners with one for-profit firm while senior faculty members are consulting for its competitors.[15] The essential issue for colleges and universities remains that of upholding their academic identity and reputation for quality when partnering with a for-profit firm. Brand is important in higher education, and especially critical in online distance learning as offerings and competition increase.[16]

Academic collaborations with for-profit firms continue to expand in continuing education and specialized degree programs, but they have as yet made little headway in core undergraduate and graduate curricula.[17] The most interesting and potent partnerships today are to be found in MBA and non-degree business education programs, involving the top-rated as well as other business schools. How these partnerships fare and evolve in the next several years will help determine the overall prospects for academic/business collaboration in online distance learning.

Notes

1 Such criticism is by no means new. In 1908, economist Thorstein Veblin stated that "business principles" were changing US higher education into "a merchantable commodity, to be produced on a piece-rate plan, rated, bought, and sold by standard units, measured, counted and reduced to staple equivalence by impersonal, mechanical tests." Quoted in Press and Washburn (2000: 39–54). For current critiques of online distance learning, see Feenberg (1999) and Myers (2000).

2 Estimates from International Data Corp., "The US Corporate eLearning Market Forecast, 1998–2003" (quoted in Sambataro, 2000).

3 OnlineLearning.net was acquired by Sylvan Learning Systems in July 2001.

4 The need to redesign content has been necessary with every new medium. Many early television productions were essentially 'radio with pictures' – a problem we seem to be repeating in the transition to the new digital media.

5 Textbooks are typically written by academics who are leaders in their fields, and then used in courses taught by other faculty members and more junior instructors at many institutions. The (usually for-profit) publisher provides editorial support, quality control of content through peer review, manufacturing, marketing and distribution. In some cases, the publisher's editorial staff participates in writing and/or revising the text. Developing instructional content for online distribution will involve similar arrangements; but because the up-front costs are higher, firms are likely to play even stronger roles than they do for textbooks.

6 See www.ftknowledge.com and Excelsior College (2000a).

7 Babson College (2000). The sub-heading on this press release stated: "Deal Redefines Corporate Role in Curriculum Development with Program that Combines Online and Onsite Instruction."

8 A similar agreement between the Kenan-Flagler Business School at the University of North Carolina and Quisic (formerly University Access, Inc.) to produce and distribute a Corporate MBA foundered when the company ran into financial trouble and decided to focus its efforts on non-degree corporate training.

9 This collaborative model, in which the academic institution or one of its administrative units contracts with a for-profit firm, is to be distinguished from consulting arrangements or contracting with a firm by individual faculty members to develop courses or provide instruction.

10 Knowledge Universe, in which Michael Milken, his brother, Lowell Milken, and Oracle CEO Larry Ellison are the principal investors, own 20 per cent of UNext.com (McGeehan, 1999).

11 However, UNext.com and Cardean, primarily through Michael Milken, have ongoing business relationships with senior faculty and administrators at affiliate schools, including Nobel Laureates Gary Becker of the University of Chicago and Kenneth Arrow of Stanford University.

12 For example, see Carr (2000).

13 For example, see University of Illinois (1999).

14 As one example, the San Diego State University Faculty Senate has adopted a distance learning policy that states explicitly: "Full-time faculty members must not be replaced by part-time distance education instructors." (Carnevale, 2000a).

15 This question has recently been raised in connection with Columbia Business School's alliance with UNext.com/Cardean (see Huffstutter and Fields, 2000).
16 As one participant in the UCLA Extension courses offered through OnlineLearning.net remarked, "I picked UCLA because their classes looked good and their interface was impressive, ... [but] the name recognition doesn't hurt" (Confessore, 1999).
17 One exception directly targeted to undergraduate education is the early-stage collaboration between Global Education Network and its academic partners at Brown University, Wellesley College and Williams College. See also Taub (2000).

13 Distance education provision by universities

How institutional contexts affect choices

Oliver Boyd-Barrett

The organizational issues discussed in the previous chapter are important elements in influencing the outcome of a distance education initiative, which is most likely to be sustained if it fits well with the policies and cultural attitudes of both the University in which it is being introduced and the broader political setting. This chapter seeks to assist educational planners and practitioners by further refining descriptions of the variations in distance education approaches. Boyd-Barrett draws on practical experiences in the USA and UK to identify six models of distance education which capture some major differences within and across nations. The models are based on a classification scheme which focuses on criteria affecting broad 'macro' contexts, such as whether distance education is a core or peripheral activity of the institution. He explains how a good understanding of such dimensions has significant implications for vital practical 'micro' issues, such as the range of courses which will be given institutional support.

Key institutional and political characteristics affecting distance education

The institutions and political systems within which distance education initiatives take place provide a 'macro' context with vital implications for detailed 'micro' implementation issues. For example, strategic planning decisions can determine whether or not complete degree programs will be provided; what the balance should be between credit and non-credit courses; the extent to which a university or department originates or outsources distance learning activities; and the number of full-time staff responsible for day-to-day course development and teaching.

In this chapter, I identify six models of distance education which indicate how different institutional contexts affect the choices made by planners and practitioners. These models are based on my analysis of distance education practices and policies in a number of institutions in the USA and UK. The models are classified according to three *primary* 'macro' dimensions:

- *Private or public:* This includes the mix of private and/or public sources of funding and the degree to which the institutional mission favors the public good or private profit.
- *Dedicated or incorporated:* Distance education is undertaken as a *dedicated* activity when it is a University's sole or most important activity. Alternatively, it may be *incorporated* within a conventional campus environment, or as an extension of the campus.
- *Strategic or non-strategic:* Distance education is a *strategic* activity when it is governed through a 'whole-institution' philosophy that penetrates everyday culture. It is *non-strategic* when it is added on incrementally by particular departments.

I have also identified three *secondary* characteristics, which contribute significantly to the 'look and feel' of distance education:

- *The mix of technologies employed:* The role of face-to-face encounters is an important constituent in this blend.
- *Financial and production models:* These include options such as: treating distance education separately from campus education, possibly as a self-sustaining profit-center; investing substantial extra up-front funds in distance education – or nothing at all; using an individual academic expert or multi-professional team to originate material; and establishing dedicated ancillary staff positions to promote excellence in technology and instructional design.
- *Target student market:* Important variables here include the location of students on- or off-campus, as well as their age, education, gender, occupation, and geographical profiles.

The identification of these characteristics underlines the dangers of focusing exclusively on technology in analyses of distance education. It also offers valuable guidance at 'macro' and 'micro' levels. For instance, government officials and university strategists can learn from the crucial differences between the outcomes of a carefully planned, centralized, well-funded and publicly scrutinized initiative, such as the Open University in the UK, and the incremental, fragmented, under-funded and perhaps under-scrutinized initiatives that characterize many online initiatives at US universities. University staff developing and implementing courses can apply their understanding of influential contextual factors to assess whether a particular approach is likely to succeed in a given setting.

In the remainder of this chapter, I explore how I have used my analysis of distance education contexts and practices to characterize six models (Table 13.1). I have extensive experience in managing, preparing and teaching such courses within three of these, at the Open University, Leicester University and California State Polytechnic University, Pomona.

Table 13.1   Six models of distance education

Model	'Macro' characteristics	Exemplars
1	Public, dedicated, strategic	Open University, UK
2	Public, incorporated, strategic	Leicester University, UK
3	Public, incorporated, non-strategic	California State Polytechnic University, Pomona, USA
4	Private, incorporated, strategic	University of Phoenix, USA
5	Public/private, dedicated, strategic	Various clearing house brokers, USA
6	Private, dedicated, strategic	Jones International, USA

Model 1: 'Public, Dedicated, Strategic'

The opportunities created by the Open University

The British Open University (OU) is the best known example of this model. It has been a general inspiration for distance education in many countries because of its dedication to 'open' distance learning in making higher education available to everyone, on demand. I will therefore describe it in more detail than exemplars of other models. To understand its success, I have supplemented my own experience at the OU by drawing on accounts by the University's first Vice-chancellor, Sir Walter Perry (1977), and the Vice-chancellor from 1990 to 2001, Sir John Daniel (1998, 1999, 1999a).

The Open University was launched in 1969 by a Labour government and its first students were enrolled in 1971. It took root in a conservative society which was divided by social class, where the academic establishment revered elitist Oxbridge traditions derived from Oxford and Cambridge universities. At the time, correspondence teaching was widely deprecated as an activity of grubby, huckster institutions exploiting the educational pretensions of unworthy lower-class losers. By the twenty-first century, the University had so overcome this ideological challenge that it could boast hundreds of thousands of graduates, international expansion and consistently high ranking in official league tables of teaching, research and funding.

The Open University model was the calculated response to prevailing problems of the time. It enabled government to expand higher education for less money. It responded to anticipated demand for education throughout life, allowing adults to maintain jobs and support families as they acquired university education. It harnessed media to education, a reassuring countervailing influence to government-sanctioned commercialization of television.

The University pioneered the remarkable concept of open access, on a 'first come, first served' basis, *regardless of previous qualifications*. This commitment to those who had little other realistic opportunity to achieve higher education, notably adults of modest income and with family commitments, challenged the rigid 'ladder' principle of educational advancement by giving weight to factors such as world experience and motivation. Students pay relatively modest fees for admittance; average cost for a whole degree in 2001 was £4,100 (about $6,000). Despite fears that its openness would lower standards of teaching and learning, the OU compares well with conventional universities, as its high ranking in national teaching and research league tables consistently demonstrates (it has been within the top third over all, and top ten in many subject areas). It has also pioneered many educational innovations, such as a course portfolio covering four levels, which introduced modular 'a la carte' higher education to England and Wales.

Until the 1980s, the University did not compete against conventional higher education for the latter's main market – the under twenty-ones. Many of the early students were teachers up-grading their teaching certificates to degree level, in a profession which was then converting to graduate-level entry. Largely content with their experience, these students became a source of word-of-mouth endorsement. Teachers today constitute only a small proportion of total students. The University's subsequent success is indicated by its growth to approximately 200,000 students studying with the university in 2001 (over 40,000 studying postgraduate courses), with a total of over two million graduates since it opened in 1969. Daniel (1998) calls it a 'mega-university', whose size yields significant economies of scale to facilitate high-quality education for relatively modest student fees.

Cautious international expansion, to serve students in over forty countries, has included collaboration with other large-scale quality providers, including the Institute of Management in Singapore and the Open Learning Institute in Hong Kong. The OU provides consultant support to distance learning ventures around the world. It had more than 25,000 non-UK students in 1998, and these included 17,000 from the former Soviet block (Daniel, 1999). The Open University of the United States, incorporated in Delaware in 1999, built on collaborations with the state university systems of Florida and California (Blumenstyk, 1999), but was phased out from 2002.

How Open University courses are developed and delivered

The Open University provides 360 undergraduate and postgraduate courses in arts, modern languages, social sciences, health and social welfare, science, mathematics and computing, technology, business and management, education and law. It is the principal originator of its own courses, with full-time faculty staff responsible for course development, in collaboration with professional broadcasters and consultants. Faculty staff are required to be productive in research as well as teaching. Some original planners thought the University should be managed by a consortium of existing adult education units. This probably would have relegated the practice of distance education to a marginal bureaucracy of non-prestigious departments.

Arrangements for local face-to-face teaching by 7,000 part-time associate lecturers address the needs of students for day-to-day contact and tutorials. Part-time staff, who undertake tutorials and marking, mainly work as full-time lecturers for other institutions. Tutor marking is monitored by central academic staff. Approximately £1.5 million (about $2.2 million) a year is spent on training for associate staff.

The University is supported by central government funding and tuition fees, supplemented by sponsorship from foundations, industry and other sources. Its total budget in 1999 was £215 million (around $310 million), including a government subsidy of well over £100 million (about $150 million). Its headquarters was built on a 'green fields' site in central England (near the new city of Milton Keynes). There are thirteen regional centers that run 300 study centers throughout the UK and 30 study centers in the rest of Europe. The regional centers organize sites for the taking of examinations, but the examinations are set and marked by the national center. The British

Broadcasting Corporation (BBC), which is sub-contracted to produce and broadcast radio and television programmes for students and the larger 'listening-in' audiences, lends further prestige. Independent media companies also help to produce audio-visual course support.

So that students can achieve degrees entirely 'at a distance', a wide mix of technologies is employed by the University: print, audio-visual programming, face-to-face tutorials, computers, the Internet and CDs. In addition, important face-to-face tutorials are held on a fortnightly or monthly schedule. Course development gets substantial preparation time (at least two years) and investment, estimated at over £1.2 million (about $1.75 million) for a full-credit course even in the early 1990s. Courses are produced by multi-disciplinary groups of academic experts working alongside pedagogical advisers, designers, audio-visual production personnel, developmental testers and other experts. Although the University exudes a public service ethos, specifically entrepreneurial programmes date from the late 1970s with the introduction of a self-sustaining MBA programme.

Reasons for the Open University's success

The open-entry policy is a fundamental aspect of the University's achievements. By the 1990s, approximately one-third of its graduates had entered without conventional university entrance requirements. Using the BBC as a broadcast channel provides invaluable promotion through the airing of the University's material, including associated publicity and listings in newspapers and guides. This is reinforced by the high-quality professional production values that the BBC instilled from the time the OU was formed, and which are still maintained now that greater use is made of professional independent media-production companies.

For many courses, BBC broadcasts are secondary to the principal learning components: printed course units easily deliverable through a reliable nationwide postal service and, increasingly, through the Internet. Courses typically comprise voluminous, thoroughly-vetted original works consisting of specially prepared course units, externally-published course readers, set-books, broadcast notebooks, audio and video cassettes. They often represent daring new conceptualizations of whole academic disciplines, drawing on faculty expertise and other specialists around the world. The University's 'popular culture' course in the 1980s was one of the first higher education courses of its kind. Its course readers and set-books fostered ties with publishers and bookstores, and were adopted widely throughout higher education.

Printed texts did not challenge conventional ideas about teaching quality in the same way as television-led learning, and their successful use cautioned against precipitate enthusiasm for newer technologies. Videos were incorporated after evidence showed that most people had easy access to players. A similar attitude prevailed towards computers: most courses now have online tutoring, with about 150,000 online students in 2001. Although 150 courses out of 300 undergraduate and postgraduate courses use information technology in 2001 and some 62,000 students are taking courses that require a computer, only fourteen are delivered via the Internet. Some courses allow for electronic submission and marking of assignments. Easy visibility of high-standard course materials provides reassurance to the general public as to standards, but exposes controversial materials to wider scrutiny, and has even occasioned ministerial intervention.

Strong, consistent government sponsorship has been critical to the OU's success. Initial hostility from the Conservative Party yielded to respect when it formed the government for much of the period between 1970 and 1997. Conservative, and later Labour, educational policy promoted self-sustainability for all universities through entrepreneurship, and has seen government funding fall from 80 per cent in the 1970s to about 60 per cent in the 1990s. The University must therefore balance its books, while sustaining many courses that are uneconomic in order to maintain breadth of choice.

The co-option of part-time tutors from higher education institutions contributed positively to the OU's image, establishing a basis of collaboration rather than competition with other universities. The regional model endorsed the University's service commitment to the UK as a whole. Its degree system, using a credit structure adopted from the Scottish university tradition, has also been responsive to student needs and interests. Eight credits are needed for an honours degree (six for a pass degree). Foundation courses that require week-long residential summer schools initially had to be taken in two disciplinary areas, but there is now no longer an absolute requirement that students take such courses.

The University's Rolls Royce model of course development may have over-compensated to convince a skeptical public that distance education was not a third-class education for the poor. Large course teams do not displace department or faculty structures, but constitute strong work groups with lives of two to three years; once a course is in presentation to students, it is managed by a much smaller, core course team. Programme development contracts from government agencies in fields such as health, social welfare and education have enhanced prestige. For instance, in 1995 the University started the first government-recognized teacher training qualification in the UK delivered by distance learning.

An American model of foundation courses and credit structure would have provoked sharp criticism in a country which considered its own system more specialized and demanding. A 'non-rigid uniformity' of operations, standards and practices has governed the length of courses, layout and design, pre-course evaluation and quality control. This helped to construct a distinctive brand image and reduced the temptation to constantly re-invent the wheel.

The insistence that faculty staff must undertake research has emphasized the University's commitment to scholarship and under-mined attempts to dismiss it as inferior. The University has also greatly expanded its postgraduate programmes, including a taught educa-tional doctorate. These attract substantial numbers of students, including the University's own graduates.

Summary of Model 1

The Open University is committed to a public ethos of dedicated distance learning within a holistic strategy. It takes a broad view of the technologies used to reach its all-inclusive market, including mass dissemination media and face-to-face meetings. A diverse range of experts from within and outside the University develop courses. Entrepreneurial activities are also encouraged, within the generally publicly funded framework.

Examples from the USA of such 'public, dedicated, strategic' distance learning initiatives do not approach the scale of the OU. They are generally more restricted in the range of subjects, media mix and target audience; many are associated with conventional campuses. Such initiatives include Regents College (part of the University of New York), which enrolls 8,600 learners a year, including many members of the American military; the Thomas Edison State College of New Jersey, whose students mostly pursue nursing degrees; and the Fielding Institute of Santa Barbara, California, specializing in clinical psychology.

Model 2: 'Public, Incorporated, Strategic'

Postgraduate distance education at Leicester University

Leicester University is located 100 miles north of London. It is mostly a conventional campus, with over 17,000 students, of whom approximately half study postgraduate courses. Senior administration encouraged the wide establishment of postgraduate distance learning degree courses following successful recruitment of several hundred students in South East Asia to an MBA-by-distance that started in 1989. By 2001, the range of distance education programmes included postgraduate certificates, diplomas, and masters courses in archaeology, business, management, finance, marketing, human resources, training, sports, applied linguistics, primary education, educational management, international law, mass communications, museum studies, psychology and security management. A distance learning PhD in archaeology or ancient history was introduced in 2001. These programmes exist to make surplus revenue, which most of them do.

There was some initial faculty resistance to distance teaching, as it was perceived to be demanding, time consuming and 'different'. To overcome this, many short-term appointments were made specifically for distance education, including clerical and other office staff for each programme (but some departments gave existing faculty time to develop distance learning programmes). New staff worked under considerable pressure while exposed to market risk, yet were subject to similar or less attractive terms and conditions of employment as their colleagues on conventional courses.

How courses are developed and delivered at Leicester University

Leicester University has built on the distance education credibility established by the Open University, but with a more entrepreneurial flavor. Departments at Leicester were largely autonomous, at first, in determining the formats, content, pedagogy, marketing and advertising of distance learning courses. Oversight is now maintained by both the University's Academic Board and its specialist distance education advisory committee chaired by the Academic Registrar. The University library operates a distance learning support unit whose services include postal book loans, help with literature searches and photocopy requests. In the late 1990s, the University's central administration exerted pressure for common formatting and publicity to establish a 'brand image' and to generate efficiencies in book design, copyright issues, structures of assessment, and so on.

Distance education courses at Leicester are funded from accumulated revenues. They are sustained because they generate revenue, which has helped to finance projects the University might otherwise not have funded. Surplus revenue is shared between the University, its colleges and individual programmes. Staff appointments for distance learning are often more dependent on the viability of courses than many conventional academic appointments.

Students can study for their degree entirely by distance. By targeting the postgraduate market, the University appeals to students who are accomplished independent learners. It focuses recruitment on niche markets and professional groups, in the UK and abroad. Significant concentrations of students in overseas countries are serviced through collaboration with educational agents or overseas universities. There is careful monitoring of such collaborations to avoid abuses. At their best, agents can be more flexible and responsive than universities.

The University originates most of its distance learning course materials, although some early courses were constituted principally from 'readings' of existing texts. Course developers are full-time faculty staff, supported by some external consultants. Materials include set-books (printed and bound through university printers or external sub-contract), relatively cheap audio-visual components and online interaction. Unlike the Open University, teaching has been principally in-house, with some support from part-time staff. Most courses have face-to-face tuition, often voluntary; for example, the Mass Communications MA held occasional weekend course conferences in Britain, Greece, Hong Kong, and other countries.

Programmes require substantial up-front investment, but not at Open University levels. For example, the MA in Mass Communications developed in 1994 had a float of approximately £250,000 in 1994 (about $360,000). Course presentations to students began less than a year after start of development. Audio-visual productions were either re-recordings for which educational re-use was protected under copyright, or inexpensive in-house productions. Course teams are generally smaller than at the Open University, work for shorter periods, and meet less frequently. Another difference is that many degrees have parallel on-campus equivalents: these are both a resource and a point of reference for the maintenance of 'standards'. Courses are delivered almost exclusively in English, although many students do not have English as a first language and study in cultures quite different to that of the UK.

Summary of Model 2

Leicester fits a 'public, strategic, incorporated' model of distance learning – a conventional institution that assimilated distance learning within existing academic and management structures. At the same time, it ring-fences distance education within an environment of entrepreneurial practice that is subjected to special oversight, making the generation of surplus revenue its fundamental purpose. This is different in spirit to the Open University's philosophy, but Leicester can justly claim to make postgraduate education practical and afford-able for working adults by enabling them to achieve qualifications entirely at a distance, studying in their own time without obligatory classroom attendance. Distance learning programmes at Leicester orig-inated as incremental, departmental innovations that were increasingly subject to central strategic planning while they grew to represent multi-million dollar operations accounting for a substantial proportion of all Leicester's students.

Leicester may not reward distance learning staff for additional exposure to market risk, or distribute the burdens of risk equally; but it tends to privilege distance learning managerially by allowing programmes to operate relatively autonomous budgets. The University distance education focus is on postgraduate 'cream' rather than a broader 'public service' approach. Its emphasis on postgraduate courses for professionals appeals to conventional institutions wanting new income to offset near-permanent threats to grant income, while placating academics' fears that they are being compelled to commer-cialize.

Initiatives in the USA using Leicester's strategic model tend to have a more online emphasis. One example is the University of California online program, which by 1998 had recruited 1,400 students to 59 courses (Almeda, 1998); in 2001 it offered 200 online courses. The Old Dominion University of West Virginia runs the Teletechnet program, which uses satellite technology for interactive distance learning programs in more than fifty locations across several states, accounting for more than 15,000 student registrations. Other online courses in the USA are mentioned in the next section.

Model 3: 'Public, Incorporated, Non-Strategic'

The approach at California State Polytechnic University, Pomona

California State Polytechnic University, Pomona is one of the twenty-three campuses of the California State University (CSU). The relatively laissez-faire approach to distance education at CSU, with policy left largely to the discretion of campuses, has resulted in signifi-cant inter-campus variation. In 1997–8, just over 18,000 CSU students enrolled in courses using satellite, videocassette, cable and other means of delivery. The non-credit portion of television instruction served an estimated one million students annually. Three CSU degree programs and five certificates, totaling 3,300 students, were delivered exclusively through the Internet (California State University, 1999).

Anticipated increases in conventional enrollments to 2010 provide an incentive to use distance learning to reduce demand on space. Demographic predictions suggest to some faculty that continuing demand for traditional teaching practices is secure. At Pomona, online courses were boosted during the 1990s by digital summer schools; and in 2000, the University dedicated specific development resource for thirty technology-mediated courses, principally through release-time.

How courses are developed and delivered at Pomona

Although distance-learning approaches at CSU vary considerably, I believe the Pomona campus is indicative of the CSU's overall approach, as it represents the position of many university campuses that are still in the process of determining where they want to go with online teaching. In 2001, no degrees could be achieved at Pomona entirely online; the small proportion of courses delivered entirely online are principally for the benefit of on-campus students. There was a distance learning 'LEP-UPLINK' program leading to professional certification for teachers in bilingual classrooms, and this had recruited up to 100 students for each of its four courses. A few online courses targeting on-campus students regularly recruited up to 100 students, mostly living within or near the University's service area. Online certificate extension programs were in preparation.

Online programs are based primarily on Web-delivered text and online interaction between instructor and students, and among students. This is supported by workbooks, text books, and occasional face-to-face orientation or examination sessions. Such material is developed mainly by faculty on release time, with courses taught by single instructors supplemented by technical support and advice from the Instructional Technology Advisory Center and Faculty Center for Professional Development.

Pomona's experience is in tune with a general growth in online education in the USA, which sometimes also follows the distance education Model 2. Over a third of all higher education institutions in 2000 used, or had formal plans to use, the Internet in distance education. Many such courses have been designed for on-campus students. A large but unknown proportion of online courses available for off-campus students are non-credit. Online players include prestigious institutions such as Stanford, which began an Internet Masters in electrical engineering in 1998, and Harvard Business School which is developing online business courses. Many state college systems also offer Web-based learning, including New York (with 1,000 online courses in 1999) and the University of Maryland (with about 10,000 students taking online courses). Growing online education attracts a significant service industry, representing a process of institutional 'unbundling' of functions. Such organizations provide packages that offer access to course architecture, administration, tracking software, online faculty training courses, technical support and other capabilities. In 2000, these education-service companies included Blackboard.com, Convene International, Generation 21, Parliament Software, Real Education, and the University of Delaware's SERF. A new generation of firms such as Skillsoft began to provide content that could be used within wholly online or conventional courses.

Summary of Model 3

CSU Pomona represents a 'public, incorporated, non-strategic' context of distance education provision, common across the USA It is a fairly conventional state university that has incorporated distance learning without a substantial strategic policy or philosophy. It illustrates a trend away from satellite television and video as the favored distance learning media towards online provision. Online courses are developed by interested faculty, largely on the basis of courses they already run and the ability to secure some (modest) funding and/or release time. External funding is generally a one-off occurrence, but typically provides more substantial investment, preparation time and corresponding quality of resource than is possible through institutionally funded initiatives.

The attitude of CSU Pomona's Senate towards expansion of distance learning has been cautious. Further development may depend in part on the attitude and requirements of the university's accreditation agencies, but for the short to medium term, principal barriers are limitations of resource and shortage of motivated faculty. The situation potentially opens the door to external content providers, but no such deal has been seriously considered. Overall student numbers for Pomona's distance learning initiatives fall short of the critical mass at which significant economies of scale are achieved and infrastructure is available that routinely supports high-volume development. The students are principally on-campus and live mostly within or near the University's service area, which indicates that online education in the

USA may be a surprisingly local phenomenon, except for courses or programs from institutions with strong national brand identity.

Model 4: 'Private, Incorporated, Strategic'

Flexible higher education: the University of Phoenix

The University of Phoenix has responded to adult demand for flexible higher education in ways that other universities have not matched. It achieved considerable success and economies of scale in distance education even before the availability of online teaching. Unlike the Open University, whose predominantly 'correspondence' character would still classify it as 'technology-mediated', Phoenix initially adopted principles of flexible learning and customer-focused provision based on traditional classroom methods. This locates classrooms as near as possible to wherever there are students to be found. The University is a privately owned unit of Apollo Group Inc. which made a profit of $46 million on $391 million revenues in 1998 and increased stock by over 1,500 per cent between 1994 and 1999 (Guernsey, 1999). Net income for 2000 was $71.2 million.

How courses are developed and delivered at the University of Phoenix

The Phoenix approach to distance learning is similar to the use of extension satellite centers for the delivery of programs taught by university faculty traveling out to teach, as is common to Australian universities which send faculty to run classroom courses in south-east Asia. The University has distinctively extended this practice in terms of scale and the use of part-time faculty, many of whom are not otherwise employed in higher education. There is strong emphasis on professionally oriented certificate, graduate and postgraduate programs in business, health care, education, human services and information technology.

The University of Phoenix was accredited in 1978 and started online courses in 1989. It had 50,000 students by 1997, rising to 68,000 by 2000. Its Web site in August 2001 boasted 95,700 degree-seeking students. Approximately 16,000 of its students take online courses. The Phoenix model offers conventional classroom teaching (typically 15–25 per class), flexibly taught by part-time faculty in many different learning centers (119 sites in 34 states, Puerto Rico, Canada and London, mostly located in leased buildings near major highways). This approach aims to fit with the timetables and domestic constraints of its prime target audience: working adults between thirty-five and thirty-nine who want to earn their professional degree-level qualifications quickly. Its part-time faculty, many of whom have the qualifications to pursue non-academic industrial or professional careers, deliver courses subject to the standards and criteria established by the institution.

An undergraduate degree can be completed in as little as two years, depending on the amount of prior credit earned. Students take one course at a time, lasting five weeks for undergraduates and six weeks for graduate students, scheduled mainly in evenings and week-ends (Leatherman, 1998; Padilla, 1999). Programs run throughout the calendar year. There are 5,200 instructors, all but 150 of whom are part-time. They receive between $1,000 and $2,500 per five-week course. Undergraduates spend about 17.5 hours over five weeks in face-to-face classroom setting with a professor during a three-credit hour semester course, which is less than half the 40–45 hours spent by students in traditional face-to-face classroom settings. The deficit is made up by mandatory, largely unsupervised, weekly small-group study sessions in which students are supposed to meet independently with other class members.

Summary of Model 4

The University of Phoenix is a non-conventional private institution that has incorporated online distance learning as an increasingly significant strategic supplement to its dispersed provision of degree level programs. It is profit-driven, but succeeds because it responds to demand from adult learners in search of career-relevant degree qualifications that they can achieve with maximum flexibility and speed under accredited conditions. The University's course development is largely the product of individual faculty working in collaboration with technicians; this is regarded as requiring the higher levels of investment characteristic of the British Models 1 and 2 examples discussed earlier. Phoenix has explored the option of incorporating materials from external online training sources, such as Skillsoft.

Model 5: 'Public/Private, Dedicated, Strategic'

The clearing-house approach

One of the many models of distance education developed in the USA involves the use of organizations that acquire or broker programs from a variety of institutional providers, then add value through flexible entry and credit-transfer policies (Farrell, 1999: 8). Such clearing houses are conduits for distance programs from member institutions. They seek to overcome fragmentation of the educational market by pooling distance courses, support, marketing, and even technical infrastructure and training through consortia that can improve the overall strength and quality of their collective portfolios (Mendels, 1999a).

How courses are developed and delivered using the clearing-house model

The following are some examples of the clearing-house approach:

The National Technological University (NTU) is an accredited, degree-granting university which offers for-credit and non-credit courses delivered via what it calls 'leading-edge telecommunications technologies'. These courses are produced by a working alliance of fifty-two universities and training organizations, that include thirteen of US News and World Report's top twenty-five graduate engineering programs. NTU contracts with institutions to develop curricula and courses, which in the past have been delivered directly by satellite to the work-site and are now increasingly online. The course portfolio totals nearly 1,400 graduate-level courses, principally in engineering. Over 1,100 students graduated between 1984 and 1997 from NTU, which had a total of 1,800 students in 1997. Courses are currently offered through Stratys Learning Solutions, formed upon NTU's acquisition of the PBS Business and Technology Network.

The Public Broadcasting Service (PBS) Adult Learning Services (ALS) assists colleges to develop distance degree programs through a 'Going the Distance' project that aims to ensure students throughout the USA have the opportunity to earn their college diplomas entirely at a distance. ALS was established in 1981 to co-ordinate with 190 public television stations and some 2,000 colleges to deliver telecourses for college credit. It has grown from a portfolio of seven telecourses to over eighty, with an annual enrollment of 470,000 in 1999. Colleges pay a license to use the materials for local delivery within their own credit and non-credit programs.

Knowledge TV was established in 1987 by Glenn Jones, a cable pioneer. It is a television channel designed to meet diverse needs for education, information and instruction. It focuses primarily on for-credit, college-level telecourses, available both for registered students and a much larger 'eaves-dropping' audience. Based in Englewood, Colorado, programming comes from thirty affiliate universities, colleges and other providers in the USA. Degrees are conferred only by affiliate institutions. The channel is delivered to individuals or institutions by satellite, broadcast, cable and the Internet. Instructor contact is via telephone, mail, e-mail and periodic teleconferences (Jones, 1997).

California Virtual University (CVU) was launched in 1998, listing 2,000 courses. During its first year, CVU attracted 25,000 enrollments and about 120,000 people visited the Web site monthly (Downes, 1999). However, in 1999 control shifted back to participating universities who balked at a proposed marketing bill of $3 million over three years. Downes (1999) has argued money was not the problem (there was $6.1 million backing from the University of California, California State University and community college systems), but the different interests of the key partners. He also queries why students would want to sign up with the CVU when they would get their degrees from another institution.

Western Governors University (WGU) was founded by governors of several western states in the USA and has grown into a collaborative effort involving nineteen states and territories, based on partnerships with dozens of higher education institutions and corporations. WGU's essential role is to set and assess competency examinations, so its degrees are competency-based (Carnevale, 2001). It had attracted 100–120 students by the summer of 1999, and was reported to need 3,000 students to break even (EDUCAUSE listserve, http//www.educause.edu, August 23, 1999). Many potential students who visited its Web site may have registered directly with member universities of its consortium. In June 2001, the US Distance Education and Training Council (DETC) awarded accreditation status to WGU, which could boost student registration.

The Kentucky Commonwealth Virtual University started in the summer of 1999 with 160 students enrolled in twenty-one classes, the participation of twenty-two of the state's fifty-nine colleges and universities and an annual operating budget of $8 million (Associated Press, August 23, 1999). It enrolled 6,100 students in its first five semesters. The state planned to invest nearly $18 million over two years. The University has no professors, does not deliver its own courses nor grants degrees. Instead, it offers a directory of online courses statewide, a central online library and support services for distance learning students. The University pays for technology used on individual campuses and, sometimes, for release time for professors to develop courses. It operates a toll-free 'call center' where students can seek technical or academic help. All courses use standard software to give a consistent 'look and feel'.

UNext.com invites universities to contribute course materials that can be sold to major corporations for employee training. Participants include Columbia University's Business School, the University of Chicago, Stanford University, Carnegie Mellon University and the London School of Economics and Political Science. Its first customer was IBM, whose Lotus Development unit, called LearningSpace, is used for delivery and sales. Participating universities benefit from sales revenue, royalties and equity (Guernsey, 1999). One objective is to achieve accreditation as an online business school for MBA degrees.

R1.edu brought together fourteen large US research universities in 1999 to market their distance education efforts through a central Web directory, co-ordinated by the University of Washington (Young, 1999).

Caliber Learning Network Inc. based in Baltimore, links together five universities (Columbia, Georgetown, the Wharton School of the University of Pennsylvania, Johns Hopkins University, and the University of Southern California) with the European Training Group, a European network of IT training centers. They offer courses in business, health care and teacher training via satellite television and the Internet (Guernsey, 1999; McGeehan, 1999).

Summary of Model 5

The clearing-house model is driven by the allure of relatively modest start-up costs, economies of scale, and strong name branding. Participating institutions may or may not have a management or ownership stake in the clearing house; they may include both public and private institutions, profit and not-for-profit. Clearing houses are by definition strategic. They target both existing on-campus students who want to better juggle their timetables using distance learning options, and external students who benefit from programs that do not require physical class attendance. Course credit is generally awarded by the institutions originating the courses.

A clearing house typically has no full-time faculty of its own and courses usually result from the efforts of individual staff working in relative isolation. They are designed to maximize dissemination, but not all are effective. The model allows for a mix of technologies and delivery systems, including online; terrestrial, satellite or cable television and radio; and correspondence. By bringing together courses from different sources, clearing houses may be well positioned to construct entire degrees online. With the exception of some PBS telecourses, many of the courses have not been spectacularly well resourced, and some programs may merely reflect the idiosyncrasies of individual member portfolios.

Model 6: 'Private, Dedicated, Strategic'

Commercially-driven private educational institutions dedicated to distance delivery

Private institutions dedicated to distance delivery of education have typically been offshoots of older publishing and media interests, or have some links with conventional universities.

For example, Jones International University (JIU) is an offshoot of Knowledge TV (described in Model 5 above). It was founded in 1995 and in 1999 became the first Internet-only university to be fully accredited to grant college degrees. The decision of the North Central Association of Colleges and Schools to accredit Jones International in March 1999 was formally protested by the American Association of University Professors (AAUP). The AAUP alleged that: Jones instructors taught courses prepared by others and had little say over how material was presented; nearly all instructors were part-time; and there was little emphasis on research.

In March 1999, JIU had 950 registrations for its various courses, of which ten were enrolled in the Bachelors degree program and sixty-four in the Masters degrees (Blumenstyk, 1999a). Ten students graduated with MAs in Business Communication in 2001. At fees of $4,000 a year, Jones has to compete with the $3,200 average of a state college. In 2001, Jones announced the formation of six new Masters in education degrees.

Another dedicated private distance learning initiative was announced in July 1999 by publisher Harcourt General Inc., which said it intended to introduce a program called Lifelong Learning, an

Internet university and an Internet high school. It wanted to become the first major publishing house to offer accredited college degrees, through the New England Association of Schools and Colleges, which also certifies Harvard University and other major colleges in the region (Hechinger, 1999).

Non-accredited Internet-only institutions include Concord University School of Law in Los Angeles and OnlineLearning.net, owned partly by Houghton Mifflin, which has the exclusive rights to market non-credit versions of courses from the University of California at Los Angeles.

Summary of Model 6

The institutions of this model are largely profit-driven and some have strong commercial roots in publishing and entertainment industries. They tend to employ only as many full-time faculty as are needed for accreditation purposes, if that. Like the University of Phoenix (Model 4), they depend heavily on part-time faculty for both course development and presentation. They are dedicated to distance learning, and their approach is strategic. Their technology is online for both content delivery and interactions between instructors and students, and among students. Not enough is known yet about the up-front investment available for the preparation of individual courses, nor whether there is any significant shift away from the traditional instructor-centered approach in favor of course team operation. Courses tend to concentrate on areas of high potential revenue, inevitably strong on management and computing.

Conclusion

This chapter seeks to bring into focus a range of significant institutional and broader social contextual factors that impinge on any assessment of distance education. I have identified six models of distance education institutional provision, arguing that their production and delivery is shaped in critical ways by choices relating to three primary contextual dimensions (private/public, dedicated/incorporated, strategic/non-strategic) and three secondary aspects (technology mix, financial and production models, target audiences). Improved understanding of these environmental factors can be of assistance at three levels:

Planning and practice in universities   The primary contextual factors have important implications for secondary features, such as the amount of resources and institutional support made available; whether entire degree programs or only individual courses are permissible; and whether ventures need to be viewed as essentially entrepreneurial, or part of the normal public service mission of a university. Actual and potential distance learning capabilities should be assessed in relation to the achievement levels enabled or predisposed by the institutional and political context. An environment that has no essential commitment to the development of distance learning, no institution-wide strategy, and a lack of clarity about its institutional motive or philosophy in this area is unlikely to provide an adequate level of funding, policy support or framework of security to ensure the long-term health of any distance learning initiative.

National and local government   My highlighting of the reasons for the success of the Open University's well-planned and thought-through strategy indicates how policy makers can enhance the quality of distance learning programs, the seriousness with which they are regarded by the general public and the extent to which they contribute to options for adult educational development and the improvement of pedagogy and subject growth.

Research   Without a strong sense of the macro level, it is virtually impossible to generalize meaningfully from studies of specific instances of distance learning, or to assess their applicability for other contexts.

14 The Virtual University of Applied Sciences

A flagship German project

Rose M M Wagner

The growth in distance education is leading to increasing international competition in higher education, which in turn is affecting the direction of national educational strategies. This chapter examines an important response to this challenge in Germany, which involves new forms of collaborative relationships among universities. Rose Wagner describes a pilot 'flagship' higher education project involving ten universities of applied sciences in jointly developing online study programs. She also describes the national context within which the initiative is taking place.

The key role of national educational systems

Educational systems have always played a key role in the economic, political and cultural transformation of societies. In Germany, for instance, the education system was crucial for the successful transformation into an industrial society and provided the necessary means to transmit cultural values and key work ethic concepts (Weber, 1972; Wehler, 1989). The role that the education system should play in the current transformation from an industrial into an information society is of high public interest, especially following a talk by Federal President Roman Herzog (1997), in which he started a groundbreaking public debate in Germany by stating that modern education should be oriented toward labor market needs, and that ICTs should be rapidly employed on a large scale.

Critics argue that the education system needs reform, but that it should not be transformed into a commodity. There has been a revival of the ideas of educational reformer Wilhelm von Humboldt (1767–1835), who claimed that the aim of education (Bildung) was not the service of society or the state, but rather the cultivation of the individual (Dürr, 1997; Meyer 1998). It is precisely because the world is becoming more complex that critics maintain this kind of more wide-ranging education will be needed.

The German higher education system

Most of the 344 institutions of higher education in Germany are public institutions, funded by the state with free tuition. There were also seventy-five private institutions of higher education in 1998, many of which are also free (BMBF, 2000).

Of the roughly 1.8 million students enrolled in German institutions of higher learning in 1998, nearly half attended a university of applied sciences (BMBF, 2000). These were established in the early 1970s to answer a demand for a practice-related higher education. They offer mainly courses in engineering, social work, economics, agriculture and design; in general, they are smaller than traditional universities. Students graduate after eight semesters, after a final examination.

Germany's first and, until 2001, only distance-learning university, the FernUniversität Hagen (www.fernuni-hagen.de) was also set up in the early 1970s. Although it offers degree programs, it draws a different type of students than on-campus colleges. Generally, they are older and many of them study in parallel with their jobs or domestic obligations. About 56,000 students were enrolled in 2001. Its courses have free tuition; however, students have to pay a modest fee per course (roughly €60 or $53) for the learning material provided, such as brochures and CD-ROMs. Study centers located all over Germany are used to offer face-to-face encounters as part of its courses. Until 2001, FernUniversität Hagen used the Internet mainly for the distribution of teaching material. However, this has been changing as the university undergoes a process of major restructuring, which involves making teaching and learning much more Web-based. The future focus will be on engineering and economics, with the elimination of all previous courses in humanities.

Germany's academic institutions generally promote internationalization, but they do not welcome the strong international competition. In 1998, about 40,400 German students were enrolled at universities abroad, of which around 20,000 were in just three English-speaking countries: the USA, UK and Canada (BMBF, 2000). With English as lingua franca, the USA increasingly dominates the international education market, since ICT provides new opportunities to reach out for students via the Internet (Picht, 2001). The University of Phoenix (www.phoenix.edu), for instance, is explicitly targeting German students (BMBF, 2001).

In order to support internationalization and enhance flexibility and mobility, a number of higher education reforms and innovations were introduced in the late 1990s at both federal and state levels.[1] These included new Bachelors and Masters degree programs and adoption of the European Credit Transfer System (ECTS).[2] However, not all universities have yet adopted the measures, and many of those that have are implementing them slowly. These reforms have resulted in a paradoxical situation in which the more German institutions of higher education adapt to the American system (for instance by introducing Bachelors and Masters programs) the more opportunity there is for American institutions to enter the German market or to attract German students (Picht, 2001).

Federal and state programs

Although Germany is federal and responsibility for higher education lies with the states (Länder), one of the most important players in the field of e-learning is the Federal Ministry of Education and Research (BMBF). It held a contest in 1997, called *Exploitation of Internationally Available Knowledge for Development and Innovation* (BMBF, 1998), which resulted in the choice of three so-called 'flagship' projects. These would serve as pacemakers for innovation in higher education, and to open new educational markets. These flagship projects run from 1999 to 2003, with funding of €50 million ($44.5 million).[3]

An umbrella program launched in 1999, *Innovation and Jobs in the Information Society of the Twenty-first Century*, comprises objectives and actions that the Government regards as essential to move successfully into the information age (BMBF and BMWI, 1999). Among the ten general aims formulated in this action plan are such goals as to:

- increase the spread and use of ICTs in every sector of the economy and society, with the aim of achieving a leading position internationally by the year 2005;
- offer equal chances for all social groups in accessing and using ICT;
- thoroughly modernize the educational system.

As part of its explicit highlighting of the educational system as one of the most important fields for strategic action, the program sets an ambitious goal for Germany to become the world leader in the educational software market by 2005 (BMBF and BMWI, 1999). A key educational initiative under the umbrella program is the *New Media in Education Program*, which was started in 2000 with one of its goals being the stimulation of educational software developments.

This new-media program has federal funding of roughly €300 million ($267.3 million) for five years, plus additional financing for pilot projects from the states (BMBF, 2000a; Bulmahn, 2001). Its overall objectives are to:

- support structural change in higher education and enhancement of the international competitiveness of Germany's academic teaching; and
- introduce a new, co-operative focus of teaching and learning (BMBF, 2000a).

Funding is provided for projects that will help universities to become producers and providers of e-learning modules for academic degree programs as well as for continuing education; the latter is regarded as a new source of revenue. At first, the emphasis in the funded projects was on specific courses which were of limited scope. This has changed however, and the focus has shifted to a more systemic approach (Kerres, 2001). Now, financing goes predominantly to projects that stimulate collaboration among academic institutions and across departmental borders and furthers the development of comprehensive distance-education strategies. Above all, universities are expected to develop business plans and attain sustainability for their e-learning activities. The *New Media in Education Program*, too, underlines the ambitious goal of developing high-quality educational software, especially the kind that can build on the quality and image of German engineering ('Made in Germany') and thus be marketable worldwide (BMBF, 2000a).

A flagship project: the Virtual University of Applied Sciences

In addition to the more than a hundred projects funded by the BMBF in 2001 in the *New Media in Education Program*, the three flagship projects funded under the *Exploitation of Internationally Available Knowledge for Development and Innovation* program play an important role. Of these, the Virtual University of Applied Sciences in Information Science and Engineering and Business Administration is the most prominent, and with roughly €21 million ($18.7 million) the best funded.[4] It began officially in 1999, but its origins go back to 1997, when faculty at Lübeck University of Applied Sciences set up a working group on online education. Its ambitious goal is to form a virtual organization of ten existing universities of applied sciences from six German states,[5] operated essentially through decentralized and distributed governance.

The responsibilities of each of the universities involved are precisely defined, for example for administrative services, technology support, course development, educational software, instruction and tutorial support. One faculty member from a specific university is responsible for the design of one course, which will later be adopted by all partici-pating universities. All courses are being approved jointly. Suitable modules from commercial vendors may also be employed, provided they meet the required quality standards. The traditional unity of course design and teaching will be abrogated.

The main tasks of the project are officially defined as:

- educational methodology of virtual learning;
- structure and organization; and
- content development and educational software.

However, the emphasis appears to be on the latter two aspects.[6] To achieve its objectives, the project has set up a very complex organiza-tional scheme, with the participants of the network collaborating closely in numerous committees. A central steering committee, with the heads of all universities, decides on pivotal questions. The jointly-offered online study programs have resulted in substantial structural changes in the several institutions. For example, the participating universities must:

- create a joint virtual structure with clear responsibilities;
- agree on and introduce joint curricula and guidelines and regula-tions for exams;
- offer courses which they have not developed themselves, but for which they must nevertheless organize face-to-face tutorials at each university;
- ensure the protection of intellectual property rights for the online courses, which means drawing up contracts with the professors who designed the courses;
- develop an efficient infrastructure for the design and upgrading of online courses and applications, which will no longer rest in the

hand of a single professor (such an infrastructure does not yet exist in German universities);

- introduce new ways to measure teaching loads;
- employ part-time tutors for the face-to-face modules, thereby breaking up the current system of full-time faculty and tenured professors – which would essentially be a paradigm shift in the German educational system with its predominantly full-time and lifetime-tenure faculty.

The Virtual University's mode of operation

Each institution within the Virtual University offers the same consecutive online degree programs (Bachelors and Masters) with courses in computer science (Medieninformatik) and engineering and business administration (Wirtschaftsingenieurwesen). These were chosen because of preferences of the faculty involved, viability for distance education[7] and suitability for commercial exploitation. The American Blackboard V. Level III system is being used as the ICT platform.

The curricula are based on the European Credit Transfer System. A complete course of study, such as Engineering and Business Administration, consists of several subsidiary courses, such as marketing, accounting and logistics. It is being stressed that the approach favors student-centered learning. Examinations at the end of each course are identical at each of the universities. Each course consists of 80 per cent of e-learning components and 20 per cent face-to-face encounters. The FernUniversität Hagen and the British Open University have served as role models for one-to-one tutorial support, face-to-face components and interactive multimedia.

Participants in the Bachelors degree program, which is tuition-free, graduate after six semesters. A Masters degree can be earned after an additional four semesters, and there is currently discussion about whether the advanced Masters program, which will start in 2004, should also be free or whether tuition fees should be charged. This is a delicate political issue; tuition fees at a public institution of higher education would be a paradigm shift in the German educational system.

Enrollment is carried out via the Internet, with the first intake starting in the Winter semester 2001/2. Due to limited resources, particularly of academic staff for tutorial support and face-to-face seminars, the number of students for the first enrollment was restricted to 200 per course. There were initially discussions about whether to offer the online courses in German or English. The decision for

German was made on the presumption that there is a market for high-quality German-language online courses in computer science and in engineering and business administration, as this need was not being met by other providers at the time.

The online students of the University of Applied Sciences differ significantly from on-campus students: they are older and they have jobs and other responsibilities, such as childcare, but above all they appreciate the flexibility that e-learning provides. That is not the case with many on-campus students. Several tests, involving over 1,000 students[8] showed that they did not take advantage of the flexibility; instead, they accessed the online modules from their university's computer labs on weekdays when they attended courses, preferably during their lunch break. This might, in part, be explained by the still high costs for Internet access at home in 2001. Most of the on-campus students preferred traditional face-to-face teaching. Therefore, the study program of the Virtual University of Applied Sciences thus far does not compete with existing higher education, but rather supplements the range of teaching methods and courses available.

More than 80 per cent of the €21 million ($18.7 million) funding for the Virtual University is spent on personnel costs, mainly for additional staff to design courses and multimedia applications. Development of content and interactive educational software are extremely time-consuming. The positive aspect of the network is that not every institution has to fund and develop costly Web-based study-courses on its own. Consequently, even the medium-sized and small universities of the network will now also be able to offer attractive online study courses. However, the pilot phase will end in 2003; after that, the institutions involved have to secure the long-term maintenance of the online degree programs through their own basic funding.

The Virtual University intends to exploit commercially the developed content and educational software, including marketing them to end-user companies in German-speaking countries. Modules from the academic degree program will be repackaged for the specific demands of continuing education and vocational training, for which a for-profit subsidiary has been set up. However, it is not certain that this endeavor will be successful, particularly as cost-covering fees per course could amount to €12,000 ($11,000). The consortium lacks experience in the marketing of educational products and must identify and market to customers that are still only theoretical.

Conclusion

The flagship distance-education project described in this chapter highlights key questions about the general direction of Germany's higher education. The Virtual University of Applied Sciences will not provide all the answers, but a careful in-depth evaluation and analysis can provide many of them. The dichotomy of meeting labor market needs while not turning education into a commodity is at the heart of the issue. Another fundamental question is: Should public institutions of higher education offer courses for continuing education and, if so, should they offer them tuition-free or charge fees?

Whichever course emerges, the traditional pattern of academic activity in universities will definitely change profoundly through the uncoupling of teaching and content production, and the homogenization of learning content. However, across the board acceptance is unlikely, given the absence of a central government authority to order such changes, the inertia of traditional institutions, vested interests of faculty in the status quo, preferences of students and, finally, critical intellectuals. The kind of qualifications and skills labor markets need in the long run, given the growing importance of non-substantive, process-oriented skills (see Agre, Chapter Eleven) is also open to question. In this context, a blend between the ideals of Humboldt and labor market needs is a plausible outcome of the debate.

Notes

1 At the federal level, for instance, the law (*Hochschulrahmengesetz*) has been changed in order to give the states more leeway in modifying their own higher education laws, as well as to allow for more autonomy and economic activity by universities and to introduce Bachelors and Masters degrees. Previously, final examinations at universities were 'diplom', Magister Artium or teacher's certificate. Another major and very controversial change is a new federal law (*Dienstrechtsreform*) which will in future profoundly change the income of professors by tying performance and salary. It will also practically abolish the 'Habilitation', an in-depth post-doctoral qualification – mainly in humanities – for those who intend to pursue an academic career, which usually takes four to six years to complete.

2 The European Credit Transfer System, developed by the European Commission, operates by means of exchange of transcripts of records between home and host universities in different countries.

3 The winners were the Virtual University of Applied Sciences, Networked Chemistry Studies (www.vernetztes-studium.de) and VIRTUS, which stands for the development of publicly accessible web-based working environments for entire departments (www.virtus.uni-koeln.de). VIRTUS gets

additional funding from the Bertelsmann Foundation and the Heinz Nixdorf Foundation.

4   The official project Web sites are at www.vfh.de and www.oncampus.de. This description is based on a telephone interview with the project manager Professor Rolf Granow on 11 September 2001 and Granow (2000).

5   For a list of participating universities, see www.vfh.de.

6   This may be in part due to the fact that the University of the German Armed Forces at Hamburg (Universität der Bundeswehr), which is to conduct an evaluation study, has not yet published a report.

7   Historically, 'Engineering and Business Administration' was one of the first subjects to be taught in distance education.

8   The University of the German Armed Forces at Hamburg has conducted several studies on the initial trial projects with on-campus students. For a list of relevant publications describing the results, see their Web site www.unibw-hamburg.de/PWEB/paebbp/veroef/zimmer.html.

15 Virtual learning and the network society

Martin Harris

The complexity of the relationship between ICTs, knowledge and organizational structure is reflected in a diversity of values and rationalities embodied by learning institutions. This has resulted in a wide variety of vital organizational structures and technologies becoming associated with distance education and distributed learning. In this chapter, Harris compares the UK's two largest such initiatives – the Open University and University for Industry – as well as exploring developments in the USA. He uses this analysis to help identify four models of educational virtualization. The chapter is particularly useful in connecting the debate over new media in education to more general theory and research on the social shaping of technology.

The advent of new techno-organizational forms in higher education

Enthusiasm for new ICTs has generated much commentary about how the technologies could be used to create distance-education and distributed-learning environments, sometimes referred to as the 'virtual campus'. Many proponents of virtualization argue that ICTs and multimedia have the potential to transform the process of learning and the institutional space where learning occurs. Such use of digital technology in education parallels the changes in the management and organization of service delivery which has occurred in other public sector settings.[1]

Debate on the virtual campus has been heavily influenced by three highly distinctive intellectual perspectives. First, neo-liberal thinkers have welcomed the possibility of intensified competition between providers in education. A second, more recently established, body of comment is concerned with the threat to the traditions of the scholarly 'enquirer' within the academy. This perspective is characterized by discussions of 'academic capitalism', the 'postmodern university' and the 'end of knowledge'. Finally, a number of commentators – drawing on the work of neo-Schumpeterians such as Freeman (1990) – argue that ICTs and devolved organizational structures will combine to create entirely new techno-organizational forms. They expect these emerging forms to introduce a new and highly flexible paradigm based on knowledge and information networks. Manuel Castells (2000) has emerged in recent years as the most influential proponent of this view.

While stimulating much speculation, the debate on the virtual campus has been short on empirical investigation. There has also been little discussion of specific institutional or organizational choices. This gap in our knowledge is all the more remarkable when one considers how much of the research on the new technologies has been influenced by social-process and social-shaping perspectives (MacKenzie and Wajcman, 1985; Dutton, 1996).

The virtual campus debate: three intellectual perspectives

Neo-liberal commentators have argued that digital media and information networks will undermine the position of the academy as the *locus classicus* of knowledge production and dissemination (Hague, 1996, 1996a; Handy, 1995; Negroponte, 1995). For example, Gell and Cochrane (1996) point to the digitized galaxy of educational content available online, while arguing that universities are increasingly out of touch with the learning needs of society. Nicholas Negroponte (1995) depicts a world of deregulated markets populated by a myriad of educational service providers. Douglas Hague (1996a: 22) follows Negroponte's Hayekian logic, by arguing that people will increasingly use knowledge "where it is, and not where it can be institutionalized." This leads him to a particularly uncompromising stance on free markets in education that will mean the collapse of traditional structures of learning.[2]

David Noble (1998) is the leading radical critic of these perspectives, as he has argued that the virtual campus is a direct consequence of global competition and the consequent need for management to exert greater control over the production and dissemination of learning. For him, the advent of virtualized 'diploma mills' is synonymous with managerial control, the commodification of intellectual goods and the de-skilling of academic staff. Noble (ibid.) documents the struggles for control which have attended the virtualization of courses at the University of California at Los Angeles (UCLA) and at York University, Toronto. He also draws attention to the ways in which educational software platforms are being directed by industrial consortia made up of companies such as Kodak and IBM. Noble's analysis is in line with wider perspectives on globalization and the rise of the "entrepreneurial university" (Slaughter and Leslie, 1997; Smith and Webster, 1997).

Castells' (2000) account of the "network enterprise" resonates well with the new techno-organizational forms exemplified by the virtual campus. The network enterprise refers to the devolved structures which replace bureaucracy and to the more flexible organizational forms associated with ICT. The network enterprise is decentralized, loosely coupled, flexible, non-hierarchical and fluid, operating more on vertical and horizontal networking than 'command and control' principles. Castells relates the emergent new techno-economic paradigm to the concept of "informationalism" (ibid.: 215–16) – the process whereby information technologies and networks create a new medium of exchange, generating productivity rises and increase in the "circulatory sphere." He anticipates that the "vertical bureaucracy" is being transformed into the horizontal corporation, which he describes (ibid.: 178) as a "dynamic and strategically planned network of self programmed self directed units based on decentralization, participation and co-ordination."

Two significant examples of virtualized forms of educational organization

These three intellectual perspectives offer highly distinctive readings of the part played by ICTs in creating more devolved 'virtualized' organizational forms, such as the virtual campus. However, they share a certain abstract quality, and the debate on the virtualization of education has not thus far been grounded in the specific choices faced by institutions in moving towards new techno-economic forms. This will be the task of the following sections, which examine the organizational structures and online learning technologies adopted by the two major distance-learning initiatives in the UK: University for Industry (Ufi) and the Open University.

The University for Industry and learndirect network

The concept of 'a university for industry' was initially conceived by the British Labour Party in the early 1990s and the idea was shaped over the next decade by the active involvement of the educationalists, open learning specialists, the telecommunications industry, trades unions and employers. Labour also believed that the UK multimedia industry would be substantially 'pump primed' if national 'brand leaders' – such as the BBC, the British Council and the Open University – could establish themselves as leading players in the emergent world market for educational software and digitized learning. When it was elected in 1997, the Labour government developed and implemented Ufi as its flagship project for lifelong learning, beginning its early stages of implementation in late 1999.[3] In addition to Ufi, other government 'learning age' initiatives include a multimedia National Grid for Learning (NGfL), with a plan to link every school, college and library to it by 2002.

From its initial conception, Ufi has been aimed at creating a new kind of electronic public space drawing on private sector resources to provide both infrastructure and services. It has focused on offering access to learning facilities on an 'anyone, anytime, anyplace' basis, in order to help adults in four priority learning areas where there is seen to be large scale demand: basic skills; ICTs; small and medium sized businesses; and specific industrial sectors, such as retail, environmental technology and automotive components.

Ufi is co-ordinated through Ufi Ltd (www.ufi.com) and is based on a network of 'e-learning centers' – known as learndirect (www.learndirect.co.uk) – operated as 'Ufi hubs'. The centers are run by local authorities, companies, trade unions, universities, colleges and community development trusts. In late 2001, there were over 1,300 learndirect centers and about 187,000 learners at the centers, with a total of more than 410,000 course registrations. The long-term target is for 2.5 million users of the Ufi information service and approximately 600,000 people a year to pursue learning programmes. A study commissioned by the UK Department for Education and Skills (DfES, 2001), concluded that Ufi compared favorably with over thirty other equivalent providers around the world, particularly in terms of factors such as its commitment to both social and economic agendas, scale of operation and encouragement of universal access to learning opportunities.

The flexible learning promoted by Ufi depends crucially on organizational innovation, with ICTs and multimedia used in a supporting role. Ufi's key role is essentially a brokerage function: to maintain control over quality and to act as a conduit for online materials, educational programs and services to homes, workplaces and local learning centers. Individuals can access high quality materials, plan and record their learning and be assessed online in ways that are integrated with conventional learning modes.

Labour policy makers in the 1990s identified three possible roles for the state in stimulating the demand for educational content. The first of these, the traditional option of state intervention, required policy makers to predict the content and means of delivery for future learning, and to establish a new institution which would work with hardware and software suppliers. However, this dirigiste approach was rejected because it was viewed as likely to be costly and inflexible. The policy document which supported the launch of the Ufi (Hillman, 1996) argued that the objective is not to forecast, but to provide a framework for people to choose. Learning will be provided 'on demand', in response to the combinations of skills identified by learners themselves, at times and places convenient to them. The alternative, laissez-faire approach would be to treat education and training as goods like any other, allowing the market develop at its own pace. This report argues, further, that:

> The risk of the laissez-faire approach, is that provision remains piecemeal and haphazard, with development at a slower pace than in other countries. Moreover, groups of potential learners would continue to be excluded or hindered, particularly in the absence of substantial demand side subsidies.
>
> (Hillman, 1996: 32)

Labour's preferred option – less expensive than dirigiste, but more interventionist than laissez-faire – can be equated with the emergence of a 'third way' (Giddens, 1998) in providing electronic public goods within a policy environment where training, employment and industrial policy issues converge with questions of media regulation, ICT infrastructures and the establishment of 'knowledge utilities'. The structure of the Ufi training initiative has been informed by the commissioning model adopted in UK broadcast television by Channel 4, where a central body validates and contracts out the supply of content, leaving production to a myriad of small suppliers (Hillman, 1996). The adoption of this 'third way' involves government in 'market making', co-ordinating and accelerating the nascent market for multimedia and other learning technologies by franchising the supply of approved courseware and services.

The OU and technology-based learning

The OU combines a commitment to high-quality research and teaching with the pursuit of 'scalable growth' and open access for adults who do not hold conventional pre-entry qualifications (see Chapter Thirteen in this collection for more background). The OU is one of twelve distance-learning institutions enrolling over 100,000 students in degree-level courses which Daniel (1998) defines as "mega-universities."

The OU has become increasingly internationalized and commercialized, with many students – particularly in other EU member states, the former Soviet Bloc, Hong Kong and Singapore – taking OU courses outside the UK. This internationalization is combined with a commitment to the principle of individualized tutorial support in its overseas operations.

A former OU Vice-chancellor, Sir John Daniel (1998), has argued that the University should continue to prioritize the high-quality interaction between students and tutors over screen-based learning and the use of electronic assessment. The University is now selectively integrating the use of the Web into the organization and resourcing of teaching, while continuing to reserve judgment on precisely how these new technologies will be used. A number of courses are based on multimedia CD-ROMs, with trials showing that students can retrieve information with speed and flexibility. Self-assessment is also being selectively introduced. In addition, there are plans for multimedia expansion; the most successful large-scale application of new media appears to be computer conferencing.

Understandings drawn from comparing the Ufi and OU cases

The Ufi case provides an account of the formulation of policy and planning concerned with shaping the digital environment for learning in ways that would avoid the extremes of markets and state intervention. Ufi has been conceived and implemented as a genuinely 'virtual' form. It has no physical infrastructure or permanent faculty. The 'university' coinage is something of a misnomer, in that Ufi might be viewed more accurately as a learning utility, which uses information networks and 'networked' organizational forms to provide 'mass customized' access to vocational learning material and courses. The OU also uses a range of technologies to provide open access to education for large numbers of learners, but it combines this with a commitment to high-quality research, research-led teaching and permanent faculty staff. While the OU has decades of experience in operation, Ufi is as young as the twenty-first century, emerging from a complex policy milieu and debates that embraced previously separate spheres, such as industrial policy, media regulation and the reform of training.

The global market in distance learning is dominated by a number of the 'mega-universities' that recruit large numbers of students. This market is characterized by relatively low costs, economies of scale and by a substantial element of price competition. However, most commentators agree that learning institutions need to realize the economies of scale associated with low-cost mass provision while differentiating themselves on the basis of high-quality offerings made to specific student markets. This "productivity innovation dilemma" (Hayes, Clarke and Lorenz, 1985; Hill, Harris and Martin, 1997) is typically managed in ways that reflect particular institutional values, strategies and competencies.

The Ufi–OU comparison shows the ways in which separate approaches to the dilemma help to explain the different forms that virtual learning can assume. Ufi aims to maximize student numbers and deliver 'virtualized' learning material on a fully asynchronous basis, while the OU seeks to balance mass student markets and online learning with its commitment to one-to-one tutorial support and a strong research base.

Comparing these two approaches helps to identify two further possible routes to virtualization. One is that of conventional universities, which seek to differentiate themselves by building on their existing competencies. These institutions may consider adopting an intermediate position which takes some advantage of the economies of scale and flexibility offered by the new technology, while retaining conventional modes of learning. Another approach by some traditional institutions is to attempt to insulate themselves completely on the basis that superior 'branding' will guarantee survival in high-cost, highly-differentiated niche markets.

Ufi and the OU challenge some conventional assumptions of debate on the virtual campus. Neo-liberal commentators, such as Negroponte (1995) and Hague (1996, 1996a), celebrate the capacity for digital technology to provide low-cost, instantaneous access to information and knowledge. The favored imagery is of a myriad of small providers offering a galaxy of choice to online users. However, this picture of the digital learning environment is at odds with emerging developments in both the OU and Ufi. The effectiveness of both initiatives, largely dependent on their potential for 'scalable growth', has been realized by the UK government either through direct intervention (as with the OU) or, in the case of Ufi, through 'market making'. Moreover, the OU has evolved in ways that combine bureau professionalism with innovation in educational technologies and competition in world markets.

In contrast, radical commentators have been generally concerned about the effect of market values on universities and 'disinterested' scholarship. The labour historian Noble (1998) has argued that the virtual campus phenomenon is a direct consequence of global competition and the concomitant need for management to exert greater control over the production and dissemination of learning. This chapter acknowledges the cogency of this argument by highlighting the ways in which developments in the 'branding' and management of intellectual assets are deeply implicated in the structures and controls of multimedia corporations. However, the radical preoccupation with control underestimates the diversity of possible outcomes at the level of particular institutions.

Resolving the productivity-innovation dilemma

Distance-learning institutions such as Ufi and the OU are centrally concerned with large student numbers and with economies of scale. The International Center for Distance Learning (ICDL) estimated that the world's largest distance-learning institutions educated three million students in 1995 (ICDL, 1995). Daniel (1998) estimates that the annual cost per student across these 'mega-universities' averages less than $400 compared to over $10,000 in the UK and the USA. Daniel (ibid.) argues, further, that world-class players in the distance-learning field need to realize economies of scale associated with low-cost mass provision while differentiating themselves on the basis of high-quality offerings in specific student markets.

This type of 'productivity-innovation dilemma' has been observed in export-led manufacturing industries (Hayes, Clarke and Lorenz, 1985; Hill, Harris and Martin, 1997) and in knowledge intensive services (Quinn, 1992: 241–92). Universities engaged in distance learning are likely to resolve the dilemma in ways that reflect particular institutional values, strategies and competencies. Table 15.1 summarizes some of the main elements of the OU–Ufi comparison and shows that the need to balance mass provision with offerings aimed at specific learning constituencies may be resolved in ways that produce a number of separate approaches to virtualization.

As a provider of low-cost 'mass customized' vocational training material, Ufi has been designed to maximize student numbers through the remote delivery and assessment of teaching material. Ufi thus operates as a 'learning utility'. This can be contrasted with the more diverse range of teaching modes adopted by the OU, where the commitment to reaching large numbers of students is balanced with

Table 15.1 Resolving the productivity-innovation dilemma: four models of virtualization

Model	*Key characteristics*
Learning utility (Ufi)	'Virtualized' learning aimed at maximizing student numbers. Learning material delivered and assessed asynchronously. Fully virtualized service provision operating without faculty.
Networked bureaucracy (OU)	Commitment to scale balanced by one-to-one tutorial support. Innovative use of learning technologies combined with a strong research base and permanent faculty.
'Insular' model	Very small numbers taught without technology. High-cost/highly-differentiated market position.
'Interstitial' model	Investment in new learning technologies combined with conventional methods. Flexible access to courseware combined with low-risk approach to technology investment. Strategic 'hedging' produces diverse mix of distance and conventional teaching modes.

the need to maintain tutorial support. The OU is also committed to using ICTs to enhance "learning productivity" (Daniel, 1998), but it combines this with a strong academic ethos and commitment to research embodied in its academic staff. Although the OU continues to operate according to many norms and structures of a conventional university, it combines this with advanced learning technologies and strategic alliances. The OU can thus be seen as a 'networked bureaucracy'.

Table 15.1 identifies two further possible approaches to virtualization. A minority of institutions – particularly those teaching very small numbers of students – could conceivably operate in ways that circumvent questions of productivity and new learning technologies. Following this 'insular' path would presumably require a highly differentiated, high-cost position in the market. Many learning institutions are likely to adopt a more equivocal 'interstitial' stance, which combines selective investment in new media and/or information networks with traditional methods. These universities will typically seek to combine the economies of scale and flexibility offered by ICTs with a low-risk approach to investment in online learning. This strategic 'hedging' has also been observed in various industrial settings, for example, those observed by Sabel (1991); it produces a very diverse mix of options in combining traditional methods with remote access.

Assessing the neo-liberal and radical critiques

The neo-liberal view finds its clearest expression in the 'anti-bureaucratic turn' in economic management and in the rise of a 'service delivery' culture in public-sector organizations. These elements are clearly reflected in the flexibility and consumer choice offered by the 'virtual campus'. My investigation of Ufi, and the comparison with the OU, produces a number of difficulties for the neo-liberals.

The first, and most obvious, is that large-scale initiatives have been supported by government either in the form of direct intervention or, in the specific case of Ufi, by means of 'market making'. Secondly, the OU has evolved in ways which combine bureau professionalism with innovation in educational technologies and competition in world markets. This produces a third difficulty for the free marketeers. Learning institutions have creative organizational choices about how they assimilate virtual learning into their existing operations (Child, 1972, 1997). The question of organizational choice is explored below in the context of the radical perspective.

Radical commentators have been generally concerned about market values and their potentially corrosive effect on the university as the custodian of 'disinterested' scholarship. The virtual campus is seen by Noble (1998) as a direct consequence of global competition and the consequent need for management to exert greater control over the production and dissemination of learning. These aspects are congruent with the view that the 'virtual corporation' has emerged out of the very tangible need for organizations in a wide range of service settings – for example in banking, broadcasting, healthcare or education – to manage their core competencies more effectively in line with the need to "do more with less" (Harris, 1997). Noble

(1998) also takes more specific issue with the ways in which the rights to learning material may be controlled by private enterprise. This concern seems to be borne out by the ways in which a 'converged' and deregulated multimedia environment may provide universities with compelling reasons for emulating the strategic behavior of broadcasters or publishers. Some players have reacted to these pressures by collaborating with third party partners who act as service providers under license to disseminate 'branded' courseware.

This scenario is being played out by world-class universities, such as the London School of Economics and Columbia University who have joined with Cardean in making mutual online offerings. Universities in Canada and the USA have established strategic consortia comprised of collaborating institutions and electronic publishers. UK policy makers have recognized for some time that the supply and distribution of electronic courseware will best be served by self-governing consortia made up of learning institutions, commercial publishers and broadcasters (DfEE, 1998). These private/public sector groupings are likely to include leading players from the 'edu-tainment' sectors of the multimedia industries. The emphasis on strategic alliances and complementary intellectual assets is redolent of the work of Quinn (1992) who has researched the moves towards disaggregated forms in organizations whose core business is knowledge- intensive services. [4]

Content providers who wish to recoup the development costs of multimedia offerings seek to develop export potential and access to wider markets. They are also using the core characteristics of the new media to create online payment mechanisms, marketing tools and distribution chains. Branding across previously separate markets and genres helps to secure market presence and consumer recognition. The above developments underscore the broad relevance of the radical perspective, and they offer some support for Noble's arguments about commodification and control.

The main weakness of Noble's critique is its tendency to underestimate the diversity of possible outcomes at the level of particular institutions. Twenty years of empirical research on ICT-related organizational change suggests that outcomes are driven not by a single logic of digitalization nor even by the control strategies of management, but by specific institutional histories, social choices and the active involvement of agents on the ground (Dutton, 1996a; McLoughlin and Harris, 1997). The strategic choices facing those universities who occupy an interstitial position are particularly complex.

Castells' network enterprise thesis

Castells is the latest in a long line of thinkers who believe that society is undergoing a shift to a new techno-economic paradigm (Castells, 2000: 178). Castells argues that all forms of production and exchange are becoming subject to the increasingly pervasive use of information technologies and 'networked' organizational forms. These forms are associated particularly with knowledge intensive services: the network form functions in ways that allows it "to generate knowledge and to process information efficiently" (Castells, 2000: 188). The shift to the networked form will be based on 'informationalism' – the process whereby information technologies and networks create a new medium of exchange, generating productivity rises and an increase in the "circulatory sphere." Each of these aspects resonates strongly with current developments in the virtualization of education. The question of information networks and the imputed link with radically new structures can be clarified by distinguishing 'strategic' networking – for example long-term collaboration between partner organizations – from the networking of operations allowed by ICT. The analysis which follows has been carried out with this distinction in mind.

The OU is strategically networked to other institutions and businesses, such as the BBC, whose markets and assets are complementary. Operationally, it has made considerable advances in the use of electronic conferencing and is gradually assimilating e-mail into student–tutor interactions. Ufi has been designed in ways that will make it, strategically and operationally, the more dispersed organization of the two. The 'networked' character of the new institution is reflected, at the operations level, in the ambitious scale of its 'anyone, anyplace, anytime' delivery of learning material – but the networked form is also apparent, at the strategic level, in the radically devolved institutional structure that separates the production of content from its commissioning.

The disaggregated organizational form offers a direct correspondence with Castells' depiction of network enterprise and the logic of informationalism, expressed in the view that ICTs are expected to form the basis for all transactions, the production of content will be outsourced where possible, and mass customization creates the economies of scale and expansion of demand. For its part, the OU has evolved a highly distinctive, radically decentralized approach to teaching over the last thirty years. A central feature is that educational technologies and course organization are combined in ways that support one-to-one tutoring. Senior decision makers are, however, equally concerned with learning productivity, cost effectiveness, market share and the tradeability of intellectual assets (Daniel, 1998). Various new media and e-mail are being used to augment the older educational technologies (TV broadcast, audio and print) in ways which promote asynchronous learning. Daniel (1998) records that the OU earmarked substantial funds for investment in logistical support systems and business process re-engineering in 1999. This suggests that the OU is also following the logic of information processing, combining enhanced service delivery with further 'scalable growth' in student numbers.

However, these operational concerns cannot be equated with either the core knowledge or the strategic use of networks. The OU case shows that some of the more utilitarian aspects of distance learning may be compatible with the bureau professionalism found in conventional universities. The OU maintains a substantial knowledge base embodied in its courses, a permanent faculty of over 800 full-time staff, and research programs. Nevertheless, it has diversified and taken on elements of the 'networked' form at the structural level by establishing commercial subsidiaries, joint ventures and strategic alliances with other players whose intellectual assets complement or extend its own offerings in world markets. This corroborates the insights developed by Castells' "networked enterprise," but the OU is best seen as a 'networked bureaucracy' that is committed by charter to open learning and to the inculcation of academic modes of inquiry. Ufi, in contrast, is a learning utility operating as a broker of high-quality learning materials. Here, the core expertise is not the production of knowledge, but the *service competencies* which allow the new institution to relate the learning needs of employers and individuals to a diverse array of courses and learning packages.

Organizational theory helps to illuminate some of the political controversy which has surrounded Ufi, where the networked form is used to control quality and co-ordinate the supply of learning material in order to try to overcome the problem of market failure. However, the Ufi case shows that the network solution may entail a number of inherent disadvantages which highlight the possibility of network failure. One major source of criticism is that the initiative lacks institutional coherence and that the public will be confused by the labyrinth of access points, structures, providers and learning modes.

Ufi has also been criticized on the basis that (Harris and Corrigan, 1996): the costs of training are passed on from the state and employers to consumers; moves to learning 'on demand' may not provide a sufficiently focused and directed national solution to the problem of skills shortages; and remote and asynchronous learning needs to be complemented by direct contact with tutors. The Labour government has avoided any suggestion that employers will be compelled to subsidize training through levies.

The preferred way forward, indicating the scale of the government's commitment to Ufi, is to establish an 'individual learning account' for every adult learner in the UK, probably eventually based on smartcards. Learning accounts may be supplemented by contributions from trainees and – in principle – also from responsible employers. The ambiguous attitude of many employers has become one of the pivotal issues in the progress of the initiative. Organization theory suggests that there is an inherent tendency for the advantages of the networked solution – flexibility and low cost – to be won at the expense of accountability and control.

With respect to the network enterprise thesis, the OU and Ufi comparisons suggest that the relationship between information networks, knowledge base and organizational structure are more complex and variable than is assumed by the network metaphor, or by the idea that a single defining technology forms the leading edge for the 'paradigm shift' from one industrial era to another. Information networks may provide learning institutions with new infrastructures, and these may even be regarded as universal in their application across various settings. However, the OU and Ufi are defined by quite distinct 'networked' institutional structures. The knowledge base of the OU has been institutionalized according to the cultural and structural norms associated with academia and university bureaucracies – the 'networked' elements in its structure relate more to diversification and strategic alliances than it does to ICT.

The detailed OU–Ufi comparison, and the four-part typology featured in Table 15.1, suggest that we can expect a wide variety of forms to emerge. This diversity can be squared with the network enterprise thesis, in that radically different social objectives and agencies may make use of the network form. But the evidence suggests that there are good reasons for regarding the use of information networks for information processing as quite separate from the 'strategic' networked structures. Networks are compatible with – and may be used to complement – market-based and bureaucratic modes of organizing production. Networks and markets may both be *conditioned* by bureaucracy. However, networks do not, as is suggested by the 'paradigm shift' perspective, exist in a relation of binary opposition to markets or hierarchies.

The above analysis suggests that one might question Castells' (2000: 188) view that the purpose of networks is "to generate knowledge and to process information efficiently." Collaboration with strategic partners may certainly be seen as a way of sharing knowledge, which can be justified mainly as a matter of realizing economies of scale and/or scope. Yet, as I have sought to show in this chapter, the primary function of these alliances is to extend the operations of learning institutions in ways which reduce market uncertainties. A number of studies suggest that the key issue in network formation is not simply the diffusion of knowledge through the network, but how this knowledge is framed and institutionalized in accordance with the surrounding uncertainties (see, for example, Fransman, 1990; Howells and Hine, 1993). From this viewpoint, Castells' account of the network enterprise may have underestimated the complexity of the relationships which link technology, institutionalized knowledge and organizational structure.

Strategies to balance productivity and innovation requirements in higher education

Analysis of the OU and Ufi shows that the core elements of the virtual campus are 'scalable' growth and the use of technologies that offer the possibility of asynchronous delivery of teaching. Universities are currently concerned with balancing creative choice and innovation with automation and mass provision. This is redolent of the productivity-innovation dilemmas and the strategic 'hedging' observed in other settings (Hayes, Clarke and Lorenz, 1985; Sabel, 1991; Quinn, 1992; Hill, Harris and Martin, 1997).

However, this study suggests that learning institutions have considerable room for maneuver in balancing these two elements, and that there is a particular value in less than maximum scale in the interests of maintaining tutorial relationships. For example, the analysis reveals four main approaches to virtualization, reflected in the 'learning utility', 'networked bureaucracy', 'interstitial' and traditional or 'insular' positions (Table 15.1). Many universities will opt for a mixture of different elements, such that we can expect a wide diversity of variants across the typology. Learning institutions have a wide degree of choice about how technology should be assimilated into conventional teaching.

These conclusions can be contrasted with both neo-liberal and radical commentaries, which tend to assume a single logic of virtualization that is analytically blind to the ways in which the virtual campus is being defined by an extremely diverse spectrum of rationalities, social choices and organizational priorities. Noble's (1998) concern with questions of ownership and control are corroborated by the current moves towards learning consortia, many of whom operate on a multinational basis. Homogenization of learning content is a risk in these developments. The virtualization of learning can to very large extent be seen as a revolution in service delivery. The new media are characterized, on one hand, by their inherent plasticity and potential for experimentation; at the same time, they are also being used to create a new symbolic environment which appears to be inherently suited to commodification. This is reflected in the use of these media to create online payment mechanisms and marketing tools.

Similarly, these two cases suggest that there may be a need to modify Castells' network enterprise theory, which is centrally concerned with the disaggregation of production, the ubiquity of information networks and productivity in services. While Castells anticipates a number of key developments associated with the virtual campus, his account underestimates the diversity and reflexive choice associated with network formation. Castells' account of the digital revolution has been very substantially articulated around a belief in a historically decisive paradigm shift away from bureaucracy towards entirely new networked techno-economic forms. The evidence presented in this chapter suggests that this oversimplifies the relationship between technology, knowledge and organizational structure. The strategic networks which are being adopted by both the OU and various learning consortia should be seen as a complement to, and not a rejection of, the bureaucratic form. And the radically devolved structures associated with the virtual campus need to be understood not simply as conduits for the transmission of knowledge, but as dynamic responses to the pervasive uncertainties of the new environment.

Notes

1   Dutton (1996) identifies electronic networks with five categories of service delivery applicable to both education and local/central government services: dissemination of information to the public; online access to public documents and records; transaction processing; asynchronous communications through public forums (e.g. bulletin boards and e-mail); and synchronous communications (e.g. teleconferencing).

2   Hague (1996, 1996a) offers a Hayekian attack on the British university system, by putting the case for knowledge entrepreneurs and the virtual campus. For a counter-attack, see Harris and Howells (1996).

3　The Learning and Skills Act 2000 (DfEE 2000) was derived from earlier official proposals (DfEE 1998, 1999) and these, in turn, were based on policy discussion and consultations which ran more or less continuously from 1993 until Labour formed the government in 1997.

4　Quinn (1992: 283–92) records that, when they saw that basic entertainment hardware was moving towards commodity status, Sony and Matsushita used vertical integration to appropriate expertise in major 'software' (film and distribution) companies relevant to their equipment.

16 The informational view of the university

Neil Pollock

This chapter explores a different kind of 'virtuality' tied to ICTs than that understood in the context of distance education and distributed learning. Through an empirical analysis of the introduction of an enterprise-wide information system at a large British University, Pollock explores how the rolling-out of a rather mundane administrative support system turned into a large, complex and almost mythical model of a 'virtual university' based on 'information' as a new resource and forged by the project's mantra of the 'provision of timely and accurate information'. He explores the tension and conflicting perceptions between the older 'chaotic' and 'irrational' view of a university and the supposedly more ordered 'virtual' informational model, and explains how this new model translates all issues into rationalized information issues against which the 'real' university can be criticized.

Introducing a new informational model of a university

It has become something of a commonplace to say that new ICTs are transforming higher education. To date, much of this discussion has interpreted such change as something being added, as in the introduction of new actors, new forms of learning provision, new technologies and so on. However, while these technologies are – in an obvious sense – about the introduction of something new, they are also about the redefinition of many existing actors, activities and processes within universities. The example being used here is 'information':

> Currently most UK universities and colleges of higher education
> ... are re-evaluating the way they gather, process and disseminate
> information for teaching, research and administration, for many
> this will mean radical change.
>
> (Allen and Wilson, 1996: 239)

Information has always been attributed a crucial role within institutions; however, it constitutes one of the aspects that – through a process of redefinition – has now come to take on an importance out of all proportion to the past (cf. Agre, 2000). There are, for instance, increasing pressures for institutions to think of themselves as 'modern organizations' (cf. Lockwood, 1985; Barnett, 2000). Key in the emergence of this organizational view of universities is a demand for clearer roles, relationships and responsibilities, as well as more efficient work practices. Underpinning many of these changes are new forms of large-scale institutional computer systems and, of course, information. Indeed, a high-level report by the Joint Information Systems Committee (JISC), the body responsible for university computing in the UK, stated that information systems and, particularly, information have become the lifeblood of higher education institutions (JISC, 1995). As a resource on a par with labour, the JISC report commented, information should be considered as part of the infrastructure of universities. So central is information that JISC argue for the conflation of the role of information with the very 'vision' of the university.

In an attempt to analyze critically the information issue, this chapter reflects on an information system project being carried out at a university in the UK,[1]which I refer to as 'Big-Civic University'. Narrowly defined, this project is concerned with the implementation of an Enterprise Resource Planning (ERP) System, typical of those widely used by large corporations around the world. Recently, many universities in the UK and elsewhere have also turned to ERP as a means of replacing existing management and administration computer systems (Pollock and Cornford, 2001).[2] I will call this system 'Enterprise'. It includes a number of modules dealing with particular functions or aspects of the University, such as finance, human resources, project management and, eventually, student records. Enterprise replaces a number of software technologies grouped around the University's existing Management & Administrative Computing (MAC) system. The project involves a wide range of actors, including the University's management and central administration, the software vendor itself and third-party consultants. At the heart of Enterprise is a very large and complex relational database that will eventually contain and, importantly, integrate information on the status of staff, students, buildings, equipment, documents, and financial transactions (cf. Davenport, 1998).

Particularly relevant to this chapter is the way in which the Enterprise Project Team has come to conceptualize its task or mission, and to represent that mission both to itself and the rest of the University. At one level, Enterprise is solely concerned with the provision of timely and accurate information throughout the University. Whilst it might be argued that this aim is hardly surprising – the provision of information is, after all, the central purpose of information systems – at another level there are further, more interesting, even sublime, aspects to the Enterprise project. In point of fact, such is the nature of the mission being built around Enterprise that some have come to think of the system as a kind of 'virtual university'.

It is seen as 'virtual' for two reasons. First, within the system there is a large and complex model that has the form of a university, but without the thing itself. Instead of the heterogeneity of an organization full of competing goals and interests, in the Enterprise model every issue seemingly equates to an informational issue (cf. Pollock and Cornford, 2000). For some within the Project Team, the informational model embodied within the system comes to represent the actual University. Second, at a more analytical level, the 'virtual' notion captures the idea of different models or worlds that co-exist in a relation/tension, or that one 'abstract' model can affect power through describing how that world 'ought to be' (Carrier and Miller, 1998). It is because of the introduction of the new model, in other words, that the old is seen as problematic. The interesting theoretical move, therefore, is in tracing the implementation of Enterprise as it begins to contribute to a shift from an old to a new model of the University. Indeed, it is through the very construction of Enterprise that a difference between the old and the new is achieved: the implementation of the system is simultaneously the construction of the new model and the destruction of the old.

The material for this chapter was gathered during a participant observation carried out over a two-year period. As well as sitting in on meetings, presentations and talking to members of the project team and users of the system, I collected and analysed various documents concerning the Enterprise project. A number of focus groups were also conducted with the users of Enterprise.

Insights from Actor Network Theory

The argument I shall put forward is that Enterprise is able to replace MAC successfully because various actors around the University began to accept the problematization as set out by the Project Director (particularly the notion that there is now within the University a new requirement for information). Importantly, I want to show how this is part of a larger discursive reorientation of the university as an 'information institution', where actors involved come to accept the inevitability of the model being offered (the informational model). To demonstrate the process by which everyone begins to speak – and think – in terms of 'information', I will be drawing on insights from a strand of thought that has emerged out of the sociology of science and technology known as Actor Network Theory (ANT).

According to ANT, to understand just how a technology becomes (or fails to become) a success we must follow and observe various innovators as they attempt to enroll others into their 'networks'. Such enrollments are typically based on one actor raising problems about the identity of another. Callon (1986a), for instance, discusses how environmentalists in the 1970s began to problematize assumptions held by a major car producer that consumers, increasingly motivated by environmental concerns, would still want to drive petrol-engine vehicles. They achieved this by outlining a scenario where new forms of battery-powered cars would be the only acceptable means of transport. In *Science in Action*, Latour (1987) characterizes successful innovation as what happens where one actor accepts and takes up the problem put forward by an innovator. In other words, the targeted actors have their goals and interests 'translated' to fit those of the emerging network. According to Callon then, the car producers shifted their interest from their current technology to those that were already being investigated by the environmentalists. For ANT, a technology – such as the battery-powered car – becomes a success when a sufficient network has been built for it, based on those who are willing to support it. Indeed, as Rudinow Saetnan (1991) points out, without such networks a technology is said to only 'partially exist'.[3]

The utility of the ANT approach is twofold. First, it assists with 'redefinition': the process by which certain seemingly stable actors and entities are problematized and begin to take on new roles and identities. Second, it allows us to move beyond overarching general notions, such as technological determinism, to explain the way universities are changing. Rather, as is the purpose of this chapter, it helps to show some of the intricate ongoing work that makes it possible for one actor to convince others of the need for the university to change – and to modify its mode of working. Indeed, the mechanism by which one model of the university comes to dominate or replace another is related to the very practical work of loosening some associations (i.e., rendering ineffective or problematizing an existing network) and the simultaneous introduction and production of others. This shows how the construction of one new network is simultaneously the destruction of the old.

One of the key sources I draw on in my analysis is 'Information Mythology', an article by the historian of technology Geoffrey Bowker (1994). In describing the early geology of some of the unexplored areas of Venezuela, he reveals the intricate socio-technical processes whereby scientists are able to turn local, unstructured knowledge about soil into "global scientific information," which could then be read back in the labs of the Schlumberger Corporation. His argument is that the process whereby everything can be constructed according to the properties of information is not "a preordained fact about the world" but "it becomes a fact as and when we make it so".[4] This is the method by which certain actors come to accept the 'need for information' – or, indeed, the process by which a 'space for information' is constructed (cf. Porter, 1994). In this chapter, I explore how such a process works in relation to the Enterprise system.

The reasons given for replacing the previous system

Big-Civic had been using a system developed through the University Funding Council's MAC initiative. This had been implemented in the early 1990s as a large-scale attempt to put in place, in a number of different institutions, a computer system capable of handling both the needs of universities and the production of standardized information that could be used to report to the UK government, which is the main funding body (Goddard and Gayward, 1994). In 1995, the University engaged the services of a well-known firm of management consultants to carry out a technical review of the state of the MAC system. This produced a document which, in common with the standard mode of consultancy reporting (cf. Bloomfield and Vurdubakis, 1994), combines technical detail with a 'context'. For instance, before mentioning MAC's limitations, the preamble talks about the increases in student numbers, the advent of auditing, extreme competition for research funding, and so on. The document details how all of this is leading to demands for efficiency gains, and that the role of the computer system is no longer solely the presenting and accounting of the University to funding bodies. There is a now a direct pressure to spend more effort on management and administration, and to provide more data and information on relative performance.

The importance of all this lies in the fact – and this is before reaching any of the technical detail concerning MAC's limitations – that the document can be read as an effort to signal that the University is working in a changing terrain, and that it should reconfigure itself – and its systems – in relation to this. The extent to which the notion of a 'changing terrain' was accepted as sufficient reason to replace MAC with a new system is made evident in the following extract. Here we are listening to the Project Director during an away-day meeting providing the history of Enterprise to the Project Team:

> I'd like to say a few words about where we've come from ... [T]he World was changing, but I think the view [here] was – well, we hoped it would go away and it wouldn't change. Historically through the eighties, we under-invested in management information systems. Then MAC came along and it was seen as a panacea. It turned out not to be the magic bullet that many people had hoped, partly because the whole context in which MAC had been conceived was in the old model of higher education. The main funder was the government, and it was a 'command and control' system of reporting to government. Culturally and, also, probably technologically, it was an old model of the higher education system. And when we started moving into this new requirement for much more flexible information, MAC just didn't come up to scratch.

Interestingly, the Project Director is depicting a scenario in which there is an effortless shift from "the World" and its external pressures, to the University, the model of the higher education system and, finally, to the MAC computer system itself – and a requirement for "more flexible information." To be precise, the picture he is painting here is actually not one of a seamless shift, but a series of disjunctures. The University is out of step with the external situation (the rest of the World): the assumptions embodied within MAC are based on an "old model" of the higher education system – a model that is no longer appropriate for today's climate. All this has been highlighted since the University moved to this new need for flexible information. The response is apparently a straightforward one: bring all these factors into line through changing the system.

The interesting issue here is how the story that all of this can be provided for through the implementation of a simple management information system seems to make – at least in the institution where it was voiced – perfect sense.

The mantra shaping the move from MAC to Enterprise

The management consultant's technical review document produced in 1995 was so wide-ranging in its criticisms of the MAC system that it was generally accepted by all as the definitive nail in MAC's coffin. The document's lengthy listing of MAC's technical and other limitations included failings such as that: it appears "old-fashioned;" is slow; lacks "system bridges" between the center and the faculties; and does not compare well to commercial software with which people are already familiar. However, it was not until at least a year later that the 'real' reason why MAC was to be replaced eventually emerged. A senior member of the Project Team describes in a newsletter how:

> [Enterprise] software was chosen because it best suits our needs. It is flexible, easy-to-use and will provide *timely, accurate and accessible information* ... MAC does not give us what we need to run efficient administrative and information systems ... [j]ust one example is that it does not provide financial reports online to give people responsible for controlling budgets a real-time picture of their expenditure, instead they have to rely on paper reports, which are inevitably out of date. The difficulties this presents are well and widely understood. The advent of [financial devolution from the center to departments] makes access to *accurate, timely information* even more important (*my emphasis*).

This was confirmed in the same newsletter by an end-user seconded into the Project Team:

> My job is made more difficult by the fact that we have two systems in the department, each carrying account information that does not match ... One of our big problems is not knowing our exact financial position. For example, there are always accounts which have been paid but have not yet shown up in the budget. Obviously this hinders planning ... [the new system] will give us the opportunity to improve the way we manage our money and our people – and from what I have seen it looks very promising. For me, the biggest single advantage of [Enterprise] is its ability to provide *timely and accurate financial information* on research projects. I believe it offers significant improvements (*my emphasis*).

The recurring theme coming from these two accounts is that simply listing MAC's limitations is insufficient to explain why the system is to be replaced. It is seemingly not enough to say that the system "does not provide financial reports online," or that it cannot "give people responsible for controlling budgets a real-time picture of their expenditure." Nor is it adequate just to say that while using MAC nobody knows his or her "exact financial position," or that account information "does not match." One way of addressing this is to say that such limitations are not convincing enough; in terms of enrolling others, they offer what Latour (1988) calls little "explanatory power." In other words, in order to understand the outcome of all of this it is necessary to consider the relational context in, and through which, the story moves (cf. Woolgar and Cooper, 1999).[5] Conceptually, this means that just what is to count as a sufficient explanation can only be understood as a result of 'usage': the way explanations of the reasons for change are accepted and taken-up by others. So, just how do others use this story?

Whenever we are presented with MAC and its limitations, the story is always centered on the aims of the new project; these appear to manifest themselves in one single phrase, script or mantra that is repeated over and over again. The 'provision of timely and accurate information' mantra continuously appears as the rationale, mission and justification for the project – in internal project documents, consultancy reports, communications from the team to the rest of the university and in team discussions. Ever-present, at every meeting and in every document, this phrase has become, as it were, a member of the team, an actor.

What is more, the phrase is widely used within the team's strategy for communicating with the rest of the university, when discussing the move from MAC to Enterprise. Through its repeated usage, this very phrase has come to stand for the reason for the replacement of MAC. For instance, to repeat the words from above: "The advent of [financial devolution from the center to departments] makes access to accurate, timely information even more important." Similarly, "the biggest single advantage of [Enterprise] is its ability to provide timely and accurate financial information on research projects." The important question that needs to be asked here is: How is it that the aims of the Enterprise project were taken-up so straightforwardly?

How the Project Team used its mantra to drive Enterprise

There is little doubt within the Project Team as to just what Enterprise is about. In internal meetings, for instance, when discussions concern the goals of the project, or when questions come up about just 'what' they are trying to achieve, we invariably hear the repetition of the mantra. In one meeting, a senior administrator involved in the project was asked what she expected her department would gain from the implementation; she replied that Enterprise would provide her staff with "information which is timely and accurate." Another senior administrator articulated how such things as the "production of the annual accounts and the [Higher Education Spending Authority] returns [should] hopefully become easier because [Enterprise] should facilitate better information and more timely." This would help those out in faculties or departments who "will get more timely information looking at their own accounts and plans against actuals."

Enterprise is conceptualized according to a set of priorities that are 'known' and seemingly 'understood' by everyone within the team. Here, in contrast to the less convincing limitations belonging to MAC, the power of explanation of the mantra is strong. It holds in place the relationship between MAC and Enterprise as well as, arguably, the University, the model of higher education and their relationship to 'the World'. Indeed, such was the mode of use of this particular mantra that it was sometimes able to absent itself partially: the acceptance of the goals of the project were such that, at times, there was often little need to articulate the full vision, for instance by just stating that the project is concerned with the "... provision of all this timely and accurate etcetera, etcetera ...".[6] In terms of ANT, this could be described as a 'successful translation' because everyone is saying the same thing about the Enterprise system, and everyone has accepted the problematization of the MAC system, i.e., that it does not provide the right kind of information. It must be asked: why could the informational mantra work so well?

My suggestion is that the phrase operates well because of the very 'resonance of information' within the University, in that it appeals equally to what Bowker (1994) terms the "mundane" and the "mythical." In using these terms, Bowker is pointing to the way in which some information-society theorists have attempted to redefine all human history as the history of information processing. This view redefines in terms of information processing the most prosaic bureaucratic processes, the nature of society and, in some cases, the very meaning of life (i.e., living systems as information processors). Analogously, I want to suggest that there is a discussion within Big-Civic University that characterizes Enterprise as both a simple information system and as the University itself. To exemplify what this means, we can return to the Project Director. Here, at the same away-day meeting, he is reading from a document containing a number of bullet points:

> I would like to spend a few minutes on the missions of the project ... the first point: 'To provide consistent and timely information'. So this really is an information project. It is about information to run the business ... Just going on to the various subheadings there so: 'Support the day to day'. The word day-to-day is an important word there. This is an information system that which is also concerned with routine activities. There is still the basic 'running the business', which needs to be informed by, supported by, information systems.

Here, the Project Director is talking about the administrative processes you might associate with any large organization. He continued, emphasizing that information is concerned not only with the day-to-day running of the business:

> The second bunch of points is about the structure of the organization: 'bind together a decentralized organization'. Well this is the whole idea that the whole is more than the sum of its parts, that the University is not just a sheltered workshop where academics pursue their particular interests. It clearly has to be a supportive environment where people can do their own thing because if you really turn off those people then you are dead in the water. But, increasingly we're in a situation where we've both got to be entrepreneurial, but ... good management is essential such that we do have processes which bind these entrepreneurial people into something which is the University of [Big-Civic]. And it's really a very important point where people have to have some sense of identity with the institution as a whole and some engagement, and agree to operate on the basis and principles that are there.

Here, we are witnessing the taking apart of one 'physical' model (the centralized administration) and the construction of another seemingly 'virtual' model. Once the project is implemented, much of the administrative activities currently carried out centrally will be 'devolved' to departments; central administration is apparently not conducive to the entrepreneurial activity that is required. However, the worry is that once the administrative center disappears, the University becomes nothing more than a "sheltered workshop" for academics who are there only to purse their own particular interests. Hence, the need for a "supportive environment" – a "something" – to "bind these entrepreneurial people" into this entity called the University. But what is this something? Seemingly, it is informational processes. Academics are increasingly doing "their own thing", the physical institution being for them nothing more than a constraint. Here, the University is (re)made according to the needs of these actors. Thus, we have a definition of Enterprise as both a mundane system that processes information, and the basis for a new model (mythology?) of the university, a 'place' – or, rather, a set of processes – with which certain people can identify. The resonance of information is thus this causal link from the banal to the sublime (cf. Bowker, 1994).

A second move leads from this. Not only is it a case of these "entrepreneurial people" identifying with a university composed of informational processes: the actors themselves – and their relation to each other – are similarly constructed in terms of information. Indeed, according to the JISC report mentioned above, universities can be thought of as completely composed of 'Information Groups' (i.e., students, buildings, projects), 'information items' (i.e., teaching materials for a course) and 'information standards' (i.e., the attributes of Groups and Items).[7] What is more, these are also all 'performative' roles.

According to an internal document: "Almost all organizational units, Faculties and Departments as well as central administration, will be collectors and generators, providers as well as customers of data and information." This means that actors are conceptualized not in traditional terms (i.e., according to hierarchies) but according to their new 'de-layered' duties towards information. This signifies that actors across the university (whatever their existing allegiances) can – in principle – align with everyone else according to the 'nature' of information. In other words (picking up on what was being suggested by the Project Director), these new informational roles are 'integrative': they act to "... bind together a decentralized organization." What this is suggesting is that the hierarchy and nature of engagement of actors in this network are reconfigured; information has become the unifying principle in the University, the basis around which all actors are ordered.

The transition from an old to a new model of the University

Once established within the realm of the Project Team, the real work of implementing Enterprise began. This entails extending the mantra out into the University, which requires a stronger explanation to help the Project Team connect its mission with a straightforward outcome. The assumption is that the Enterprise system will enable the University, with all its problems, to move unproblematically towards the new model.

In terms of capturing how actors construct the existing model, the following conversation is illuminating. It is a conversation between the Project Director and the Projector Manager (again taken from the away-day meeting). The Project Manager begins:

> Here people are very, very parochial, and if we are deciding whether we should be putting in an extra bit of a finance system as opposed to an extra of a student system, [the Finance Director] is going to vote for a finance thing and the student guys are going to vote for the student bit

The Project Director follows up by agreeing, stating how he accepts: "absolutely the part about being parochial, I think that's the way it has been but in a way we've got to get away from this us and them model."

The Project Manager replies: "The problem I found when I was on the [University's Information Technology] Committee was that you had a whole raft of people who had their own vested interests, and actually chaos was the one word I would hate to mention."

According to the Project Director, in place of this parochialism, vested interests and chaos, Enterprise will: "[g]uide the internal decision making at all levels." By this, he means that the University will "move into a situation where people make decisions on the basis of information rather than prejudice, hunch, rumor [and] all those other things by which we currently run the business." From an analytical point of view, the key in all of this is the attempt to construct the University through the image of chaos. Information – it seems – will permeate "all" aspects of the University, rendering decision making increasingly more visible and therefore subject to some form of internal bench-marking. This increased visibility is expected to displace, or translate, the chaotic and parochial university, the assumption being that through the increased provision of information some form of 'order' will rise from the chaos.

It is clear that all of this needs substantial unpacking.[8] Berg and Timmermans (1997) argue that disorder, for instance, does not precede order, but is constituted alongside order as a "necessary and un-erasable parasite." The argument is one of the co-construction of problem and solution, meaning that the process is not the bringing forth of an established problem but the act of producing the problem with an eye to its eradication. In other words, through imposing the model onto the actual university, the order/disorder distinction is made possible. Within a university where information is seemingly freely and widely available, a "whole raft of people" are readily seen as operating according to "vested interests." The model, by its very presence, makes the University appear disordered or, in other words, every order by necessity embodies its own disorder (cf. Berg and Timmermans, 1997). It follows that to be wrong in this university, that is to be considered parochial, or chaotic, or self-serving, and so on, is to take decisions that are not based on information – and, more importantly, not based on information made visible according to the Enterprise system.

Living in the space and time of the Virtual University

Reconfiguring the University

If we were to take at face value the notion that the introduction of information will begin to permeate every aspect of the work done, then a question that might arise would be this: how might the new network space – where information is everything – begin to reconfigure this University? In order to benefit from all this timely and accurate information certain forms of compliance would be demanded (Wildavsky 1983). One example concerned with administration is the processing of paperwork. In a new way of working – which entails that information is always timely – forms cannot be left to pile up on desks until the end of the week or month, to be dealt with at a later convenient time; instead, all data must be entered when and where it is produced.

An example of what is meant by this can be seen in the attempt to automate the student admissions systems. According to the Student System Manager, the system: "will provide a workflow functionality so that we can get applications [for postgraduate study] in, we can scan them, we can send them around departments, selectors, selections teams, whatever. A decision can be put on which can be automatically coded." Therefore, under the new system, applications: "should be acknowledged automatically and at the same time applicants should be advised of response times for the notification of decisions." This is in contrast to the MAC system, where:

> ... there is no clear process. Every department does things differently. There are long delays. There is the old argument 'do we lose postgraduate students because we don't turn decisions quickly

enough and this kind of thing?' So you put a system in like this, provided you could monitor and control it, is one of the benefits that you turn around decisions more quickly. Do we actually increase our recruitment?

According to this, the old model is without a clear process, and this leads to 'long delays'. If we were to turn around decisions in a real-time fashion, apparently we might actually increase recruitment. More conceptually, here, we are being presented with two images: the 'slow to react' student process versus a real-time system. What we are seeing here is the creation of a difference between the processes carried out under MAC and those that will be in place with the new system: this is achieved by explaining the former according to what might be said to have caused it (delays, every department doing thing differently, etc.), and the latter in terms of what might be thought to result from it (quicker decision making, increase in recruitment, etc.). This is interesting because it assumes that a consequence of the introduction of Enterprise is that the old approach to time will move straightforwardly towards the new real-time, and that each form of working practice is mutually exclusive. Further, it trades on the notion of Enterprise's diffusion into the University as akin to something like a 'blanket cover', when it would be more usefully thought of as one space, or network, co-existing with others.

I shall now expand on this as I think it offers some interesting insights into the relation of Enterprise to the rest of the University, or how one model is in tension with another.

How Enterprise extends itself throughout the University

In one important sense, Enterprise does begin to extend itself throughout the University when the users also begin to acknowledge that there is a need for a new system that produces more timely and accurate information. One might imagine that repetition of the mantra would be voiced with varying levels of commitment, enthusiasm or, perhaps, irony. Nevertheless, whenever we were present at meetings, the mantra was still repeated.[9] In other words, in perpetuating the mantra, the users begin to perform in this network. However, their commitment to the system is more ambivalent, as they do not perform the role that is expected of them. For example, the next quote is taken from a focus group, where a member of the support staff, having attended some of the initial training courses, is beginning to think how the system will work in her own department:

Now when [Enterprise] comes in, the academics are going to have to conform to quite a lot of rules and regulations that they don't now. How on earth I am going to get my lot to do it, I do not know. Whether the center has realized this, and is just not telling us what they are going to do about it, whether they are just going to trust to luck and hope that it works I just don't know. But, I am quite concerned about that. I mean it does create bad feeling if you are saying to somebody look you just can't just make an order of the phone, I won't pay for it if you do. It must come through the office, that's the system ... And I can see that they are going to start screaming, as soon as I say to them 'sorry, you can't do that anymore you have got to do that now, that's what the system is supposed to do'.

What we have here is a powerful description of the way in which the Enterprise project is conceptualized as a mere mechanism for change, with the administrator portraying herself simply as a conduit for that change. The order embodied within Enterprise is expected to be reproduced throughout all departments – displacing existing modes of working with lots of new rules and regulations. While this type of account should not be disregarded, it seems that things were very much more interesting than this in practice.[10] In one department, for example, it appeared that many of the new rules and regulations were themselves 'worked around' in order to slot into existing practices, rather than to reconfigure existing networks.

In the case of purchasing (i.e., stationery requirements, new equipment and travel tickets) the procedures had always been to obtain a new item or service through the production of a number of forms. In urgent cases, the practice would be flexibly adapted so that travel tickets, for instance, could be purchased first, with the appropriate forms raised later. This ad hoc practice is impossible under Enterprise, as all suppliers have received written instructions allowing them to supply goods and services only for those orders which are both printed on an appropriate form (i.e., the one generated by Enterprise) and bear an Unique Order Number (again, generated by Enterprise).

In urgent cases, therefore, the administrator would generate the paperwork, and a ticket, for instance, could be bought the same day. When the administrator is not available, however, the remaining support staff are faced with a problem. However, the administrator has circumvented this by designing on her word processor a copy of the Enterprise order form, which can be printed out at any time. This can be used when adorned not with the Enterprise Order Number, but with something she calls a "pseudo number" or the "Secretarial Requisition Number" (a physical list of numbers kept by other members of the support staff). After this workaround has been carried out, the administrator is free to process the order through Enterprise in her own time.[11]

The significance of user workarounds

What do these workarounds tell us about what is going on?[12] At the very least, they teach us that the implementation would not be possible without such ad hoc modifications. At most, they indicate the nature of the new model and its relation to the old: that the real-time University where information is always 'up-to-date' is very much a performative notion. On the basis of what it knows and is told, the center believes the departments are working according to the real-time procedures; and as long as the users maintain these intricate workarounds, the University might as well be considered real-time. Thus, while the work of implementing Enterprise has involved both the production of a new model and the seeming destruction of the old, in many ways the established routines and practices (the old model) carry on as before. However, this is not to say that the University is the same as before.

To describe what this means I want to turn again to Bowker (1994), particularly his description of the building of a network of roads and pipelines through jungle country by the Schlumberger Company, as it searched for oil in Venezuela: "The old state was often a mass of impenetrable jungle: the network rendered it, at key points, visible and accessible to the oil companies" (ibid.: 243). He goes on to describe how, within this network space, the companies were able to produce a "local order" in the disordered space of the old state; this meant that no global picture was possible, as the scientists were only able to understand "small pockets" of the jungle. Also, because the local order existed only in the places where the roads and pipes were physically located, this network would throw into stark contrasts everything around it (so, from the point of view of the road, all the rest really was a jungle).

If we apply this to the Enterprise example, it might be said that the system, through the requirements that all decision-making activities are represented as information processes, is making the University, and the way that it works, visible and obvious to everyone. Further, because of the presence of the system, everything not already included within the system appears disordered – or much like a jungle (based on 'prejudice, hunch and rumor'). By establishing the informational model throughout the institution, it is therefore possible that all activities, practices, and processes not carried out according to the system will be found wanting in various ways.

Is the university to be redefined as an 'information institution'?

While world-wide changes to higher education as a result of new ICTs are increasingly researched and reported, we still understand very little of the particular dynamics associated with the implementation and use of mundane information systems – particularly the well established, generic and corporate computer systems. Arguably, the use and adaptation of these systems have implications for the reshaping of institutional, organizational and individual identities. In particular, this chapter has attempted to show the means whereby a university can be redefined as an 'information institution'. In doing so, I also wanted to demonstrate that the processes by which a large institution begins to think, talk and redefine itself according to the properties of information is not a fact about universities – but becomes a fact "as and when we make it so" (Bowker, 1994).

Empirically, I have focused on the replacement of one management information system with another, the reason for its replacement being that one does not provide the same type of accurate and timely information as the other. However, I argued that it is only through bringing together people disciplined enough to repeat an informational mantra that a difference between the two systems is actually achieved, and a new information model is established throughout the University. While the complexity of the implementation allows for a certain amount of flexibility in how the users take-up the various parts of the system (hence the discussion of workarounds as the continuation of the old model), now that the new model is established all activity will be measured against this – and (of course) found to be wanting. Through the process of bringing everything together under the metaphor of information, Enterprise has therefore seemingly begun to allow the production of order in the chaos of the University.

Notes

1 This research was supported by the UK's Economic and Social Research Council's Virtual Society? Programme.
2 While, as yet, there is little available systematic research on the spread of ERP systems to universities, more anecdotal evidence suggests that many

institutions across the globe have invested in, or are contemplating investing in, some similar form of industry standard computer system. For example, SAP, the large German ERP supplier, is working with universities from Belgium, South Africa, Canada, the UK and the USA, to build the 'Campus Management' system which can be integrated alongside other more established ERP modules, see Pollock and Cornford (2001).

3   In other words, ANT views technology as a network made up of technical and social elements. For a good example of a technology that only partially exists, see Latour (1996).

4   His argument is that soil does not naturally translate in information terms but was constructed as such by scientists.

5   Woolgar and Cooper draw on Latour (1987: 29) here and his so-called First Principle: "the fate of what we say and make is in later users' hands."

6   This was the Project Manager. After finishing his sentence with "etcetera etcetera," there is a brief silence before he finally adds "...information to make business decisions at all levels."

7   Within Enterprise, staff are conceptualized according to the supposed attributes of information as 'informational actors'. For instance, where we might have once thought about the university in terms of the Vice-chancellor, administration, academics, support staff, students, and so on, we are now encouraged to think in terms of the 'information manager', 'information custodian' or 'information users'.

8   A further example of what is being suggested here can be found in *The Control Revolution* by James Beniger (1986), who argued that the world is chaotic unless managers impose order on it through various technologies. Thanks to Phil Agre for bringing this work to my attention.

9   See the paper by Brown and Capdevila (1997) for a fascinating discussion of the repetition of the phrase "the customer is king." The only occasion when we were able to hear someone elaborate on the genesis of the phrase was during a conversation with a senior member of the project team. He decries how the mantra originally started with the Project Director.

10   The previous quotation is taken from someone just about to implement Enterprise in her department. We also conducted research in a department where the system was already being implemented.

11   This is a classic example of some of the 'interfacing work' carried out by individuals who span differing networks (cf. Gasser, 1986).

12   For a detailed discussion of workarounds, see Pollock (1998).

Part IV

Governing digital academe

Management and policy responses

17 'Information Society' as theory or ideology

A critical perspective on technology, education and employment in the Information Age

Nicholas Garnham

The clarion call for universities to rise to the challenge of providing higher education which is appropriate to the needs of the emerging 'knowledge economy' or 'information society' can be heard across the globe. The link between higher education and the demand for a growing pool of 'knowledge workers' forms the basis for politicians and policy makers to argue for an expansion in the provision of higher education. In this chapter, Garnham critically explores the validity of such widely-promoted assumptions about the need to keep pace with the 'information revolution', explaining why he believes this view is predicated on false beliefs. He also warns that such beliefs can act as a smokescreen for more deep-seated conflicts over the role of higher education, such as the attempts to utilize new media primarily to increase productivity in higher education – rather than improve quality.

The ideological basis of 'information society' visions

Thinking about the practice and future of education in general, and higher education in particular, takes place increasingly within the context of a specific vision of our economic and social future. This vision is commonly termed the Information (or Knowledge) Society. This is illustrated by the following comment from Hamish McRae, a respected British economist and economic commentator:

Rule five is: educate, educate, educate. We have very little idea of how e-commerce will develop over the next five years. The browser – the key invention that enabled the internet to become a commercial reality – is only five years old; look how far we have come since then. What we do know is that human capital – how clever we are, how well educated, how inventive and how flexible in our ideas – has become a more important element in the commercial mix. Other inputs, such as finance and factories, have become relatively less important. Education is, to some extent, still in the power of governments. It will become less so, as we come to educate ourselves more and more by downloading packages over the Net instead of being taught in conventional educational establishments. But basic education, the skills that enable us to access more specialized education later on, is the responsibility of government. Simple things, such as handling the Qwerty keyboard, should be standard skills for everyone, not just the young.

This emphasis on education is not just to make us more efficient or more able to garner a bigger share of the global e-commerce cake. It is to reduce divisions in our society. The Net is inherently a democratizing technology, in that it makes available to the many what was previously available only to the few.

(McRae, *The Independent*, 14 October 1999)

In this chapter, I want to suggest that the term 'Information Society' is not helpful because it has become largely meaningless and the vision bears very little if any relation to any concretely graspable reality. It therefore operates not as a useful concept for theoretical analysis but as an ideology. Rather than serving to enhance our understanding of the world in which we live, it is used to elicit uncritical assent to whatever dubious proposition is being put forward beneath its protective umbrella. Indeed so widespread is its casual and careless deployment in policy discourse and in what passes for serious journalism and business and economic comment that it reminds me of nothing so much as those medieval outbreaks of mass flagellation. One can only hope that it passes without causing too much permanent damage.

In studying the growth and propagation of this ideology one becomes a connoisseur of the inane. Its use is particularly distressing coming from those in higher education who should know better, and whose special responsibility it is to maintain standards of critical intelligence. Let me give two recent examples of what I mean culled almost at random from the UK. The first is the professor of education at Cambridge University reviewing Alan Ryan's (1998) defense of the liberal university:

> Nowhere in the book does Ryan address the dramatic changes in the educational landscape that are likely to occur over the next two or three decades. The modern knowledge economy will force most people in work to renew their skills and even change jobs every few years.... In knowledge economies, training will continue throughout our working life and will be a blend of vocational and liberal education that supplies transferable intellectual and social skills, especially the capacity to locate and evaluate knowledge in an information-soaked world.

Notice here how a view of the world and an educational response to it is presented as both unquestionable fate and as new. Thus any critical questioning of the propositions advanced is set up as both old-fashioned and unrealistic.

My second example comes from the address by Howard Newby, Vice-chancellor of Southampton University and ex-head of the UK's Economic and Social Research Council (ESRC), to the annual meeting of the Committee of Vice-chancellors and Principles of which he is President: "We are no longer an ivory tower separate from society, but an integral part of the knowledge based economy and central to it".

The reality beyond the ideology

In the light of the prevalence of this ideology I want to ask what are the real world phenomena to which they think they are referring? Is there, in fact, any good evidence that they actually exist and what implications do they have for the current and future role and practice of universities? I think we can break down the impact of Information Society thinking on higher education into two key components:

The first is illustrated by the quotation from McRae above. It is an argument about human capital formation that sees such formation as central to economic growth and international competitiveness, and which then argues for investment in higher education and its reorientation on the grounds of the particular skill shortages and labor market dynamics supposedly associated with a shift to a knowledge economy.

The second is the possibility of raising the productivity of higher education through the use of technologies of educational delivery. Associated with this line of thinking is the issue of the commoditization of knowledge and education and the question as to whether technological and economic developments mean that private corporate providers will increasingly compete with the inherited national institutions of public higher education on a global basis. Another related question is whether, in search of the economic growth of a tradable information or creative industries sector, such a development might be positively desirable. It is here that the Information Society debate meets the globalization debate. I am equally skeptical about many of the claims made for globalization but I will not, for reasons of limited space, address them.

I want to suggest that thinking about either of these two issues in terms of the Information Society is less than helpful.

The production of knowledge in an Information Society

The term Information Society refers to a number of distinct trends and arguments that we need to uncouple. First, there is Daniel Bell's (1999) well-known Post-Industrial Society argument that organized knowledge was becoming the key ingredient in value-added, and therefore in economic growth. It is important to stress that for Bell it was not information or knowledge in general that was the key, but the application of Weberian rationalization to the production of knowledge itself. This is important because it then led on to his incorporation of the ICT revolution into his scenario as a technology that enhanced the planned nature of knowledge production and its productivity. From an economic perspective this is a Chandlerian and not a Schumpeterian view. However, what is crucial for my analysis here is that, on this basis, Bell argued that a shift of power was taking place (because the terms of trade were altering) between capital owners and knowledge producers. In this scenario, it is universities and industrial research labs that become the core institutions of capitalism, not banks.

Two things need to be said about this version of the Information Society argument. The first is that the relation between organized knowledge as a force of production and the university sector is not new, but goes back to Germany's success in the second industrial revolution and the resulting exporting of the German university model with its associated PhDs to the USA and elsewhere at the beginning of the twentieth century. The second is that Bell's exercise in social forecasting has not stood up well in the face of actual historical developments. I want to suggest that we are where we are today precisely because the terms of trade have gone in precisely the opposite direction to that predicted by Bell, and that so-called knowledge workers in universities everywhere have experienced increased subjugation to capital, what some – for instance Halsey (1992) – have not hesitated to describe as proletarianization. There are good reasons for this, as I shall argue later.

The shift from an economy based on producing goods to the production of knowledge

A second Information Society argument, of which there are also elements in Bell, is that the center of gravity of the economy has increasingly shifted from goods production to knowledge production. This version of the Information Society argument is captured in the terms 'weightless economy' or 'frictionless economy', and in Negroponte's hyperbolic claim that increasingly economic activity is focused on shifting bits rather than atoms (Negroponte, 1995). Here, it is important to disentangle carefully the shift from manufacturing to services – with which manufacturing remains confusingly entwined – from an increased level of knowledge intensity across the economy as a whole. This is particularly important because this confusion often underpins the argument about skill shortages and the changing role of human capital and thus of education.

Two distinctions need to be made: between the role of services and of knowledge intensification within the goods producing sector itself; and, within the service sector, between personal and knowledge-based services. Once we make these distinctions two things become clear. First, that the production, distribution and marketing of goods remains the dominant sector of the economy (perhaps 64 per cent of total employment) and the key sources for rises in productivity and employment growth. Second, that developments within the personal and knowledge-based services have been and will continue to be very different. This is important because, contrary to a widely held view, the projected rise in employment growth is in personal services such as in health care, rather than knowledge-based services. In addition, the types of knowledge or skills required will differ with the result; for instance, an Australian study showed that it is the demand for interpersonal rather than cognitive skills that has risen most markedly (Sheehan and Tegart, 1998). From this perspective, capitalist economies have been knowledge economies for a long time; for the Information Society thesis to hold up, we would need to establish a large step-change in what are long-term trends. In my view, to lump very different sectoral trends and dynamics together as though they were one phenomenon under the rubric Information Society or knowledge economy is not helpful.

Thus, if we look at so-called e-commerce, the growth of which is now touted as the key indicator of the knowledge economy, what we see is the application of Internet-based communication technologies either to somewhat enhance the efficiency of the business-to-business supply chain or to shift the nature of the information search and transactional mode within the retailing of goods and services. In goods retailing, the efficiency savings to be made are relatively small. In the service sector only some services – those with a relatively low level of necessary human input – can exploit the advantages. Again it is not clear how an overall Information Society approach is useful in the analysis of these different developments. Similarly, therefore, higher education needs to be clear about its specific functions and the best mix of organizational forms, skills and technology for the fulfillment of those functions, before it launches itself on any development path in the name of the Information Society.

Changes tied to ICTs

The third version of the Information Society argument focuses on ICTs and their impact on productivity, and firm and market organization. It is this version we find in Castells' (1996) 'network society' and in advocates within the USA of the so-called New Economic paradigm (such as Rifkin, 2000). The main empirical problem with this approach remains the celebrated 'Solow paradox': the continuing failure of positive results of investment in ICTs to show up in actual productivity figures, as highlighted in the quip, 'You can see the computer revolution everywhere except in the productivity statistics'. (Triplett, 1999) This is important because the human capital formation argument in part rests on its supposed contribution to productivity growth.

The USA, the supposed prime exemplar of the New Economic paradigm, has consistently lagged behind other developed economies in productivity growth since the 1980s. While US productivity has indeed increased recently, it is only now returning to the between 2 and 3 per cent rates of growth that were the norm in the 1960s and would appear to be around the long-range rates of sustainable productivity of industrial economies.[1] The rates of productivity growth were in fact higher during the Reagan boom of 1982–6, which were not sustained. So there does not appear to be any good evidence as yet in the productivity figures for a new paradigm.

The real remaining questions are these. Why have US productivity growth rates been so low in recent years compared with the long boom of the 1950s and 1960s? And why, contrary to a technologically determined vision of the knowledge economy, has the USA had such persistently low real wage rates combined with relatively low levels of unemployment – perhaps associated with a shift from capital to labor intensity? The US real wage remains low. The wages of the average worker were only just reaching their 1989 level at the end of the 1990s and are about 10 per cent below the level reached in 1973 (Madrick, 1999).

Productivity and technological change in education

I think the best way of understanding current pressures on education in general, and higher education in particular, is to view the new media from the perspective of the productivity problem. In common with much of the service sector, education – especially higher education – generally suffers from Baumol's disease: in which the relative costs of education rise because education is labor intensive and the general real wage level is rising across the economy, driven by growth in productivity in technology-based areas of production and distribution. Coupled with a general concern to cut or at least restrain state expenditures, this creates very heavy pressures to attempt to raise productivity through the adoption of what are hoped to be labor-saving technologies. Indeed, one pervasive way of reading the Information Society thesis going back to Bell is as a general attempt to harness the computer to raise levels of productivity in services to the levels of that in manufacturing. The problem, in my view, is that this has not happened – and cannot realistically be achieved.

In order to understand why not, we need to look more closely at the issue of productivity and technological change. It is clear historically that the introduction of the capitalist mode of production, first in agriculture and then in manufacturing industry, massively raised the level of productivity and set in motion a process of continuous productivity growth. This step-change in productivity released increasing numbers of human beings from the fate of subsistence and the unremitting toil that accompanied it, thereby releasing resources – crucially including time – for increased levels of consumption, including the consumption of education. Capitalist economies are human-energy and time-saving economies. This could be said to be the point of capitalism and this is why raising productivity remains important. But in the context of a debate about the role of information, it is important to stress that this was – and is – an essentially thermodynamic process. At base it was an energy transfer between humans and nature. For all the talk of 'a move from atoms to bits', it is therefore the exploitation of the globe's material resources, in particular fossil fuels, that remains at the core of economic growth – however much knowledge is applied to that process.

Even if there have been modest recent increases in productivity due to the harnessing of computer power, the evidence and background show they nowhere approach the levels of productivity growth achieved by previous revolutions in technology and associated organizational changes in the system of production, for instance the impact of the internal combustion engine. Robert Gordon (1997), perhaps the most authoritative recent analyst of the impact of computers on US productivity, has argued that computers are largely involved in a zero-sum game of shifting wealth competitively between corporations rather than creating new wealth. There is an important reason why computers are not likely to raise long-term productivity trends:

The computer has made production and distribution faster and cheaper. But it has also changed the nature of competition. In the age of standardized products and mass production, size and speed mattered most. Fewer workers were needed to make products. But today, businesses constantly need new, varied and upgraded products, as well as managerial methods to compete. The premium is on innovation, and this requires human skills such as creativity and imagination in tandem with the computer. They are not skills that the computer can replace as rapidly as mass production once replaced workers. Today the great growth in jobs is in 'business services', such as those provided by consultants. Thus in my view there has indeed been an important technological transformation in America, but not necessarily one that will lead to more rapid productivity growth. The new economy is a return to a contemporary version of a craft economy, where the most valued contribution is the skill of the worker. The new crafts workers are business managers, consultants, and marketing and financial experts, as well as scientific and technical researchers and computer specialists. Or to put it differently, in an age where information is so widely available, it is not the information that is valuable but what is done with it (Madrick, 1999).

In my view there is a more profound problem: What in the production and use of information would an increase in informational productivity actually mean? Those who have studied the economics of information know that there are major problems in relating the value of outputs in any but a random sense to either the costs of production or to market prices. There are good reasons for this.

For example, it is unlikely that the harnessing of ICTs and the new media will enhance productivity to any great extent, however it is defined, because the value of the information produced is – as it has always been – dependent on the application of human brainpower and imagination, a process to which the computer is of only marginal assistance. Yes, I can increase the efficiency of my information search via the Internet. But this increase is largely or entirely nullified by the amount of largely redundant information I then have to search through and assess. However, even leaving that aside I doubt whether it enhances the resulting quality of the ideas or analyses made. Indeed, one can see persuasive evidence to the contrary in the very subject area we are discussing. It is hard to believe that the ideology of the Information Society could have survived if it was the case that this technological revolution had produced an enhancement in the productivity and quality of intellectual labor.

What does seem to have been produced is lower levels of efficiency, such that the common experience is increased working time for those involved in the so-called information economy and a pervasive sense of information overload. The problem is that the intangible nature of the output and of its contribution to either productivity or value added gives us no tools for distinguishing between the increased overhead costs produced by these developments and the genuine contributions to productivity growth and thus economic welfare.

Can capitalism survive in a 'weightless economy'?

I would like to end this discussion of the 'ICT impact' version of the Information Society thesis by floating another approach. Let us suppose for a moment that the prophets are right and that we are rapidly shifting from an economy dominated by material production to one dominated by the production of intangibles. The question that is then posed in my view is whether a capitalist market economy is sustainable under such conditions. To answer that, we need to return to a rather unfashionable concept: the labor theory of value.

Why did the classic political economists from Adam Smith through to Marx place the labor theory of value at the center of their analysis of the capitalist mode of production? Because some stable common denominator of relative value has to be found, both for a system of exchange to sustain itself over time and to enable an analysis to be made of the dynamics of such a system. You can sustain a mercantile trading economy with more or less random value relations based on temporary relations of scarcity and need. Such a system has no built-in dynamic of growth and is subject to constant speculative booms and busts. But for a growing, investment-based mode of production, the system of relative values must be relatively stable and calculable over time – otherwise there is no incentive to store value in monetary form or to invest for the future. The risk is simply too high. The effects of the absence of such long-term stability of relative values can be illustrated by the effects on economic activity of hyper inflation. It is this lack of a stable calculable relationship between the value of inputs and outputs that lies behind the historical difficulties in commodifying information. The labor theory of value was an attempted solution to this problem, a solution that continues to work well in an economy based, as I have argued, on the measurable increase in the productivity of human work-time and especially on the saving of human energy inputs through the substitution of natural energy sources.

In an economy dominated by information production and transfers, any stable relation between labor and value breaks down. I don't think we have begun to think through the implications of this. It is for this reason that intellectual property is such a central and contentious issue. From the early days of an information economy with the development of printing and publishing, it was recognized that the economic relations within this sector were peculiar. The result was the intervention of the state, at a time when laissez-faire policies were increasingly taking over from mercantilism, to establish the conditions for the creation of knowledge by granting an artificial monopoly to authors. But we also know that the social productivity of knowledge is enhanced by the free flow of that knowledge unencumbered by copyright and other related barriers to its use and exploitation. In my view, this contradiction is inherent and goes to the heart of attempts to turn universities into knowledge selling corporations.

The changing nature of the firm and role of knowledge workers

The fourth theme in Information Society thinking relates to the changing nature of the firm and the status and power of knowledge workers. In Castells' (1996) version of the Information Society – or as he calls it, significantly, the Network society – the key element is the rise of the so-called network firm and an associated new class of 'networkers'. I would not wish to deny that the development of efficient global communication networks has led to changes in the organization of the firm, both directly and also indirectly. In some sectors this has been done by increasing competitive pressures and making global co-ordination easier, faster and cheaper; but this increase in competition can be exaggerated and has to be balanced against the increased chances for oligopolies to develop. Nonetheless, structures of property ownership set clear limits to this reconfiguration of the firm. Given the current stress, not to say obsession, with share-holder value, I think it is hard to sustain the argument that a new breed of freebooting networkers are wresting economic power away from the ultimately hierarchical management structure that share-holder ownership entails.

Indeed, we can see this in universities themselves. I can remember the phase in the late 1970s and early 1980s when management gurus, following a broadly Information Society line of thinking, were arguing – and being paid large sums for arguing – that firms should model themselves on universities by introducing plural, independent project teams linked within a collegial leadership environment. Leaving aside the question of whether this was ever a good picture of actual univer-sities, what is striking is that precisely the opposite has taken place as corporate managerialism increasingly dominates universities.

The key educational challenges faced by policy makers

I would now like to focus on the main education, employment and technology issues facing policy makers. Much of the talk and planning in relation to higher education and the impact of the new media stems from the same source as the managerial thrust I have been describing. It comes back to Baumol's disease. The problem for policy makers is not in fact to improve the educational process in order to meet the needs of the knowledge economy – the skills shortage, human capital argument. The problem is to cut or at least control the cost of a labor intensive service sector. It is doubtful whether this is likely to improve the quality of the output, assuming we could measure it. Here we need to separate out two issues. And neither in my judgment has anything to do with the Information Society.

First, networked computers and forms of so-called multimedia can in some instances enhance the learning experience, although this needs to be assessed on a case-by-case basis. But these are extensions of old technologies – the book, the over-head projector, the film projector and, in the field of distance education, the mail, radio and television. As we have learnt from painful previous experience with educational technologies, in most cases they enhance rather than replace tradi-tional modes of small-group teaching and are usually cost-adding rather than cost-reducing. I have lived through several cycles of educa-tional technology, distance learning and the policy debates surrounding them. In each case, they have failed to deliver on their original promise and each cycle has ended with those with a vested interest in continuing investment in the field arguing for just one more push. In my view the interesting sociological and policy question is why, in the face of evidence and experience, this faith remains so persistent.

The importance of capital formation and skills shortages

The other main issue here is that of human capital formation and skills shortage. Crudely, the argument now mobilized by both politicians and university administrators to justify both the expansion of higher education and tax-payer expenditure on higher education goes: the knowledge economy requires an increased cadre of knowledge workers; the relative competitiveness of countries depends on the availability of this human capital and thus on educational investment; that a major cause of unemployment is the low skill levels of job seekers – crudely that the manual workers required by a muscle-based economy are no longer required; and that, therefore, these workers have to be retrained for knowledge work.

There are a number of problems with this argument. First, the relationship between educational investment and economic growth seems weak, more a matter of faith than evidence; indeed, the relationship seems more likely to go in the other direction – rich economies can afford higher levels of education and can afford to keep people out of the workforce for longer periods. Second, the skills shortage is a myth – and a particularly cruel one at that.

The situation in the early 2000s in the UK and the USA of normal economic growth and a general tightening of the labor market seems to make the supposed skill-shortage barrier to employment disappear. From a low skill/high skill perspective, studies do not appear to show a change in the skill composition of the labor market, at least in the USA. In his review of such studies, David Howell (1994) notes: "the share of low-skill jobs was remarkably stable from 1983 into the 1990s. Rather the real shift was away from higher wage jobs."

A study by Susan Wieler showed that the dispersion of skill requirements was unchanged in the 1980s, even among technologically advanced industries.[2] Moreover, in terms of employment growth in the USA between 1985–95, high-skill jobs grew by 2.1 per cent and low-skill by 2.4 per cent. If the aim is to tackle the problem of increased wage inequality through education, the trend actually seems to be to de-link skill and wage levels with rising skill requirements and falling wages for comparable jobs. Gottschalk (1998) shows, in addition, that measures such as changes in education reflect changes in supply of skills rather than in demand – a skill premium. It has been projected that a maximum of 29 per cent of US jobs will require university-level qualifications by 2005 implying excess capacity and thus falling rewards. This in itself is likely to pose a problem for higher education since at present both in the USA and the UK the increased economic burden being placed on university students and their parents is justified in terms of the positive future economic rewards of such education. But with costs rising and salaries for graduate-level jobs likely to fall, this may look an increasingly less attractive offer.

In addition to this relation between overall skill levels and the labor market in general, we also need to investigate the type of skills required. This leads us to see that the whole concept of the knowledge worker and knowledge economy is incoherent. We need to distinguish between types of skill – all require knowledge, and perhaps training, but of different types.

If we distinguish between motor, cognitive and interpersonal skills, it is true that we find the need for motor skills has declined. But the growth in the demand for cognitive skills – those usually seen as central to the knowledge economy and to the formation of which higher education might claim a distinct contribution – has been outstripped by that in the demand for interpersonal skills. Some have associated this with the feminization of the work force. What certainly seems to be the case is that the centrality of interpersonal skills is supported by projections of occupational growth. In the US Bureau of Labor's 1998 projection (see stats.bls.gov/ecopro) of the ten largest job growth occupations between 1996 and 2006, only systems analysts and, possibly, general managers and top executives could be classed as classic knowledge-economy jobs. The remainder are dominated by cashiers, registered nurses, sales persons, retail, home-health aides, teachers aides, receptionists and truck drivers. In the fastest growing categories, health workers (873,000 jobs) is only just outnumbered by computer scientists, computer engineers and systems analysts (1.04 million).

Thus, we need to distinguish between both specific types of skill and specific job markets. We need to ask whether, in fact, skills short-ages exist and, if so, whether universities are the appropriate institutions to provide such skills. It is certainly the case that previous attempts to combine labor market planning with university curriculum planning are not reassuring. But the crucial point is that this is not a new problem related to a so-called Information Society.

Trends in generic information-skills requirements

We are then left with the more generic – or, in the current jargon, 'transferable' – information skills. As we have seen, current labor market trends do not appear to demonstrate a growth in new information-intensive sectors which require a qualitatively different range of skills or type of human capital formation. On the one hand there is a growth in high-skilled white-collar work, reflecting the growth in business services where it is not clear that the information skills are either different or more intense than those always needed for management or the associate specialist skills of accountancy, law and so on. For instance, if we look at the big growth in management consultancy it is far from clear that we should be impressed by either the level or novelty of their intellectual endowments compared to those traditional socially-acquired skills more accurately described as 'chutzpah'.

On the other hand, we find the growth of classic service occupations, especially health care. Here technological change has nothing much to do with it. They are jobs based on human-to-human relations. While in some areas some part of that can be intermediated by communication and information technologies, the skills required are interpersonal and humanly embedded. Such jobs have been central to our economies and societies for a long time. Their growth is better captured by the classical analysis of the growth of a service economy and by Perkins' (1990) notion of professionalization rather than by the newly minted Information Society. The great revolution was the development of systems of public education that are largely publicly funded, with their accompanying culture of certification. Ernst Gellner has called this "exo-training", explaining:

> A society has emerged based on a high-powered technology and the expectancy of sustained growth, which requires both a mobile division of labor and sustained, frequent and precise communication between strangers involving a sharing of explicit meaning, transmitted in a standard idiom and in writing when required ... the level of literacy and technical competence ... required of members of this society, if they are to be properly employable and enjoy full and effective moral citizenship, is so high that it simply cannot be provided by the kin or local units.
>
> (Gellner, 1983: 34)

Future roles of universities

Universities have three main functions in society:

1 To provide certified general training appropriate to a growing range of professionalized roles and tasks where formally acquired knowledge can be applied.
2 To provide a social filter with an associated range of interpersonal and networking skills for a range of higher and intermediate 'management roles'. The operation of this social filter then has significant effects on ideological/political struggle within the society, since it is used to justify social arrangements in the interests of this elite, for instance structures of remuneration, taxation and so on.
3 To develop and transmit from one generation to another the culture – or, perhaps more accurately, the critical intelligence – of a given society as a general social resource.

The Information Society does not, it seems to me, serve as a useful starting point for analyzing the present position and future development of universities along any of these three dimensions.

What we are now witnessing is not a shift to a new type of economy, but a development of a very old struggle: between what Gellner (1983a) has referred to as "the Plough, the Book and the Sword" – or Runciman (1983) as the modes of production, persuasion and coercion – along each of these dimensions over the role of higher education. The Information Society is a concept with no objective correlative in the real world. Used as an ideological mantra it merely and dangerously distracts – as is often intended – from the real issues.

Notes

1 Productivity in the USA grew by more than 2 per cent annually on average between 1870 and 1970, and by nearly 3 per cent a year in the 25 years after the Second World War.
2 A useful overview of Susan Wieler's research along with other work on this skills-technology 'myth' is provided by David Howell (1994).

18 New information technologies and the restructuring of higher education

The constitutional view

Sandra Braman

The legal context in which educational institutions operate may facilitate or constrain the strategies and actions adopted by universities, for example in terms of their degree of autonomy in reconfiguring their geography and internal and external relationships. In this chapter, Braman explores these issues through the first comprehensive survey of every US Supreme Court case dealing with an institution of higher education. Her analysis of this constitutional law suggests that the university in the US is in a strong position to move forward on initiatives that may require it to assert its rights. She also warns of threats to the traditional role of universities in the public sphere.

The legal background

Issues relating to new information technologies

University use of new information technologies raises a number of legal issues – from the need to protect institutional identity on the Web, to ownership of Web-based courses, to surveillance of faculty and student communications via campus networking infrastructure – that are of constitutional status in the United States. While constitutional law will certainly not be the only factor determining the ultimate resolution of such issues, it does provide a context within which economic, social, political, organizational and other factors will play themselves out.

Higher education is an information industry that has historically filled a constitutive role for the nation-state. As a constitutive force, higher education contributes to state formation processes and to 'capacity' – the ability of the nation-state to act on its intentions. That these constitutive roles are critical is made clear by the treatment of universities within constitutional law, the self-reflexive process by which the United States considers the way in which society should be structured and the processes that should be permitted within and between elements of that structure.

Pressing constitutive issues currently face universities, for themselves and for the nation-state, as they struggle with the effects of the use of new information technologies. The questions come in pairs, reflecting the fact that every policy question has two faces, one internal to the entity asking it and one external:

Autonomy: How autonomous is the university from the nation-state? And in what ways does – and should – the university serve the nation-state?

Economics: What are the constraints upon universities as economic actors? And what are the constraints upon faculty members as economic actors?

The public sphere: How does the university community participate in the larger public sphere? And how does the university operate *as* a public sphere?

Many, though not all, of these questions involve issues that have been addressed as matters of constitutional law by the United States Supreme Court. This chapter summarizes a review of the entire body of US Supreme Court opinions dealing with higher education, from the Court's foundation in 1790 through to June 2000. The review describes the constitutional context in which higher education questions will be addressed, as well as specific constitutional principles available for use. Some questions are old, such as how much the government can intervene in university affairs, but have answers that need continuous re-examination. Others, such as whether establishing a university includes a commitment to a particular place, take on new dimensions in a distance-education environment. And some are new, such as how to deal with the extraordinary growth in the relative presence of outsiders to the university within Web-based university conversations.

Higher education and the US Supreme Court

The US judicial system is unusual in that constitutional issues can be addressed at any level of the court system. Thus, a number of higher education issues are resolved at levels of the court system below that of the Supreme Court but are not included here; analysis of these cases can be found in traditional casebooks on constitutional law and education, such as that of Olivas (1997). There is also not sufficient space in this chapter to discuss Supreme Court decisions that deal with other types of public institutions and therefore have implications for higher education; analysis of these cases may be found in the *Chronicle of Higher Education*.

Cases dealing with primary and secondary education are not explored in depth here but do provide insight into how education in general is viewed from the constitutional perspective. Such cases at the Supreme Court level have demonstrated: a sensitivity to the relationship between information and socioeconomic class (*Plyler v. Doe*, 1982; *Martinez v. Bynum*, 1983); shown awareness of the multidimensionality of access (*Hendrick Hudson v. Rowley*, 1982); and defended the speech rights of students (*Tinker v. Des Moines*, 1969), as well as the right of schools to restrict those speech rights when necessary in pursuit of educational goals (*Bethel School District #403 v. Fraser*, 1986; *Hazelwood School Dist. v. Kuhlmeier*, 1988).

Because the Supreme Court is reactive by mission and process, it can deal only with those important social issues that a party chooses to fight all the way up through the court system, an extremely costly process; thus, all issues of import that will arise for universities as a result of the use of new information technologies do not necessarily appear in analysis of Supreme Court decisions. Finally, decisions intended to accomplish one thing may instead, or in addition, do quite another. This discussion therefore looks not only at points of law, but also policy principles and conceptual frameworks.

This reading of the entire body of Supreme Court cases dealing with higher education looks first at the cases, and then at their implications for issues arising out of the use of new information technologies.

The US Supreme Court cases

The Supreme Court first dealt with institutions of higher education in its earliest years. The waves of cases over time mark the emergence of new types of questions as they have arisen out of experimentation by universities with their capacities, and out of changes in the nature of the nation-state and the economy.

Autonomy

Education first articulated itself as a set of institutions distinct from those of the nation-state over the course of the nineteenth century. The government added new informational activities to its repertoire and deepened its engagement with others – Richards (1993) refers to the nineteenth-century nation-state as the 'archival' state. At the same time, other informational activities were spun off to institutions either under the purview of the states or in the private sector. Indirect public and private demands for the training of workers also influenced university curricula by the turn of the twentieth century – the industrial world needed not only the literate laborers produced by mandatory primary and secondary education, but also engineers, managers and clerks. Thus, institutions of higher education developed autonomy but did so under conditions which ensured that they continued to serve the nation-state. The complexity of the situation is revealed in cases dealing with the autonomy of decision-making, liability and accountability, relations with the nation-state and possible 'special features' of universities as institutions.

Decision-making

The question of whether or not colleges and universities would be able to exist at all independent of the government was at issue the first time the Supreme Court faced a higher education case (*Dartmouth v. Woodward*, 1819). Education was considered public service; therefore many argued it was the responsibility of government. While the Court held that this important public function could also be served by the private sector, in the end this decision demonstrated how very difficult it is to predict what the effects of any particular decision or policy might be: *Dartmouth* did encourage the growth of private institutions, it also delayed the launch of public universities for half a century (Olivas, 1997).

The Court in general protects the right of institutions to make decisions regarding their internal standards of performance (*University of Michigan v. Ewing*, 1985), though it is assumed different standards and procedures will be used for administrative as opposed to academic matters (*Board of Curators, University of Missouri v. Horowitz*, 1978). The Court has repeatedly taken the position that course content, not institutional affiliation, determines whether a college or university is religious or secular – though it has been reluctant to examine course content in detail (*Hunt v. McNair*, 1973; *Tilton v. Richardson*, 1971;

Witters v. Washington Dept. of Services for the Blind, 1986). (The question of whether a university is religious or secular is of fundamental importance in the US because of the constitutional separation of matters of church and state.)

While the Court's general position is that funding does not justify government restrictions on academic freedom (*Roemer v. Maryland Public Works Board*, 1976), the nature of a funding arrangement can make a difference. In *National College Athletic Association (NCAA) v. Smith* (1999), it was ruled that receiving federal funds did not make that organization's activities state action,[1] but in *Regents of the University of California v. Doe* (1997) it was held that a university was not liable for breach of contract if an individual fails to pass a security clearance needed in order to work on a particular government-funded project. Federal funding for non-educational purposes, such as the Medicare at issue in *Thomas Jefferson University v. Shalala* (1994), cannot be used to cover costs shifted to the educational side of a mixed-purpose institution.

Accountability and liability

While colleges and universities pursued autonomy overall, at times they have also sought to bring themselves closer to government in order to cloak themselves with its immunities. This issue arose first in 1911 in *Hopkins v. Clemson Agricultural College*, when the Court refused to let a college escape liability for flooding neighboring property through its assertion that the immunity claimed by many state governments also applied to a college established under state law. In 1988 university dismissal of a coach for breaking National Collegiate Athletic Association rules was deemed not to be state action in response to a similar claim applied at the federal level (*NCAA v. Tarkanian*). However, in the critically important recent case *Florida Prepaid Postsecondary Education Expense Board v. College Savings Bank* (1999), a financial entity established by the state to help finance students' higher education was held to be immune from prosecution for copyright violation based on the same immunity logic rejected earlier.

Service to nation-state goals

A specific argument for devoting university resources to nation-state goals was offered in *Hamilton v. Regents of the University of California* (1934), where the Court upheld the right of the institution to require student participation in the Reserve Officer Training Corps (ROTC), since the state government perceived its own survival – and therefore that of the university – to be dependent on such activities.

In 1978, the Court upheld the Veterans' Administration's (VA) right to refuse to provide GI Bill[2] support to students attending colleges with innovative curricula (*Cleland v. National College of Business*). This decision was justified by explicit deference to the VA's concern that an entire new category of institutions was coming into being simply to take advantage of the new students entering college on the GI Bill. The VA also refused to support branch institutions within a certain distance of their mother institutions (often where innovative curricula were located), as well as programs in which the number of students attending on federal support exceeded a certain percentage.

Special status

Universities have gone back and forth on whether or not they should have any special status as a result of their social function. In *Minnesota Board for Community Colleges v. Knight* (1984), the Court emphasized that serving in the state higher education system did not affect the First Amendment status of faculty members who have no more right than others to insist that the intended audience for their speech *listens* to what is said. In *National Labor Relations Board (NLRB) v. Yeshiva* (1980), the Court rejected the notion that any specific employment status attached to those serving on faculties of academic institutions; rather, the question of whether faculty members are management, employees or contractors must be determined on a case by case basis. Students, too, have at times tried to assert a special status, as did the plaintiff in *Culver v. US* (1926) when he claimed he should have received extra flight pay from the military – even though he was in military-assigned classes rather than flying during the disputed period (the Court disagreed).

Economics

Most important among the ways in which universities achieve autonomy from governments is through the ability to generate and control capital and property. One of the most dramatic trajectories visible in the history of Supreme Court decisions dealing with colleges and universities has been the steady expansion of the range of types of property over which universities may exert control and the ways in which they can do it. In addition to setting parameters for universities as economic actors, the Court has addressed a variety of types of property: money, land, cultural property, intellectual property and intellectual capital.

Parameters

Parameters for the behavior of public universities as economic actors were laid forth in two Supreme Court decisions from the beginning of the twentieth century. In *Thomas v. Board of Trustees of Ohio State University* (1904) and *Speer v. Colbert* (1906), the Court used analysis of a land-grant question to specify the powers available to universities. These included the rights to sue and be sued; contract and be contracted with; make, use, and alter a common seal; and to receive a variety of types of property through a variety of means.

These parameters have been revisited recently as universities experiment with the new ways of structuring themselves internally and relating to other institutions made possible by the use of new information technologies. In *NLRB v. Yeshiva* (1980), *Florida Prepaid Postsecondary Education Expense Board* (1999) and other decisions, the Court supported the broadest definition of the ways in which universities are permitted to structure themselves as well as to operate economically.

Money

Fees, gifts and bequests have been treated separately. The decision in *In re Pennsylvania College Cases* (1871) established that colleges could accept payment for classes and that those payments would be considered contracts. The question of whether or not other ways of acquiring property were acceptable was addressed in *Board of Public Works v. Columbia College* (1873), in which it was held that commitments to colleges are as important as other kinds of financial commitments, and that resources so committed, as a result, cannot be withdrawn in favor of other needs. Universities do have to follow specific conditions set by gifts or bequests (*Mayer v. American Security & Trust*, 1911), but testators and donors need not be technically precise in their description of intended uses for funds (*Taylor v. Columbian University*, 1912).

If a university sets up a foundation incorporated in another state, the use of its funds is determined not by the jurisdiction in which the university sits, but by the jurisdiction in which the foundation was incorporated; thus, a University of Arkansas foundation incorporated in Texas was prohibited by Texas law from spending funds on a

University of Arkansas medical facility in Arkansas (*Arkansas v. Texas*, 1953).

The Court has also supported entrepreneurial activities on the part of universities. The importance of sports to the income of many universities, for example, was at the heart of the decision in *NCAA v. Board of Regents, University of Oklahoma* (1983) when the Supreme Court would not permit an injunction against broadcasting football games while broadcasters were under investigation for antitrust violations.

Land

The land-grant process[3] raised issues both of property ownership and of the relationships among higher education institutions, state governments and the federal government. The process itself was complex, with numerous opportunities for abuse. The commitment to public higher education had to be reinforced in cases that supported the right of states to establish the financial arrangements necessary to translate funds from the federally-granted lands into capital with which to build state universities (*Bier v. McGehee*, 1893; *Keane v. Brugger*, 1895; *Montana ex rel Haire v. Rice*, 1907); acquire further land (*Cavanaugh v. Looney*, 1919); and decide for themselves which institutions would receive land-grant funds (*Wyoming Agricultural College v. Irvine*, 1907).

Not all land owned by a university is necessarily used directly for educational purposes. Once the Court held that taxable and non-taxable activities of universities could be treated distinctly for legal purposes (*Jetton v. University of the South*, 1908), it became easier to defend the right of the university to rent out land or other property (*Osborne v. Clark*, 1907; *Taylor v. Columbian University, 1912*), or use it for other non-educational purposes (*Millsaps College v. City of Jackson*, 1927; *Seton Hall College, et al. v. Village of South Orange*, 1916).

Cultural objects

Ownership of cultural property by museums, archives, and universities, one of the most urgent of contemporary cultural policy issues, arose as a question first at the constitutional level as early as *Onondaga Nation v. Thacher* in 1903. Plaintiffs (leaders of the Iroquois Confederacy and the University of the State of New York) accused an individual of stealing four wampum belts that allegedly belonged to the university, to whom rights as 'wampum keeper' had been transferred both through tribal ritual and bill of sale. Lower courts had claimed no commonality of interest among individual members of the tribes, and therefore denied that the tribes had the ability to sue. The Supreme Court declined jurisdiction as well, arguing that the suit was cast in terms of tribal, not constitutional, law. Through contemporary eyes, this position appears to reflect a lack of respect for tribal sensibilities; today it is not uncommon for museums and archives to return property to tribes that claim ownership according to tribal, if not US, law.

Intellectual property

Intellectual property rights were at issue in *Florida Prepaid Postsecondary Education Expense Board v. College Savings Bank* (1999). Here, a state governmental entity that offered prepaid annuities to state parents seeking to finance their children's education was accused of infringing upon the software patent of a bank. The Court upheld the university's claim to immunity from lawsuit under cover of the state's blanket. The enormous impact of this decision makes it likely that a related case will again work its way to the Supreme Court so that the issue may be revisited.

Intellectual capital

Aware of the relationship between socioeconomic and informational class, the Court has supported the role of higher education in the formation of a variety of types of intellectual capital beyond that embedded in intellectual property. The right of a professional association to require a degree from an institution of higher education in addition to passing an examination for certification purposes was upheld in *Graves v. State of Minnesota* (1926); Aid for Dependent Children (AFDC) funds must be provided not only to 18–20-year-old students attending vocational schools, but also to those attending colleges and universities (*Townsend v. Swank*, 1971); and access questions, such as those affecting students with disabilities, are considered of constitutional status (*University of Texas v. Camenisch*, 1981).

All of these cases deal with the accumulation of intellectual capital by students. Oddly enough, when the Supreme Court came to the question of the intellectual capital of faculty, it was less sure of the value of knowledge – in *Ollman v. Evans & Novak* (1985), the Court held there was no libel case because there was no defamation when nationally syndicated columnists Evans and Novak described a professor as being without stature and having a research program that is 'hooted at' by his colleagues!

Public sphere

While the Supreme Court has not been using the language of civil society and the public sphere, it has repeatedly addressed questions arising out of the participation of higher education institutions in the larger public sphere and as venues within which public sphere activities can unfold.

The university in the public sphere

The Court has dealt both with questions of just what the public is for any given university, and of what members of the university community may do within that sphere.

The issue of a geographic locus for a college first rose to the Supreme Court in a fascinating 1871 case, *In re Pennsylvania*. Complaints were put forward by students when a college to which they had committed moved as part of a merger process intended to save the institution's financial life – they claimed their prepayments were contracts for educational services in a particular locale. Though the Court acknowledged that the move added to the cost for some, it took the position that the commitment was to an educational process, not a place.

In 1894, the question was again raised as to whether college administrators could move the college from its original site – and again the Court defended that right, noting this time that geographic location was irrelevant to the relationship between the college and the church that had established it (*Bryan v. Board of Education of Kentucky Annual Conference of Methodist Episcopal Church, South, et al.*, 1894). In the 1970s, however, the Court used government funding to justify the position that geographic limits by the Veterans Administration (VA), which administers the GI Bill, were acceptable. The legal home, rather than the infrastructural home, of a university determines its geographic location for such constitutional purposes.

In *Board of Regents v. New Left Education Project* (1972), the question was whether a state institution's public was local or statewide and, if the former, just what 'local' meant. The Supreme Court believed a University of Texas rule prohibiting a student from selling a newspaper on campus was potentially unconstitutional, but that further examination of the specific facts was needed to determine whether or not this was the correct analysis of the case. Rather than remand the case to the same state-level District Court that had earlier ruled in favor of the university, though, the Court wanted to send it back to a local-level Circuit Court that seemed more likely to be friendly to the First Amendment issues at stake. In order to justify this, the Court argued that University of Texas issues were merely local to those few communities in which state university institutions were located. While this may have been tactically appropriate given the political tensions of the times, Justice William O. Douglas vigorously dissented, arguing that the public of a state university system is by mandate the entire population of the state itself. Because the US judicial system relies heavily on precedent – dependence upon prior decisions at the same and superior court levels – Douglas' fear was that, irrespective of the momentary utility of the Court's position in this one case, a dangerous precedent had been set for all time.

Whether or not to include transient students within voting area populations for purposes of district boundary definition has also received Court attention. It held that it is constitutional not to include foreign students who do not in any event have voting rights (*Summers v. Cenarrusa*, 1973), but unconstitutional to exclude black students who do have voting rights (*Symm v. US*, 1979). In *Hadley v. Junior College District* (1970), the conflict was over bounding districts for the purposes of higher education itself.

The university as public sphere

Cases involving the make-up of the university community and constraints upon discourse within that community pertain to the university as a public sphere.

The diversity of the student body has been supported in a number of categories, including:

* gender (*Cannon v. University of Chicago et al.*, 1979; *Iron Arrow Honor Society v. Heckler*, 1983; *Mississippi University for Women v. Hogan*, 1982; *US v. Virginia et al.*, 1996);
* race (*Bazemore v. Friday*, 1986; *Bob Jones University v. United States*, 1983; *US v. Fordice*, 1992);
* citizenship (*Kleindienst v. Mandel*, 1972; *Toll v. Moreno*, 1982);
* obesity (*Salve Regina College v. Russell*, 1991);

- tax status (*Toll v. Moreno*, 1982; *Kimel v. Florida Board of Regents*, 2000); and
- percentage of the population receiving aid (*Cleland v. National College of Business*, 1978).

Regents of the University of California v. Bakke (1978) and decisions in lower courts of recent years, however, suggest this trend may see reversal. Educational disabilities not addressable within a particular institution are legitimate grounds for denying admission (*Southeast Community College v. Davis*, 1979).

The Court has upheld the right of universities to make evaluations of students and decisions regarding their participation in academic programs based on those evaluations. It importantly distinguishes between disciplinary and academic reasons for dismissing a student, emphasizing that due process applies to the former but not the latter (*Board of Curators of the University of Missouri v. Horowitz*, 1978).

It was held that students cannot be denied the First Amendment right to associate with others in a case involving the left-wing group Students for a Democratic Society (SDS). Here, the Court held that mere membership in an organization does not necessarily entail other specific commitments or behaviors; however, students could be denied the right to associate with particular organizations within the university environment if they refuse to abide by university regulations or will not disavow violence (*Healy v. James*, 1972).

Students do have speech rights even if content is:

- obscene (*Papish v. Board of Curators of the University of Missouri*, 1973);
- religious (*Widmar v. Vincent*, 1981);
- offered by someone on academic probation (*Papish*); or
- espouses unpopular causes or positions (*Norton v. Discipline Committee of East Tennessee State University*, 1970).

Conditions may be put on a campus seeking constitutional acceptance of a speech restriction (*Barnstone v. University of Houston*, 1980). The Court has several times declined to deal with issues involving speech on campuses by students (*Jones v. State Board of Education of Tennessee*, 1970; *Ratchford v. Gay Liberation*, 1978) and non-students (*Princeton University v. Schmid*, 1982), though Justice William O. Douglas vigorously argued that all such cases should be taken by the Court in his dissent in *Zwicker v. Boll* (1968).

On the faculty side, a university may refuse to renew a non-tenure track contract without explanation (*Board of Regents v. Roth*, 1972; *Perry v. Sindermann*, 1972), but may not prevent a person from seeing confidential peer review documents in cases of unfavorable tenure review (*University of Pennsylvania v. Equal Employment Opportunity Commission [EEOC]*, 1990). Constitutional protections for the First Amendment right to associate with others, threatened by oath requirements for faculty employed by public universities, were slowly built in a group of cases: *Sweezy v. New Hampshire* (1957) specifically linked academic freedom to the building of democratic capacity by the state; *Shelton v. Tucker* (1960) ruled it unconstitutional to ask about those with whom faculty members associated; oaths were declared unconstitutionally broad and vague (*Baggett et al. v. Bullitt et al.*, 1964); and the effort to distinguish between seditious and non-seditious speech that is an inevitable part of judgments regarding those with whom faculty associate was deemed dangerously chilling[4] to education (*Keyishian v. Board of Regents*, 1967). *Keyishian* distinguished between knowledge of aims of a group with whom one associates and the intention to help further those aims; the term 'subversive' itself is also difficult to interpret, and therefore should also not be used as a basis for personnel decisions (*Whitehill v. Elkins*, 1967).

The Supreme Court upheld a decision by the Attorney General to waive his right to prevent a Belgian journalist and Marxian theoretician invited to speak at an academic conference in the US from entering. There were grounds to do so because on an earlier visit the invitee had spoken at places not listed on his visa application. The Attorney General chose not to do so in order to protect the right of US citizens to receive information, a First Amendment right traceable in the courts to the early 1940s (*Kleindienst v. Mandel*, 1972).

A public university is a limited public forum (*Rosenberger et al. v. Board of Visitors, University of Virginia*, 1995; *US v. Irwin*, 1942), meaning that, while it is public space, an institution may balance free speech rights with its own right to protect the efficacy of the educational environment. Thus, an institution can restrict an activity on campus either with respect to its content or its location.

Implications of the cases

Several constitutive questions faced by universities were raised at the opening of this chapter, each affected by the use of new information technologies. The constitutional law reviewed here addresses many, though not all, of those questions. These cases provide the context within which these activities take place and can be used as weapons or tools at any time. This section looks again at the Supreme Court cases dealing with higher education to see what they have to say in response to each of the constitutive questions.

Autonomy

The use of new information technologies raises a number of questions for the autonomy of the university from the nation-state revolving around ownership of intellectual property rights, degrees of freedom available to universities seeking to restructure themselves, use of universities as an arm of the law, constraints on university activities that may derive from governmental contracts, and the role of universities in serving national economic development through training of the labor force. Legal constraints interact with economic issues in determining the actual relationships between the two, for the relative proportion of government funding of public universities in the United States is significantly reduced from the dominant position it has held historically.

The relationships formed by the long-standing US tradition of government support for university-based research are coming under stress as both institutions of higher education and the government seek to maximize the value of their intellectual property. The government, for its part, is increasingly interested in retaining intellectual property rights over the products of government-funded research, though frameworks for doing so are still emergent and contested; one recent step in this direction could be seen in legislation requiring greater public access to data generated by such research projects. Under these conditions, the reliance of public universities on protection from copyright infringement suits because of their relationship to the government, provided in *Florida Prepaid* (1999), may ultimately prove unfortunate. The tension between universities and the government in this area is likely to be one of the most provocative in coming years, and on this point the constitutional record must be described as ambiguous.

The growing interest in Web-based courses for both distance education and on-campus uses has exacerbated the trend away from tenured faculty towards non-tenure-track full- and part-time staff, and encouraged many universities to believe they can reduce the number of personnel through a restructuring of their activities. While such moves are strongly opposed by most faculty members, the Supreme Court has consistently upheld the freedom of universities to restructure and relocate at will, including the ability to redefine relationships with their employees. In this area, universities appear to be on firm constitutional ground to do as they wish.

Because universities provide computing and communication infrastructure for its faculty, staff, and students they in essence serve as Internet Service Providers (ISPs). Thus universities must abide by the Digital Millennium Copyright Act (DMCA), which requires ISPs to shut down e-mail addresses of those accused by copyright owners of infringing upon intellectual property laws. The DMCA dramatically changes the balance of power in cases of alleged copyright infringement, for it treats the accused as guilty until proven innocent; historically, in fulfillment of the US historical presumption of innocence until guilt is proven, those accused of copyright infringement were not treated as guilty until and unless they had lost their case in court. The DMCA also reduces university autonomy from the government, using that institution like others as extensions of the government's law enforcement capacity. Just as journalists have successfully relied upon constitutional law to resist being forced to serve law-enforcement functions through turning over information gathered to the government unless specific criteria have been met, universities in future may judicially resist the DMCA in order to protect free speech, as well as university autonomy, from the government.

Government funding in itself cannot constitutionally justify intervention into university activities, but government contracts for research in the area of new information technologies and for development of training programs and curricula are another means by which university autonomy may be constrained. Even First Amendment rights can be abandoned through voluntary acceptance of terms of a contract. Though the Court long resisted examination of course content in order to determine the constitutional status of an institution, *Cleland* set a dangerous precedent by sustaining indirect intervention into curricula through its lack of financial support for student participation in innovative courses. Growing government interest in the intellectual property rights of research products suggests the trend towards use of government contracts and research funds as a means of intervening internally in universities – with constitutional support – may be on an upward swing.

An unspoken issue lies beneath the rush of universities to incorporate the use of new information technologies into their curricula as well as their operations: the societal – and therefore governmental – need for a labor force skilled in, and comfortable with, these technologies. In the same way that the nineteenth century required a print-literate labor force, so the twenty-first century appears to require a computer-literate labor force. This justification for the transformation in the nature of higher education in the USA has solid constitutional support.

Economics

Throughout the history of US Supreme Court treatment of institutions of higher education, it has consistently upheld the right of universities to expand their domains of economic activity, to use economic arguments to justify internal decision-making and to reorganize at will. The use of new information technologies provides a number of temptations of these kinds, as universities identify possible new products (e.g., Web-based courses that can be marketed in their own right without further involving a faculty member), markets (e.g., via distance education) and means of cutting 'production' costs (e.g., restructuring in ways newly enabled by innovative technologies). In all three of types of efforts, universities have strong constitutional support.

Some very old developments in constitutional law have new applications in these areas. The nineteenth-century Supreme Court decisions that upheld the right of universities to create and control the use of their own seals, for example, may well come into use in the courtroom in Web domain-name appellations, as universities seek to protect both their individual identities and the general sector of higher education on the Web. The latter has come into play in debates over whether or not community colleges, for example, should be allowed to use the coveted '.edu' in their Web and e-mail domain names.

Many universities – traditionally non-profit organizations in the USA – are creating spin-off for-profit entities to engage in additional information industry activities, such as marketing to the public software and research-based patents. Like many other types of organizations, universities are also beginning to turn internal functions into products that can be marketed outside the organization. For example, just as law firms are marketing word processing functions externally, universities are marketing their ability to efficiently acquire intellectual property rights for course reading packets, which enable instructors to compile a set of published articles for their students to purchase, so that other universities do not need to develop that capacity themselves. Again, the Supreme Court has consistently supported treatment of universities as an organizational mixture, including both for-profit and not-for-profit functions and serving both educational and non-educational missions – though historically the latter has always been justified through the support it provides for the former.

The use of new information technologies has exacerbated the trend towards struggles over control of cultural property because it makes it so much easier to access, use, and alter a variety of forms of culture. Universities are likely to face legal problems around cultural property issues in future, not only through attacks on their ownership of cultural property in museums and archives but also through the way in which forms of cultural property are included in curricula as a means of achieving multiculturalism. Constitutional law provides little guidance in this area, since the Supreme Court declined to fully engage with the one pertinent case.

Public sphere

Despite the popularity of rhetorical claims that the use of new information technologies will expand the public sphere and ensure that a diversity of voices is heard within it, the incorporation of such technologies into universities appears to be reducing their role within the society-wide public sphere, as well as restricting discourse within higher education institutions as public spheres in themselves. The US Supreme Court has, however, used a university-based case to directly oppose one of the most significant current threats to freedom of speech: denial of protection to activities defined as information processing rather than expression (Braman, 1998).

The growing interest in for-profit activities by universities inevitably reduces their presence as critical voices contributing to discourse on matters of public concern within society at large. Here, the use of new information technologies is not, of course, the sole explanatory factor. However, it does play a contributory role in ways that have complete support from constitutional law, despite the constitutive function that higher education has historically been understood to play in the United States.

The contraction of the proportion of tenured faculty and simultaneous expansion of student numbers via distance education have had the combined effect of reducing the function of the university as a public sphere. With fewer tenured faculty staff, there are fewer voices. The vast expansion in distance education blurs the boundary between the university and the outside world, with the result that academic freedoms protected within purely academic contexts no longer have the same justifications for their defense. Quite simply, it is no longer sustainable to maintain the definition of a public university as a quasi-public forum in which speech rights are fully protected, up to the point at which the institution may constitutionally restrict them in order to serve institutional goals. In bricks-and-mortar institutions that do impose some restraints on speech, it is common practice to continue to promote the public sphere functions of the university by designation of particular places in which full expression on matters of public concern may be completely uninhibited. Finding a way of ensuring the same type of discourse space within university-based Web environments may be the most important issue raised by new information technologies that has not yet been addressed by higher education.

Denial of First Amendment rights to informational activities not specifically listed among the five in the First Amendment[5] is among the greatest threats to freedom of speech today. The Supreme Court has addressed this problem in a university-based case likely to rise in salience, *Kleindienst v. Mandel* (1972). Here the Court relied heavily on distinctions among types of information processing and communication for its decision supporting entry into the USA of a speaker invited to an academic conference whom many opposed because of his ideological position. Following an extended discussion of the ways in which different types of information processing and message transmission perform different functions – including elaboration of the reasons why the Court itself relies upon oral argument as well as written briefs and a variety of types of exhibits in order to form its judgments – the decision held that it is precisely because of such differences that protection for all were needed. The opinion concludes by making clear that the First Amendment protects the entire process of applying reason through public discussion, a definition of discourse that includes every stage of the information production, from reception through to reply.

Conclusions

As has happened during other periods of transformations of the social structure and of the economy, universities are renegotiating their identities, their internal structures, their places in the global information economy and their relations with other types of institutions, from publishers to the nation-state. Among the venues in which these negotiations take place is the court system, with the Supreme Court providing the ultimate battleground in the USA.

This analysis of the entire body of Supreme Court decisions dealing with higher education until mid-2000 yields a picture of a situation in which the autonomy of the university from the nation-state has largely been reinforced and universities are clearly free to operate at will economically, even if doing so comes at the cost to society of fulfillment of traditional educational missions and to faculty of jobs. Transformations in the nature of the universities tied largely to the use of new information technologies have weakened their roles within, and as, a public sphere – despite continued constitutional support for the public sphere, as for the educational functions.

The circumstances depicted here could alter as cases that may rise to the Supreme Court could be generated in coming years by issues such as tensions between higher education and the nation-state over ownership of the intellectual property produced by government-supported research, the extent to which production of a computer-literate labor force should dominate the mission and realities of universities, and governmental efforts to use universities as extensions of their law enforcement entities.

There will be enormous long-term cost to society of the abandonment of the public-sphere functions of universities, destruction of the circumstances that enable full-time devotion to an intellectual and scholarly life by faculty members and a turn away from traditional topics of study towards a focus on technical skills. While the use of new information technologies can facilitate such trends, and US constitutional law in large part supports such shifts, they are not legally required. Ultimately, the choices universities make as they renegotiate their relations with the nation-state, other institutions and the global information economy remain their own, as institutions with a significant degree of autonomy.

Cases cited in this chapter

Arkansas v. Texas, 346 US 368 (1953)

Baggett, et al., v. Bullitt, et al., 357 US 808 (1964)

Barnstone v. University of Houston, 446 US 1318 (1980)

Bazemore v. Friday, 478 US 385 (1986)

Bertell Ollman v. Rowland Evans & Robert Novak, 471 US 1127 (1985)

Bethel School District #403 v. Fraser, 478 US 675 (1986)

Bier v. McGehee, 148 US 137 (1893)

Board of Curators of the University of Missouri v. Horowitz, 435 US 78 (1978)

Board of Public Works v. Columbia College, 84 US 521 (1873)

Board of Regents v. New Left Education Project, 404 US 541 (1972)

Board of Regents v. Roth, 408 US 564 (1972)

Bob Jones University v. United States, 461 US 574 (1983)

Bryan v. Board of Education of Kentucky Annual Conference of Methodist Episcopal Church, South, et al., 151 US 639 (1894)

Cannon v. University of Chicago, et al., 441 US 677 (1979)

Cavanaugh v. Looney, 248 US 453 (1919)

Cleland v. National College of Business, 435 US 213 (1978)

Culver v. US, 271 US 315 (1926)

Florida Prepaid Postsecondary Education Expense Board v. College Savings Bank, 527 US 666 (1999)

Graves v. State of Minnesota, 272 US 425 (1926)

Hadley v. Junior College District, 397 US 50 (1970)

Hamilton v. Regents of the University of California, 293 US 245 (1934)

Hazelwood School Dist. v. Kuhlmeier, 484 US 260 (1988)

Healy v. James, 408 US 169 (1972)

Hendrick Hudson Central Board of Education v. Rowley, 458 US 176 (1982)

Hopkins v. Clemson Agricultural College, 221 US 636 (1911)

Hunt v. McNair, 413 US 734 (1973)

In re Pennsylvania College Cases, 80 US 190 (1871)

Iron Arrow Honor Society v. Heckler, 464 US 67 (1983)

Jetton v. University of the South, 208 US 489 (1908)

Jones v. State Board of Education of Tennessee, 397 US 31 (1970)

Keane v. Brugger, 160 US 276 (1895)

Keyishian v. Board of Regents, 385 US 589 (1967)

Kimel v. Florida Board of Regents, State University of New York, 528 US 62 (2000)

Kleindienst v. Mandel, 408 US 753 (1972)

Martinez v. Bynum, 461 US 321 (1983)

Mayer v. American Security & Trust, 222 US 295 (1911)

Millsaps College v. City of Jackson, 275 US 129 (1927)

Minnesota Board for Community Colleges v. Knight, 465 US 271 (1984)

Mississippi University for Women v. Hogan, 458 US 718 (1982)

Montana ex rel Haire v. Rice, 204 US 291 (1907)

National College Athletic Association (NCAA) v. Board of Regents, University of Oklahoma, 463 US 1311 (1983)

National College Athletic Association v. Smith, 525 US 459 (1999)

National College Athletic Association v. Tarkanian, 488 US 179 (1988)

National Labor Relations Board (NLRB) v. Yeshiva, 444 US 672 (1980)

Norton v. Discipline Committee of East Tennessee State University, 399 US 906 (1970)

Onondaga Nation v. Thacher, 189 US 306 (1903)

Osborne v. Clark, 204 US 565 (1907)

Papish v. Board of Curators of the University of Missouri, 410 US 667 (1973)

Perry v. Sindermann, 408 US 593 (1972)

Plyler v. Doe, 457 US 202 (1982)

Princeton University v. Schmid, 455 US 100 (1982)

Ratchford v. Gay Liberation, 434 US 1080 (1978)

Regents of the University of California v. Bakke, 438 US 265 (1978)

Regents of University of California, et al. v. Doe, 519 US 425 (1997)

Regents of University of Michigan v. Ewing, 474 US 214 (1985)

Roemer v. Maryland Public Works Board, 426 US 736 (1976)

Rosenberger, et al., v. Board of Visitors, University of Virginia, 515 US 819 (1995)

Salve Regina College v. Russell, 499 US 225 (1991)

Seton Hall College, et al., v. Village of South Orange, 242 US 100 (1916)

Shelton v. Tucker, 364 US 479 (1960)

Southeastern Community College v. Davis, 442 US 397 (1979)

Speer v. Colbert, 200 US 130 (1906)

Summers v. Cenarrusa, 413 US 906 (1973)

Sweezy v. New Hampshire, 354 US 234 (1957)

Symm v. US, 439 US 1105 (1979)

Taylor v. Columbian University, 226 US 216 (1912)

Thomas v. Board of Trustees of Ohio State University, 1195 US 207 (1904)

Thomas Jefferson University v. Shalala, 512 US 504 (1994)

Tilton v. Richardson, 403 US 672 (1971)

Tinker v. Des Moines School Dist., 393 US 503 (1969)

Toll v. Moreno, 458 US 1 (1982)

Townsend v. Swank, 404 US 282 (1971)

Trustees of Dartmouth College v. Woodward, 4 Wheaton (US) 518 (1819)

University of Pennsylvania v. Equal Employment Opportunity Commission (EECOC) 493 US 182 (1990)

University of Texas v. Camenisch, 451 US 390 (1981)

US v. Fordice, 505 US 717 (1992)

US v. Irwin, 316 US 23 (1942)

US v. Virginia et al, 518 US 515 (1996)

Whitehill v. Elkins, 389 US 241 (1967)

Widmar v. Vincent, 454 US 263 (1981)

Witters v. Washington Dept. of Services for the Blind, 474 US 481 (1986)

Wyoming Agricultural College v. Irvine, 206 US 278 (1907)
Zwicker v. Boll, 391 US 353 (1968)

Notes

1   The concept of state action refers to government involvement in activities. State action is required in order to trigger application of the First Amendment's protections for freedom of expression.

2   The GI Bill vastly expanded the number of students in the US higher education system after World War II by providing funding for attendance at colleges and universities by military veterans.

3   Beginning in the 1860s, the federal government passed legislation granting federal lands to states to be used or sold to raise funds for the establishment of universities. This created what is in the USA referred to as the public university system – state universities with governmental support and the mission of providing relatively low-cost higher education in subject areas such as agriculture and engineering believed by the government to be critical to the development of society. By the turn of the twentieth century these universities included in their curricula the broad range of humanities and social sciences as well as the physical and applied sciences. Today the role of state government funds in support of state universities is fast declining relative to other sources of funding, a development that is an important factor in university decisions regarding their uses of new information technologies.

4   'Chilling' is a very common term in US law. It is used to refer to situations in which the law does not directly inhibit speech activities, but it does permit situations to develop that will make it less likely certain types of speech will occur because the consequences would be so unpleasant.

5   The five rights specifically mentioned in the First Amendment are opinion (to think what you want to think); speech (to tell others what you think); press (to transport what you think to others across space and time); association (to get together with others to discuss what you all think); and petitioning the government (to ask for political change if, after the community discusses it together, change is sought). Privacy and the right to receive information are considered to be 'penumbral' to the First Amendment and other elements of the Bill of Rights. Additional information policy provisions, from establishment of the postal system to establishment of property rights in ideas and inventions, are included in the Constitution itself.

19 New media and distance education

EU and US perspectives

Alain Dumort

This chapter provides an overview of policy initiatives in North America and Europe aimed at promoting the diffusion and successful application of ICTs in higher education and learning. In it, Dumort explores the challenges posed by educational, technological and business change that need to be addressed in these policies. He also describes how ICTs are actually being introduced into education on both sides of the Atlantic, drawing lessons that indicate the ways in which new media can significantly improve the educational process through new partnerships between business and the academy.

The e-learning sector

A combination of forces in pedagogical thinking, technological progress and business models have raised new expectations for the widespread use of educational technology, such as by providing major market opportunities as in the adult training segment. This has confronted institutions across all sectors of education in the EU and the USA with the challenge of providing greater access to educational services, at the same time as they face constrained budgets and a dramatically increasing and more diverse population of students. Many public sector and private commercial initiatives for connecting schools to the Internet, first adopted in the USA, and then in member states of the EU, have met with marked success. The diffusion of ICTs in EU schools is particularly rapid, given their initially low penetration rate. If American organizations are indeed leading the development of online courses and programs in the higher education sector, European universities have now also realized the importance of investing in this field.

Over five million new students in Europe and in the USA are expected to join the higher education sector during the first decade of the twenty-first century. In this context, the benefits of developing new online and interactive content for education are gradually being recognized as one way to maintain or improve the quality of education, while controlling the cost and improving the productivity of a traditionally labor-intensive sector. The use of ICTs for educational delivery in higher education is not only expected to give scope for low-cost expansion through large economies of scale, but also to provide for new revenue or profit centers, at least in the USA.

Education, especially higher education and adult training, is seen as an emerging and potentially enormous value-added sector in which the 'e-learning' segment would play a significant role. For the USA, IDC (1999) estimated that about 1 million students were taking online courses in the late 1990s (7 per cent of the total enrolled), a number expected to reach 2.2 million, or 15 per cent of students, by 2002 (IDC, 1999). It suggested that the value of the US e-learning market was worth over $2 billion in 2001, covering over 15 per cent of the total education market and with the online segment representing as much as half of the training market. By 2005, IDC predicted the total online learning marketplace is expected to reach $50 billion. In the EU, the education market has remained smaller (about $500 million at the end of the 1990s) and more fragmented – but with a high potential for growth, given the boom in Web and Internet usage and the recent development of an international and European dimension in educational systems.

Numerous pilot experiments have been conducted in the last decade. They suggest that new media, and the Internet in particular, could revitalize the processes of teaching and learning when coupled with innovative pedagogical thinking (Lipponen et al., 1999). While the advantages of the Internet and networked learning have been a focus of much discussion (Anderson and Haughey, 1998), mainstream academic programs have not been as receptive to change as this rhetoric would suggest. One reason is that the findings of experiments to date relate to a limited range of learning outcomes, which restrain any large-scale generalization or comparison of their results. Also, educational technologies are used in most cases to enhance rather than replace existing modes of small group teaching, so they tend to add rather than reduce cost. This further limits their diffusion.

Forces driving the creation of a new educational climate

This situation I have described sounds familiar. However, a convergence of forces in Europe and the USA are driving expectations for a new cycle of media applications in education. This spread is seen, and justified, as being somehow inevitable, socially progressive and cost-effective, within the 'information society' paradigm (Lehtinen and Sinko, 1999). The driving forces behind these trends include:

- new, student-centered, pedagogical thinking that envisions learners playing a much more active role;
- decreases in the cost of technologies and services, along with special conditions for educational institutions (such as low flat-rates or large discounts in telecommunication tariffs and Internet access fees, as with the e-rate[1] in the USA);
- rapid diffusion and advancement of Internet technologies in both Europe, where 30 per cent of homes were connected in 2000 and the USA, with 45 per cent of homes connected;
- growing political commitment at national and EU levels to promote the widespread use of educational technologies through partnerships between institutions and businesses;
- new investments in campus information infrastructure to keep the university attractive and competitive;
- new thinking on the mission and 'core' functions of universities; and
- proven business opportunities in the corporate and adult training market.

Most countries have concentrated on developing ICT policy in schools, and it is only recently that they are realizing the importance of having initiatives for the higher education sector. But developments in this sector are moving ahead rapidly.

Trends in higher education

A whole new sector of higher education is emerging alongside traditional, national and state-regulated systems, through branch campuses, franchising and, most recently, by electronic means. In 2001, over 50,000 distance learning courses were proposed by universities, colleges and companies from 130 countries (see the International Distance Learning Course Finder, www.dlcoursefinder.com). The sector is mainly focused on the working adult market and still driven by American providers, such as business schools and training organizations, who can fully exploit the attraction of American universities to foreign students.

By 2001, around half the 3,000 US colleges and universities were claiming to offer some online education facilities as part of their curriculum. One-third of these institutions propose at least one complete degree, certificate or diploma (Institute for Higher Education Policy, 1999). By the end of that year, nearly 60 per cent offered some e-learning (*Business Week*, December 3, 2001). Yet only a few organizations can be defined as a 'virtual university', in the sense that their services are entirely provided online, without any campus-based activities.

Jones International University (JIU) is on the leading edge in that category as it became the first accredited cyber-university in March 1999. In 1999, it had 950 working adult students enrolled in business communication degrees entirely delivered via the Internet (the university has set a goal of 6,000 students by 2001). The University partners with the United Nations' Virtual Development Academy program. (See also Chapter Seven where Pamela Pease discusses JIU in detail.)

Existing universities have also launched online programs. The University of Phoenix (www.phoenix.com) is the largest private university in the USA. It has developed specific and diverse online courses for adults since 1978; by 2000, 10,000 students had enrolled online at the University, compared to the 65,000 enrolled on-campus. More traditional universities, including some of the most prestigious, have followed this path. These include[2]: Duke University (business); the University of California at Berkeley; University of Southern California (with USC programmes in gerontology, engineering and business); University of California at Los Angeles (through UCLA's Extension); University of Washington (Uwired programme) and University of Nebraska-Lincoln.

New commercial enterprises are being set up in partnership with some of the more prestigious universities. The UNext company brings together the University of Chicago, Columbia Business School, Stanford University, Carnegie Mellon University and the London School of Economics and Political Science, along with several Nobel prize winners (www.unext.com).

Other organizations have emerged that broker training services on behalf of a network of universities and colleges. These include the Western Governors University (www.wgu.edu) and the National Technological University (www.ntu.edu). Not all have been successful, such as the California Virtual University (www.california.edu) which, notably, was scaled back in 1999 to be little more than a Web site.

In this context of American initiatives, concerns have grown across Europe over the inertia, and capacity, of European educational institutions to provide excellent online educational facilities. The risks of not doing so would be great, including the loss of pedagogical credibility in the new networked environment, and therefore the prestige of educational institutions, as well as the loss of market opportunities in the continuing education and training segments, which could be highly profitable. Nevertheless, until 1999, the development of the virtual university was ignored by most public authorities and universities of Europe. For example, the action plan towards a European area of higher education proposed in 1999 by education ministers of twenty-nine European countries did not even mention this issue (this was a joint declaration signed in Bologna on June 1999, see the Web site of the European University Association at www.unige.ch/eua).

One reason for the EU's comparatively slow response, compared to the USA, is that almost all European universities are publicly funded. Moreover, as a public institution in Europe, education is expected to play a central role in ensuring social equality. Higher education cannot therefore be as easily discussed as a business-as-usual market, where profits can be pursued as a primary objective. Universities might have greater autonomy than many other public institutions in determining how to fulfill their mission, but they also face more severe budgetary restrictions.

That said, public authorities sense the need to re-examine the kinds of services that can be provided and how they can be delivered (Pouts-Lajus and Riche-Magnier, 1998, 1999). Most universities in Europe are planning, or are already using, Internet facilities to complement current activities. The introduction of online facilities has been partly linked to the strategy of the Open University. Five countries have created a national Open University since 1970: Germany (Fern Universität); the Netherlands (Open Universiteit); Portugal (Universidade Aberta); Spain (Universidad Nacional de Educacion a Distancia); and the United Kingdom (Open University). Other members of the EU promote open and distance learning directly through existing universities or a network of universities, such as Consorzio Nettuno in Italia and the Finnish Association for Distance Education.

Networking, brokerage and bench-marking apply at the European level as well with the European Association of Distance Teaching Universities (EADTU) (www.esc.ac.at/intkoop/eadtu.html) which aims at pooling and providing distance education programs to one million students through eighteen non-profit institutions from fourteen countries. Co-operation between European higher education institutions is driven through joint programs and common diplomas, which are provided increasingly online. One example is the MBA for executives jointly offered online to part-time students by the Institut d'Administration des Entreprises de l'Université d'Aix-Marseille and the Dutch Open University.

While current practices rely heavily on new ICTs as delivery systems, they demonstrate far fewer innovations in pedagogy, or accreditation and the certification of knowledge. Experiments are largely technology-driven and remain anchored in a traditional academic paradigm. Most of the institutions offer online courses and programs as an extension of their campus-based programs (Confederation of European Rectors' Conferences, 1999). While this model requires changes among faculty, student and administrative roles, it keeps existing institutional structures intact.

Increasingly, policy makers across Europe are concerned over how universities should respond to the new e-learning environment. Within the EU, working groups have been established in the member states, such as Finland and the United Kingdom, with a view to presenting policy recommendations, particularly on the regulatory frameworks under which higher educational institutions operate, including accreditation and quality assurance issues. The European Commission is launching a political initiative, called 'eEurope', which seeks to accelerate the use of ICTs, particularly applications of the Internet and Web, in all sectors (European Commission, 2000). One of the objectives is to constitute a Virtual European Higher Education Space through extensive co-operation between universities, open and distance institutions and training facilities.

Schools moving online

Developments in higher education are being shaped by initiatives at all other levels of schooling. By 1995, fewer than 3 per cent of schools in Europe were connected to the Internet and the availability of computers in secondary schools was over twenty-five students per computer. By the late 1990s, almost 90 per cent of secondary schools had been equipped and wired, the number of students per computer had dropped to an average of ten; crucially, every new teacher and an increasing number of on-the-job teachers were being trained in using ICTs (European Commission, 2001, 2001a). School connectivity in the USA grew at the same time from 65 per cent in 1996 to 95 per cent in 1999 with an average of six students per computer in upper secondary education (OECD, 2001).

If ICT penetration in schools within the EU and USA are converging, despite the persistence of high regional and local disparities, equipment remains less widely available across classrooms in Europe than in the USA. For example, 63 per cent of US public school instructional classrooms had Internet access in 1999 (14 per cent in 1996), compared to around 20 per cent in Europe, where preference has been initially given to more centralized computer labs. Nevertheless, the more recent take-up in Europe has meant that schools can benefit from the acquisition of more up-to-date technologies with more capacity and multimedia functionality.

These changes are significant, and a result of the implementation of action plans at the national and regional level since 1995 to equip and network schools, train teachers and promote the development of appropriate electronic content through public–private partnerships. More recent plans have been launched in France (Programme d'Action Gouvernementale pour la Société de l'Information), in the United Kingdom (The National Grid for Learning, The University for Industry), Germany (Schulen ans Netz), Ireland (Schools IT 2000), Finland (Towards an Information Society and the National Training Strategy for Education and Research), Sweden (Tool for Learning), or in Portugal (Nonio XXI Century Programme). These national initiatives have been complemented and extended at the European level, within the Commission's action plans on e-learning (European Commission, 1996, 2001, 2001a) and by the commitments of the European Council in charge of education (Council of Ministers of Education, 1996, 1997 and 2001).

While most EU countries have set themselves the target of providing all schools with Internet connection, the USA is still a couple of years ahead.

Teachers in the problem and its solution

Despite dramatic success in the spread of ICTs across universities and schools at all levels, their integration in the classroom remains a formidable challenge in Europe as well as in the USA. Lessons from early experience show that university teachers, like their colleagues teaching at other levels, often find it hard to change from traditional teaching methods. Technology itself does not improve learning automatically, nor does technology alter the teaching process in fundamental ways. New approaches to teaching and learning must be embedded in the thinking of teachers, the larger school environment and the curricula. In this context, a technological-push strategy aiming at boosting a virtual learning paradigm through a quick technological fix could lead to fundamental disappointments (Lehtinen and Sinko, 1999; Mutschler, Amor and Laget, 1999).

Recent surveys show that a majority of US and European university teachers use technologies in routine communication and administrative tasks. Few are using the Internet in their own research (only one-third of US teachers), while the actual overall use of ICTs in teaching also remains limited, with the exception of particular topics, such as statistics (Institute for Higher Education Policy, 1999; Institute for Applied Social Sciences (IASS), 1998).

The teacher's inability to integrate new media effectively into classroom instruction is therefore a fundamental block (Fisher, Dwyer and Yocan, 1996; IASS, 1998). In the UK, the British Communications and Technology Agency reported that fewer than one-third of trained teachers actually use technology in their day-to-day teaching. In a survey by the US Department of Education (1998), 80 per cent of teachers in 1998 said they did not feel prepared to integrate technology into their classrooms and 96 per cent reported that the most common training received was for basic computer skills, with almost nothing on the best ways to use the best tools to support the best kind of instruction.

This is not simply a matter of teachers resisting change. Shortage of time for teacher training and course development is one of the most important obstacles. Shortcomings in skills and lack of pedagogical and technical support are among the other common obstacles raised by teachers.

Next steps towards improving the use of IT in education

Much remains to be done in the USA and in Europe to improve the use of ICTs as a tool for learning, while also ensuring more equitable access to the products of these advances. Educators at all levels are facing the major challenge of bridging the 'Digital Divide' between and within communities, schools and universities. Access to and use of ICTs still depends on family income. Despite the high growth rate of Internet use, the gap in terms of education and income level with regard to home-based Internet access has not been reduced. Boys and men remain the main users of computers and the Internet compared to girls and women, with a focus on control devices and entertainment technologies. These social and gender differences in home-use tend to be duplicated at school for students and also teachers, most of whom are women.

The successful diffusion of educational technology depends at least in part on policy issues. One is the adequacy of financing and public investments in order to sustain the demands of educational institutions. As the level of expenditure on ICT in education has increased dramatically, serious concerns arise now over the return of investment. New educational technologies involve high development costs, and there is little evidence that ICT yet meets the promise of better education for more people at low cost. Another question of policy and practice being posed is how much should be allocated to the development of content rather than to the equipment and other aspects of the wired infrastructure.

With regard to content creation, the protection of copyrighted material is a central issue, particularly in the areas of music, movies and games. Laws protecting copyright holders are complicated and many young people – and some teachers – are unaware of the risks of sharing copyrighted content on the school's internal network. Resolving the legal issues surrounding the protection of privacy and the security of networks are critical to stimulating supply.

Beyond the economic and legal considerations, particularly for broadcasters and multimedia publishers, the evaluation of the educational and social benefit of new media raises three kinds of questions:

How can the Internet reinforce education?   The Internet has the potential to broaden both the scale and scope of content delivery at controlled cost, without sacrificing quality and the socialization of learners. However, the construction of knowledge, the process of creating common values and the achievement of mutual understanding require a sound, structured approach in order to manage and build on the flood of randomly-accessed information through the Internet.

What are the socio-economic benefits of 'tailor-made' education?   Private demand-led supply of online learning material increases the risk of inequity between people and countries in access to education and knowledge. Closing the Digital Divide is at the top of the political agenda. Parts of the solution in Europe and the USA will continue to be pro-competition policies aimed at reducing the prices of equipment and communication services, as well as universal service policies that seek to ensure affordable access to communities and public institutions such as at schools and libraries.

How can Europe best capitalize on its diversity of cultures and languages in an emerging global market?   This needs to take account of the way this market is dominated by Anglo-American content, pedagogical method, supply and technology investment.

The death of the Ivory Tower?

Are universities moving from 'brick and mortar' to 'click and mortar'? New challenges call for a better understanding of the issues at stake and for appropriate concerted decisions between all actors involved. Higher educational institutions are increasingly competing with other kinds of institutions in the production of knowledge (see Chapter Six). Technology and new private providers are challenging the authority and legitimacy of traditional universities and, to some extent, those of secondary schools (Baer 1999 and Chapter Twelve of this volume). However, the key issue is not the so-called 'end of the university', to be supplanted by the virtual university and digital library. The choice is not between revolution or collapse.

Nevertheless, the continued vitality of the university is indeed at stake. The use of ICTs in education will continue to follow a progressive evolutionary route. The university of tomorrow is more likely to offer a mix of on-campus and Internet-based off-campus courses in order to respond to increasing need for accessibility, diversity, flexibility and affordability of education services. One of the critical success factors for universities lies in their ability to address the lifelong learning market in collaborations, both amongst themselves and with private partners.

New media can enrich educational choices on a sustainable and cost-effective basis, if new business–academic partnership models can be developed. All actors need to move beyond current lines drawn between software and telecommunication companies, broadcasters and publishers, for-profit educational organizations and academic providers. These boundaries are too distinct and they are blurring rapidly.

New partnership models could enhance educational services, and therefore the emerging e-learning market, by exploiting the core competencies of all actors concerned and sharing risk and responsibility through a collaborative and competitive process. In one form of partnership, for example, the business partners would provide the Internet and communication infrastructures and the academic institutions would keep responsibility and control over course content, the selection of students and their certification. A wide variety of partnerships need to fuel any further digital initiative that policy makers may adopt in order to bring the educational benefits of new media to all categories of learners.

Notes

1   The e-rate is short for educational-rate and refers to a US federal government program that offers schools and libraries a special subsidized rate for telecommunication services (Benton Foundation, 2000).
2   The states of Kentucky and Florida are also supporting high-school initiatives.

20 The virtual university is ... the university made concrete?

James Cornford

Much empirical research on ICT initiatives in distance education and distributed learning has paid little attention to their cumulative impacts on the university as an institution. This chapter helps to explore such wider perspectives by drawing on in-depth studies of ICTs in university administrative and teaching activities in four established universities. Cornford's analysis argues that one of the often unintended consequences of the introduction of these technologies has been to generate demands and pressures for a more corporate institutional form in which goals, roles, identities and procedures are made explicit and standardized across the institution. He explains why this could mean that the closer institutions move towards the goal of becoming a virtual university, the more explicit – or 'concrete' – their institutional form becomes.

Assessing the implications of virtuality in higher education

The notion of a 'virtual university' is a potent vision of the future of higher education. This virtual university – a 'university without walls' – is seen as an institution that has torn itself free from the geographical confines of the campus, using the new communications technologies to connect learners, potential learners, teachers, researchers, alumni, employers, research funders and administrators in a flexible, ever-changing network organization. This vision has captured the imaginations of academics, university managers, educational policy-makers, corporate personnel, training managers and private entrepreneurs across the world.

302   *James Cornford*

Steps towards the creation of the virtual universities are under way in existing institutions, while a wide range of new institutions and collaborative ventures between existing organizations are being set up. But before we rush to embrace the virtual university, and all the novelty that it brings, perhaps we should look too at the wider implications of virtuality in higher education: what the move towards a virtual future means for higher education institutions, their structure and identity. As Phil Agre (Chapter Eleven in this volume) has pointed out, "information and communications technologies create incentives to standardize the world." What I want to do here is to build on this observation and argue that the pursuit of the virtual university may be having a major, perhaps paradoxical, impact on the institutional form and sense of identity of the university as it has developed in the twentieth century. Specifically, the application of the new technologies is generating a myriad of demands for re-institutionalization of the university as a far more 'corporate', one might even say 'concrete', organization.

Understanding the implications of virtuality for the university as an institution

This chapter draws on a two-year research project concentrated on the intensive study of a number of projects and initiatives at four established British universities, varying in terms of age, mission and structures.[1] Unlike much of the established research in this field, we were not concerned with evaluating these particular initiatives in their own terms, but rather with understanding their implications for the university as an institution. Informed by the work of Bruno Latour (e.g. 1987), Michel Callon (e.g. 1986), John Law (e.g. 1991) and others, we focused on the processes of constructing 'virtual university' as the building of actor-networks. This involves the stitching together, and thus reconfiguration, of various animate and inanimate actors (typically people, machines, texts and money), and the implications of this activity for the institution of the university as a whole.

We adopted a variety of research methods – including semi-structured interviews, documentary analysis, focus groups, direct and participant observation – directed at a number of ICT initiatives in teaching and learning, research and administration. Our focus has thus been on what John Law (1994) has called "heterogeneous engineering," the process by which those concerned with building the virtual university seek to enroll in their activities, and keep enrolled, various elements of the university, such as: clerical, academic and administrative staff; students; budgets and funds; computers and networks; consultancy reports; and policy statements.

The virtual and the university

What is the virtual university? How can we pin down this loose term? A range of future scenarios for the use of 'new media' in higher education are usefully provided by Cunningham, Tapsall, Ryan, et al. (1998), who describe the virtual university as follows:

> Picture a future in which students never meet a lecturer face to face in a class room, never physically visit the on-campus library; in fact, never set foot on the campus or into an institutional lecture-room or learning center. Such is the future proposed by the virtual university scenario.
>
> (ibid., 1998: 179)

What marks out the virtual university in this scenario is decomposition of the university as a particular place and its recomposition as a set of wholly mediated relationships, tied together by ICTs. As the findings of Cunningham and his collaborators suggest, few believe that this totalizing vision of a 'university without walls' is achievable. Perhaps fewer believe that it is desirable. We are not without any number of critiques of this vision of the virtual university. Newman and Johnson (1999: 80), for example, identify this vision as being based on a "naive sociology" which "ignores the role of apprenticeship and implicit craft knowledge in the generation of technical progress and scientific discovery" and the role of face-to-face interaction and group socialization. David Noble (1998b) has likened the rush to embrace the virtual university to the discredited extension colleges of the 1930 to 1950s, identifying this model as the "digital diploma mill", a commodified travesty of public higher education driven by corporate greed and the self-interest of administrators (cf. Readings, 1996). Langdon Winner (1998), pours ridicule on the whole process with his depiction of an "Automatic Professor Machine."

The notion of the virtual university is useful, not as a description of a particular type of institution, but rather as a description of a process or project which is being implemented, in different ways and with different intensity in existing universities, as well as in new institutions. Much of the excitement, exhilaration and fear (see, for example, Marchese, 1998) concerns the establishment of new institutions – 'green field' sites – with US for-profit institutions, such as the University of Phoenix and Jones International University, as the classical exemplars.

However, these institutions, influential as they are, account for a tiny proportion of the higher education sector.[2]

The bulk of the work of building ICTs into higher education is, in fact, taking place in existing and established institutions – what, by contrast, we may regard as 'brown field' sites. In the jargon of industrial economists, it is 'in situ restructuring'. Cunningham, Tapsall, Ryan, et al. (1998), for example, found little interest among media and computing companies in establishing wholly new commercial higher education service provision, virtually all preferring to work *with* established universities (as suppliers or partners). The actual building of the virtual university is, then, predominantly taking place within, and on the edge of, the well-established institutional context of existing universities, albeit sometimes in close co-operation with technology vendors. It is also important to see the virtual university project as extending across the whole of the university: the virtual university is not just a matter of 'distance' or 'flexible' teaching and learning systems but extends into administration (finance, personnel, purchasing, estates, etc.), student recruitment and alumni management, research networks, library systems and so on.

The research context: a rapidly-changing national and international university system

The context of our research has been the British university system during a period of rapid change in its national and international environment (Newby, 1999; Schuller, 1995). Expansion in the 1990s increased the number of students studying at Higher Educational Institutions (HEIs) in the UK by some 40 per cent in a decade. While student numbers have increased dramatically, increased resources have been much more modest, leading to a declining per capita resource. The introduction in the late 1990s of tuition fees for an undergraduate student has made the financial relationship between the university and the student far more direct.[3] Further, with university revenues tied to student numbers, students are increasingly being actively recruited rather than passively selected.

Expansion has also changed the characteristics of the student body (Silver and Silver, 1997): even undergraduate students are increasingly less likely to be the traditional young adults engaged on a 'rite of passage'. Central government is seeking, through the funding system, to provide encouragement for the recruitment of 'non-traditional' students, leading to a demand for different kinds of support and procedures. Finally, students, both traditional and non-traditional, are seen as coming to universities with more demanding expectations, in terms of technologies and administrative efficiency.

At the same time that universities have sought to cope with expansion, and partly in reaction to the stresses which expansion has generated, there has been increasing demand from the state for accountability for public funds and 'quality' of the teaching and research which those funds procure. The simple reporting of statistics to the central Higher Education Statistics Agency (HESA) – which itself led to the introduction of a major program of computerization in universities (see Goddard and Gayward, 1994) – has been augmented by an increasingly invasive set of audits (see Strathern, 1997). The Research Assessment Exercise (RAE) and the Teaching Quality Assessment (TQA) have systematically sought to evaluate research and teaching respectively, leading to the establishment of 'league tables'. These audits are directly (RAE) or indirectly (TQA) increasingly determining the real levels of resource in university departments. The growing professionalization of university teaching through the establishment of the Institute for Teaching and Learning in 1999, of which all teaching staff are being very strongly encouraged to become members, and the new Quality Assurance Agency in 1997, also represent responses to the demands for accountability.

In addition to increasing attempts by the British state to steer higher education, there are also pressures acting on HEIs from both above and below the national scale. At the international scale, universities are increasingly seeking to compete for lucrative foreign (non-EU) students paying a high fee (see for example Halliday, 1999) and to recruit academic staff from an increasingly international labour market. In terms of international research contracts and grants, such as those from the European Commission, British universities are in a much more competitive environment. Equally, at the local and regional scale, there is increasingly recognition of, and state encouragement for, the role of universities in the community, in technology transfer and in supporting local moves in the transition towards a 'knowledge-based' economy (Goddard, Charles, Pike, et al., 1994).

To summarize, British universities face increasing student numbers and an increasingly heterogeneous student body, declining per capita resources, increasing state demands for audit and accountability, fiercer competition for students and research funds and an increasingly complex set of regional, national and international linkages and commitments. This, then, is the external context in which ICTs are being developed and deployed, the context in which the notion of the virtual university has suddenly become so appealing.

Implications for the organization and sense of identity of universities

What does this mean for the university, for the way in which it is orga-nized, and for its sense of identity? The responses to these pressures have been widely analyzed in terms of the growth of managerialism, a transition that Parker and Jary (1995) have christened the 'McUniversity' (c.f. Ritzer, 1998) and which Shore and Wright (1999) characterize as a "new and coercive form of authoritarian governmen-tality." Yet the picture that emerges from our research is more complex than is suggested by a simple binary divide between 'the traditional university' and the 'managerial university'.[4]

Ian McNay (1995) has provided a useful map (Figure 20.1) which lays out what he calls "the four cultures of the university." He identi-fied each of the four categories by the particular characteristics of the policy-definition procedures (defined as loose or tight) and the mode of control over implementation (again defined as loose or tight):

- The *collegium*, characterized by loose policy definition and loose control of implementation, is an institution in which individuals and departments have a high degree of autonomy both in what they do and in how they do it. As an institution, the university is a weakly-articulated collection of individuals and small teams.
- A *bureaucracy*, with a loose definition of policy but a tight control of implementation, allows a high degree of autonomy for individuals in the selection of aims and objectives but within a context of precise rules for implementation. Goals or policy are typically negotiated by committees and are loosely defined, but implementation draws on standard operating procedures and practices which are generalized to the institution as a whole. The institution exists primarily as a set of rules.
- The *corporation*, characterized by both tight policy definition and tight control over implementation, rigidly constrains both goals and the means by which they can be met. This is the most rigid, or concrete, institutional form with strong centralized control promoting articulation between the parts and the whole.
- The *enterprise*, with clearly-defined central policies but having control over implementation more loosely exercised, establishes clear goals for the institution while allowing considerable autonomy in the ways in which they are met. The institution is defined primarily by its goals or mission.

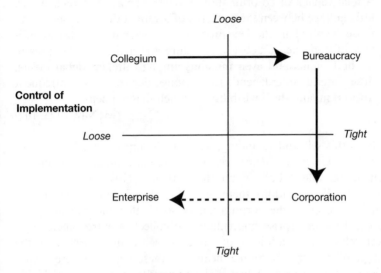

Figure 20.1 Models of universities as organizations
Source: Adapted from McNay, 1995: 106

Of course, as McNay (1995: 106) notes, "all four co-exist in most universities." Nevertheless, he sees a clear progression over the past decades in terms of the dominant culture, specifically from collegium to bureaucracy to corporation to enterprise, culminating in a "fragmented" or "atomized" institution characterized by small, task-focused work units – each having economic and managerial control over its own destiny, interconnected through "benign computer and communication links" and bonding into larger organizations through "strong cultural bonds" (ibid.: 114). In short, McNay's vision aligns closely with that of the 'virtual university'.

Our own studies of universities suggest that this image is too simple. In spite of more than a decade of managerialist reform, the collegium or the 'traditional university' remains an important self-image or paradigm for most university institutions, albeit one that is often understood to be under threat (and which may never really have existed). Many of the university administrators and senior academics in managerial positions that we have spoken to describe their own institutions in terms that uncannily echo McNay's description of "the classic collegial academy":

> A relative lack of co-ordination; a relative absence of regulations; little linkage between the concerns of senior staff as managers and those involved in the key processes of teaching and learning; a lack of congruence between structure and activity; differences in methods, aims and even missions among different departments; little lateral interdependence among departments; infrequent inspection; and the 'invisibility' of much that happens.
>
> (McNay, 1995: 105)

Given this self-understanding, where is the university as an institution? Like Gertrude Stein's celebrated remark about Oakland, it often seems that "there is no there, there." However, as McNay argues, in all institutions there are elements of bureaucracy (rules, formal roles, etc.), the corporation (co-ordinated means-ends planning) and the enterprise (individual and collective entrepreneurship). Nevertheless, the traditions of collegial self-management and the heritage of rule by committee mean that these tendencies are always held in check to some extent. 'The university' appears as a highly heterogeneous and poorly articulated institutional ensemble, which to a large extent exists in the heads of the people who constituted it, and in a myriad of locally negotiated practices and interactions. This traditional university, *as an institution*, often appears to exist only 'virtually'.

Building the virtual university in practice

In the attempt to shift to the model of the virtual university, the application of new ICTs, aligned with the imposition of increasingly short-term and instrumental policy goals by the principal funders of higher education, does not seem to be favoring the flexible enterprise model, as suggested by McNay. Rather, the technology initiatives we have studied appear to be generating pressures for the establishment of a far more 'corporate' form of organization where both policy formation and policy implementation are far tighter and where goals, roles, identities, abstract rules and standard operating procedures are made explicit and formalized. It is in this sense, then, that we can say that the virtual university may be a far more concrete organization than its predecessor. Some examples can help to illustrate this tendency in the universities we have studied.

Open University students and commensurability

The Open University (OU) is perhaps the nearest thing to a large 'virtual university' in the UK (see also Chapter Thirteen, this volume). On its own, it represents 21 per cent of all part-time higher education students in the UK. OU students interact with the University in two main ways. Courses are developed by Course Teams, predominantly based at the University's Milton Keynes headquarters. This course material is then delivered using a mixture of media, including books, television programs, video cassettes, paper course packs, and more recently CD-ROMs and the World Wide Web, with the particular mix depending on the course. The second type of interaction with the University is through course tutors (increasingly known as Assistant Lecturers), and this is organized on a regional basis. Students and tutors have traditionally interacted through face-to-face meetings and over the telephone. Some tutors are permanent members of staff (known as 'Staff Tutors'), but most work part time for the OU (often lecturers in conventional universities and colleges). Many courses also have intensive summer schools.

While the OU has undertaken a lot of work centrally on the provision of course materials, it is only more recently that it has sought to use online technologies to mediate the relationships between tutors and students. Student–tutor interaction is primarily facilitated by means of the First Class Conferencing system which gives students access to a number of conferences as well as e-mail. Assessment in the OU is generally in one of two forms: Computer Marked Assignments (CMAs) and, more commonly, Tutor Marked Assignments (TMAs). As the University has deployed the First Class Conferencing System, and made increasing use of e-mail, it has begun to adopt the practice of Electronic Tutor Marked Assignments (ETMAs) in which the student's assignment is submitted, marked and commented on electronically, before being sent to the University centrally and returned to the student by e-mail. This is, of course, a fairly mundane use of the new technology. Yet it has also had its effects, generating new demands on the university centrally. One OU Staff Tutor puts it as follows:

> As you know there are a lot of problems, a hell of a lot of problems ... now because of the technology you get a greater flow of information. So you get things like: a student gets 45 in Bristol, I got 75 in Newcastle. Then they start being able to compare. Now, this never happened before.... With the advent of ETMA (Electronic Tutor Marked Assignments) then a student has the script there marked in electronic form. So he can zap it off and

they can compare comments. "What my teacher said here, your teacher didn't pick that up".... You can try to standardize the marks, and we do that by giving pretty detailed marking schemes, ... but for comments – and our teachers are judged as much on their commentary as on the allocation of marks – ... but the commenting is from minimal to reams. Some tutors write loads and loads of stuff and they're still doing it in electronic form.

(OU Staff Tutor J, interviewed on 14 July 1999)

What has changed here? The tutor's comments are simply encoded in electronic form rather than in ink. However, the effect of this re-coding, coupled with the availability of e-mail to the students, is to make those comments far more mobile. It is this mobility that renders them visible to fellow students and thus comparable by them, which, in turn, generates demands for commensurate treatment. The effect on the University is to create a pressure to standardize not just the marking schema (which it has always done) but also the amount and format of the tutors' comments.

Indeed, as with the more traditional campus universities, staff within the OU are clear about the effects of the institution's increasing use of ICT to mediate between tutors, students, permanent staff and the administration. Another Staff Tutor describes the implications of ICTs for the Open University thus:

I think that they have found that if they suddenly say "oh, every-thing's electronic" and just let everybody do their own things, you basically get chaos. And you cannot have chaos. The only way, then, is to have structures and models. What they are trying to home into is the *kind* of structures and models: what the course team, any course team, should be responsible for, what the remit and role of the tutor is and what the remit and role of the student is. That is formalizing things to a far greater extent.

(OU Staff Tutor I, interviewed on 14 July 1999)

The key words of the corporate university are all there: structures, models, roles, remits, formalization.

Administrative systems in a large campus-based 'Redbrick' university: "That's a matter for policy!"

The demand for a more corporate response from the institution is certainly not confined to the field of teaching and learning, but extends to new administrative and management systems. For example, a large single-campus university we studied was in the process of implementing the financial, human resource, and research management modules of a new management information system provided by the German software house SAP, prior to adopting a student management module. For the Pro-Vice-chancellor in charge of the project, at least, the principal aim of the project is explicitly to "bind together a decentralized organization." [5]

The implementation is being handled by an implementation team made up of University staff and specialist consultants. We directly observed meetings between members of this implementation team and the 'faculty support team' (members of central departments, such as finance, attached to the faculty) and representatives of the departments that were going to pilot the new system. The consultants have a set of 'workflow process diagrams' which describe the proposed sequences of events by which tasks will take place within the new system, such as setting up a research account, raising a purchase order or issuing an invoice. Each step of the process is described in detailed flow diagrams, indicating the parts of the process that take place 'on the system' and those taking place 'off the system', as well as constraints on who can undertake which tasks and the order in which tasks are to be undertaken. Each of the workflow process diagrams is discussed with the departmental representatives and faculty team. The aim of the session is to clarify the workflow processes, iron out any problems which arise and identify who does what and when.

As the meeting moves through the workflow diagrams, a number of basic rules of the system are made clear, for example that two separate 'logins' are required to complete each and every external transaction – the same 'login' cannot order and receive goods. At some points, the workflow diagrams are amended to better reflect the current practice (although this amendment tends to happen more with 'off system' events). At a number of stages in the process, it also becomes clear that there is more than one way, in current practice, in which a particular step in the process can be handled. If the issue cannot be resolved one way or another, the consultant leading the meeting typically identified the issue as "a matter for policy" – a matter on which a definitive ruling must be given centrally by the university.

What seems to be happening here, as the computer system is rolled-out through the university, is more than a mere standardization of working practices and clarification of roles. Rather, the roll-out of the system makes visible the variety of local practices and, where these cannot be reconciled with the system (and thus with each other), generates a constant flow of demands for 'policy'. Indeed, from interviews with members of the implementation team we know that each of these requests for a central university policy decision was logged centrally by the team in a database and passed onto the University management to resolve. The process not only sees the tightening up of roles and procedures, but it also demands a tightening up of policy that will not apply locally, but across the whole university – in effect calling the university into being as a far more corporate institution. We might almost say that the roll-out of the system is requiring the simultaneous roll-out of a new, and more standardized, institution to host it.

(Re-)creating the institution

These pressures for a more standardized and corporate kind of university are not only happening as a result of the cumulative (and perhaps unforeseen) consequences of the move to an increasingly computer-mediated institution. In some institutions, they are more or less consciously planned as such. For instance, a large university in our study, which was formerly a polytechnic, has established a program on 'excellence' in the use of ICTs. This has a number of strands concerned with infrastructures (the Internet as a 'global campus'), the commercialization of knowledge, support services (a 'Multimedia Authoring Laboratory') and a set of experimental 'Flexible Learning' projects. There were a number of sites of experimentation with new technologies in the university prior to the start of the program, and the program was founded to link-up, support and extend this experimentation across the whole organization. The Program's Director describes it thus:

> Excellence in use of [Communication and Information Technologies] C&IT ... was a way of going right across faculty and departmental boundaries, breaking them down. And that's the whole ethos behind the project – that we want to share experience across the University rather than reinventing wheels in every little corner.
>
> (Program Director, interviewed on 13 March 1999)

A major component of the program is a number of experiments in using ICTs for 'flexible and distance learning'. The key concern for the Program Director, however, is not particularly to have a raft of successful projects, but rather to develop models of distance and flexible learning that can be scaled up to the institution as a whole. A key sponsor of the program describes it thus:

> What we wanted out of it was not some projects that in their own terms were successful and maybe glamorous in the world outside, but models that might be scaleable for the institution for distance and flexible learning, that could survive the transition from the enthusiasts – who will make it work come what may – to regular line provision.
>
> (Service Director, interviewed on 12 March 1999).

The ultimate aim is thus to establish the precise structures, roles and responsibilities necessary to implement online learning, as explained by the Program Director:

> Currently, because of the way the program is going – and it is a development program and I think that we'll stress that – a lot of the pseudo-admin work has been done by academic staff. They're doing the tracking, they're setting the things up. But to me, when you run it, as probably they will run it in the future, it would be too expensive for them to do that so the administrators would need access rights and they could do some of the humdrum day-to-day checking of whether work's come in, how many times a student has logged on etc. etc. So we will need to define, and I think rewrite, the roles and responsibilities.
>
> (Program Director, interviewed on 13 March 1999)

The familiar issues of commensurability and consistency arise. As the Service Director quoted above puts it: "We ought to be able to tell a student in Kuala Lumpur: if you become a student of the University of [name], what's the deal – and that ought to be consistent across the piece."

Once again, the key words, in this case much more explicitly coded into university policy, are to rebuild the institution around the technology. The Service Director is again clear about all of this:

> The thing that trips it up isn't that the technology doesn't work, its trying to recreate the organization so that it can usefully apply the technology, rather than crippling [the technology] so that we can do things the way we did before.
>
> (Service Director, interviewed on 12 March 1999)

314 *James Cornford*

The goal then, is to make the whole organization 'very corporate by university standards':

> rather than making a whole lot of decisions in various places and after the event hoping that they fit together, rather you co-ordinate ... All those decisions are made more collaboratively in the context of the whole .
>
> (Service Director, interviewed on 12 March 1999)

What the program seeks to achieve, then, is coherence at the center, decisions made 'in the context of the whole', 'consistent across the piece'.

Heterogeneous engineering: what is happening to the university as an institution

What is going on here? What does all this mean for the university as an institution? The process of trying to apply ICTs in the context of more or less traditional structures appears to generate demands for the construction of a new institutional structure capable of co-ordinated action with formalized roles and standardized practices into which the technologies can be fitted, and in which they can operate. These demands literally call into being a different, and more 'concrete', type of institution: one in which the heterogeneity of the institution is reduced in the sense that the various parts of the organization must be made to fit together and be aligned in the same direction. Indeed, what we have found is that attempts to build the virtual university from the bottom-up, course-by-course, without reconstructing the basic structures of the university appear to be very slow, labor intensive and highly prone to failure.

For example, we followed the progress of a number of initiatives led by the Learning Development Services department in another new university (former polytechnic) for over a year:

* a humanities degree course, where video-conferencing technologies were used to connect undergraduates based in the UK with students located in other parts of Europe, the idea being that they could present work and ideas to each other, and receive feedback, much like a traditional seminar;
* a new 'Cyber Culture' course, available for credit as a self-study module over the Internet; and
* the 'Information Skills' module taught by library staff, which had also been translated into an online self-study module.

Week after week we sat in on technical sessions and planning meetings as the academic material was gathered, the technology was developed, and the actual form of these initiatives began to take shape. Staff who were keen to be involved in the rolling-out of the projects were contacted, and possible groups of students willing to be part of the experiment were identified.

Yet, just a couple of months after everything had seemingly been put in place, each of the projects – for want of a better word – 'stalled'. The immediate reasons for this are varied: one of the partners pulled out of the video-conferencing project complaining of high telecommunication costs; only one distance student had enrolled for the Cyber Culture course; and library staff could not be convinced that the online version of the Information Skills course was sufficiently improved to warrant its introduction in place of their existing methods.

However, what is common to each of the stories from our study is the failure to enroll, or to keep enrolled, all the aspects of the university, or its partners, necessary to make the projects work, such as academic staff, students, computer services departments, libraries, validation committees and partner institutions. Further, in this case there were aspects of the University crucial for the success of the projects that did not exist, and therefore had to be built. For example, the University lacked procedures for validating online courses, slowing the whole process. Each of the initiatives was confounded by difficulties in co-ordinating a wide range of actors across a large organization made up of diverse and disparate entities (departments and service units) which lacked suitable procedures for interacting with each other. Returning to John Law's (1994) notion of heterogeneous engineering, the very heterogeneity of the university, it seems, often defeats the best attempts of the 'engineers'.

Conclusion: Information and the "view from nowhere"

I have tried to show how the implementation of ICT initiatives in a number of higher educational contexts seems to consistently generate demands for a more concrete institutional context characterized by tighter policy implementation and tighter policy definition. This is not to say that such demands will be heeded, or that if they are they will generate a response. Equally, there is no guarantee that any response will be successful in reducing the heterogeneity of the institution. There may be active, organized resistance to such attempts to re-define goals, roles and procedures.

In our work, we found remarkably little evidence of such active resistance. Alternatively, there may be a more passive kind of resistance to the introduction of more standardized procedures and formalized roles. We did come across this kind of rejection in some cases, although this must be weighed against considerable enthusiasm in other cases. Sometimes, rejection of attempts to reinstitute the university took the form of shunning or eluding attempts to establish the new order. In other cases, staff created their own 'workarounds' in order to fit the new procedures associated with ICTs into established local practice (Pollock, Chapter Sixteen in this volume).

What emerges, we suggest, is not a wholly new order, but rather a new hybrid of 'formal infrastructure' and 'local knowledge' (see Star and Ruhleder, 1996). It is not *inevitable* that more corporate or concrete institutions will emerge from the pursuit of the virtual university. This is a story about a process rather than an outcome. Nevertheless, the initiatives which we have studied do seem to consistently generate, at least, the *demand* for a more concrete university and where a response to that demand is not forthcoming, little progress will be made.

Why should this be so? Perhaps the place to start is with the notions of information and communication which sit at the root of the notion of a virtual university and its ability to abstract from, to transcend, place – the specific, the parochial. The promise of the virtual university is that, by translating the established processes of the university into information, and thus into a form that is amenable to technologically-mediated storage and distribution, these processes can be made mobile and can be re-combined in new ways and in new places. This is the vision of the fragmented, but flexible, network or virtual university with which we began. Yet this flexibility does not come without costs. The shift to a conceptualization of the university in terms of information and communications, on which such flexibility depends, contains within it a powerful incentive to formalize, to standardize, to make explicit. As Theodore Porter (1994) argues,

> the creation and use of information needs to be understood first of all as a problem of space and of scale, of getting beyond what is local, personal or intimate and creating knowledge that is, so far as possible, neutral and well standardized.

> (ibid.: 217)

"The ideal," he suggests, "is to go beyond perspective, to turn a view from somewhere into a "view from nowhere" (ibid.). Note how closely this 'view from nowhere' mirrors the promise which ICTs hold for the university: of permitting an escape from the confines of the campus, entry into a global higher education market, the possibility of being present everywhere. Further, as Porter (ibid.: 229) notes, "the history of information," understood as "knowledge detached from the skills and close acquaintanceships that flourish in local sites," "is almost synonymous with the history of large enterprises."

British universities have always been relatively large organizations, and have recently got significantly larger, yet they appear to have survived until now without much of the formal corporate structures of other large institutions. In part at least, this has been because they have been resistant to the allure of "a world of information," understood as "a world of standardized objects and neutralized subjects" (ibid.: 221). Rather, the traditional university (collegium) has seen itself as concerned with a different kind of knowledge, as a "local site where skill and intimate familiarity with people and things provide the most promising route to success" (ibid.). The price which the university may have to pay for the flexibility which information brings is a new, and harsher, institutional environment for some of those values around which it has traditionally cohered – and their replacement by more concrete means of holding the institution together.

Notes

1 The 'Space, Place and Virtual University' project was funded under the UK Economic and Social Research Council's Virtual Society? program (see virtualsociety.sbs.ox.ac.uk). It included studies in north-east England at the Universities of Newcastle, Northumbria, Sunderland and the regional center of the Open University examining ICT projects in teaching, research and administration.
2 For example, in the most developed market, the USA, new for-profit universities such as Phoenix constitute "only 2 per cent of degree enrollments" and "publicly-listed educational services companies constitute only 3 per cent by value of the billions of dollars spent on education and training in the US" (Ryan, 2000: 2).
3 The annual fee was up to £1,000 (about $1,500) in 1999.
4 These binary models strongly echo Weber's dictum: "The choice is only between bureaucracy and dilettantism in the field of administration" (quoted in Halsey, Trow and Fulton, 1971: 100).
5 Observation at Project Away Day, June 4, 1998.

21 Enhancing discourse on new technology within higher education

Michele H. Jackson and Stephen D. McDowell

Many universities have recently spent much effort in trying to react to actual and perceived educational and institutional changes tied to ICTs. However, fostering open and empirically-grounded debate within higher education on the changes taking place has been made difficult by rapid technological innovation, threats to traditional practices and institutions, and shifting perceptions of the university's role in an information society. In this chapter, Jackson and McDowell reflect on their own institutional setting to argue that nurturing such a debate would enable institutions of higher education to make valuable contributions to public knowledge and policy formation. They examine how such a debate could explore both how communications technologies are shaping our experience of time and space and, even more significantly, the kinds of choices we have about how we use ICTs and other methods to shape meaningful social and political life.

Why open and informed debate about new media in higher education is vital

Those of us working in higher education in the United States can testify to the many ways in which changes involving the use of ICTs have caught many of us unaware. Our students, our offices and our classrooms are increasingly wired. Where once we shut the classroom door to focus our students and engage in instruction, we must now ask for all cell phones and beepers be turned off – assuming, of course, that our teaching still occurs in the classroom rather than being mediated by satellite, cable or cyberspace. Our offices no longer house lots of typewriters, and professors spend hours peering into a computer screen rather than poring over manuscripts. Not only are the characteristics of our traditional environment changing, but also opportunities are presenting themselves for supplanting that environment altogether. Advertisements in current issues of professional publications, such as the *Chronicle of Higher Education* or *Academe*, are dominated by ICT providers tailoring their services to higher education: "Use our systems in your classroom!"; "Use us instead of your classroom!"; "Why worry about classrooms at all – attend a virtual university!"

In this chapter, we don't weigh in with a vote for the desirability of these changes or the likelihood of one type of configuration or another. Nor are we commenting on the need for more research on ICTs. The explosion of popular and policy attention given to ICTs is mirrored by an equally steady and expanding multidisciplinary stream of research and publications. Rather, our observations and analysis are drawn from our professional positions within higher education. We are both university faculty members, we teach and conduct research into questions relating to ICTs and we have seen our departments, colleges and universities face the challenge of responding to the growing presence and effects of new ICTs. Our aim here is simply to encourage members of higher education – our colleagues – to reflect on the experiences occurring within the university due to rapid technological change, and to reflect on the quality of our discourse about those changes.

How, then do we in the academy talk about new media to each other? Such a question is, of course, polemic. Whether or not we, as a community, engage in this meta-discussion about how to discuss ICTs, we will have to respond to them, make our decisions, adapt and cope. More precisely, then, how do we provide for a level of discourse within the university out of which a sustainable body of knowledge can emerge to direct and support decisions regarding the development, uses and regulation of ICTs?

The purpose of this exercise, pointedly, is to draw us out of the *abstraction* of the university as a place of higher learning. Instead, the aim is to conceptualize the university as a specific type of organization composed of individuals engaging in ongoing interactions and processes that serve to *enact* or continuously structure the 'university' as an institution (Giddens, 1984). The organizational members of the university – professors, students, administrators and so on – are still rather distinct from other institutions: they not only construct understandings of their own institution, but through teaching and research also have as their collective project the understanding and improvement of the larger world in which we live.

The difficulty of reflection during a period of accelerated change

Development and use of ICTs and associated reorganizations of production in the late twentieth century have brought changes in production and culture, especially those related to the reconfiguration of time and space (Harvey, 1991). Geographers have referred to the "collapsing of time and space" (Brunn and Leinbach, 1991) related to the development and use of new communication and transportation infrastructures. Similarly, political economists note that the use of new technologies follows from strategies to control (Mulgan, 1991), which organize production across space in new ways – what Mosco (1996) calls "spatialization."

These changes are wrought not only through the use of new ICTs, but also through the pace of the changes in the technologies themselves. Product cycles, once framed in terms of years to market, have shortened to months. Products themselves are often outdated within only a few years. Institutions, such as universities, wishing to keep up with these changes must act quickly in committing to a technology, even before there may seem to be adequate time to assess its appropriateness or its implications.

Through iterations of this process, we will experience further acceleration of social relations and reduction in time. As Bearman (1986) argues:

> we are living in a world in which we are inundated by huge quantities of information and are relying on interdependent information and communication services that transmit data instantaneously without regard to distance. We have much less time to cope with major conceptual changes in economic, social, and political process that are brought about by an increased volume of information transmitted at a higher speed of communication.
>
> (Bearman, 1986: 157)

We see evidence of this speed of change in higher education. Computers are purchased and computing labs are built, classrooms and dormitories are wired, students are encouraged and increasingly required to have a personal computer and administrative pressures for media-assisted instruction and for online distance learning are at a high pitch. In a challenge to our commitment to reject the theoretical stance of technological determinism, changes within this institutional context easily take on the appearance of trajectories.

These are important changes, surrounded by substantial levels of discussion. Some of that discussion is made possible, perhaps, by ICTs themselves, such as through online discussion groups or Web sites. In some sense, the collapse of space and time through ICTs works to an advantage: people who were too distant to participate are given a voice, and discussion processes themselves may become more efficient and can take place more quickly.

Yet it is this fundamental characteristic of ICTs – how they allow us to do things faster and more efficiently – that suggests to us a problem. Neither deliberative discourse nor individual reflection are necessarily improved by the communication environment created by new ICTs. Both require indeterminate amounts of time. Reflection also benefits from distance. If we value these as processes, it is at least partly because they *aren't* fast and efficient; instead, they guard against possible errors in judgment that might come from acting too quickly. Space and time are natural barriers that promote deliberation and reflection.

We do not wish to suggest that universities are necessarily places for some utopian sense of discourse. But in terms of our efforts to understand new ICTs, we do propose the presence of a paradox: ICTs both remove conditions for reflection and discourse (by collapsing space and time) and, *at the same time*, impose an increased need for such processes due to the speed with which the technologies change, and with which they change our social world.

Understanding the university as a social institution

Prior to the modern era, the university was viewed as a place for reflection and for what has been called curiosity-based research (Michael, 1986: 202). This was research less tied to the demands of specific markets or public purposes, and which would not necessarily lead to specific gains in economic productivity or the achievement of public purposes. A number of changes in the nineteenth century – primarily the US 'land grant'[1] university tie between research and agricultural modernization, and the alliance between federal funding and university research – have eroded the autonomous nature of teaching and research (Bearman, 1986: 154). Following the "almost unmarred success story" of agricultural modernization, several roles emerged for the university (ibid.: 155):

- providing a liberal education to people from all segments of society;
- striving to solve societal problems, rather than focusing only on those problems of specific interest to the scholarly community;
- preparing individuals to practice a number of professions, replacing preparation through apprenticeship and experience with academic preparation; and
- providing a center for culture to serve the community as a whole, rather than simply the students and faculty.

Meeting these roles is difficult in the information society, where intellectual products are increasingly commodified and commercialized. As Chartrand (1989) argues, the "monetarization of information" as the key ethos of the information economy clashes directly with the tradition of the search for "knowledge for knowledge's sake." In this regard, the most important new sector of the information economy is that concerned with the "buying, selling and licensing" of "abstract intellectual property rights, including copyright, patents, registered industrial design and trade marks," a conflict that "threatens the autonomy of the university" (ibid: 316–17).

In the USA, federal government support has assumed that universities serve as the major site of basic and applied research (Bell, 1988). Yet even this relationship is changing. For example, the public sector's role in the shared conceptual and physical space of the university–government endeavor to serve public purposes has been relatively easily occupied by the private sector since the 1990s. Public-sector grants have increasingly encouraged university–private sector partnerships. Business–university partnerships are seen as being more effective in closing the capital investment loop. These partnerships may also lead to the sharing of physical spaces and – as their direct shaping of the direction and content of research grows – more blurring of conceptual boundaries among the various differing objectives that might be pursued in university research.

Simultaneously, the role of the university has also been called into question with arguments that network technologies offer ways to: easily overcome time and distance; break down the physical walls and social barriers that excluded many from higher education; and improve the quality of education, while lowering its cost.

Countering acceleration: reclaiming the core issues of the shape of social and political life

A key issue we are concerned with is how a higher education environment can be created which enables and supports discourse or a standpoint that is reflective, centered not on the technology but on broader personal and civic questions. These questions should cover topics such as the quality of life, the strength of relationships and of community, and the nature of the education we should be aspiring to and enabling. The point is not just to explore how communications technologies are shaping our experience of time and space, but to debate how we wish to use technologies and other means to shape and create the time and space in which meaningful human social and political life is possible.

This type of question formation is important in all fields of investigation that play a part in public life in political communities, but especially in the nascent or developing fields of research and theory concerning new ICTs. Exploration of this question could examine the nature of discourse and research that will open up a scope of informed choice about new technology, as well as the institutional conditions that will provide the resources for this investigation.

In facing these problems, is it possible to make use of new institutional configurations and new technologies themselves to produce useful and accountable public knowledge about the implications of new communications technologies? Universities as institutions have a wide variety of forms and roles in different times and places. One theoretical approach relating communication media technology to social institutions is the medium theory approach explored and developed by Harold Innis (1951) in his essay, *The Bias of Communication*, and further explored by a number of communications scholars through historical investigations (e.g., Czitrom, 1982; Carey, 1988; Deibert, 1997).

Innis is important for our purposes because he attends particularly to the ways in which a medium configures time and space in the dissemination of knowledge. These characteristics do not imply universal effects, but must be understood in terms of the context in which they are situated:

> A medium of communication has an important influence on the dissemination of knowledge over space and over time and it becomes necessary to study its characteristics in order to appraise its influence in its cultural setting. According to its characteristics it may be better suited to the dissemination of knowledge over time than over space, particularly if the medium is heavy and durable and not suited to transportation, or to the dissemination of knowledge over space than over time, particularly if the medium is light and easily transported. The relative emphasis on

time and space will imply a bias of significance to the culture in which it is embedded.

(Innis, 1995: 325)

Innis considers a number of different examples and time periods in advancing the general historical proposition that the time or space bias of dominant media (that is, their use to carry meaning across space or across time) will be related to social and political organization. Differing media will be historically connected with dominant institutions, and groups may command a 'monopoly of knowledge' centered on the use and control of a medium of communication. Media also shape the dominant forms of knowledge in Innis' approach: "We can perhaps assume that the use of a medium of communication over a long period will to some extent determine the character of knowledge to be communicated ..." (Innis, 1995: 326).

The university and the Information Age

The connection between research and knowledge creation can be organic and institutional, or it can be mediated by property rights and market mechanisms. In the later case, the efforts of actors in markets to increase the rate of the circulation of capital and the rate of return on investments lead to efforts to tie research to economically productive and profitable outputs. This mandate will certainly shape the direction and content of institutional configurations that can find support. When considering the time and spatial context of universities, if this support is seen as an investment in a market framework there will be a clear mandate for the effort to close the capital investment-productivity-profitability loop more effectively, and to shorten the cycle between investments in research projects and clearly identifiable outcomes. The cycle or the relevant time frame for university inquiry shall be shortened as a consequence.

Universities can play a more proactive role in this situation. At present, universities may contribute to public and private knowledge formation in several ways. As institutions of the modern state or private voluntary organizations, universities are loosely configured to serve some public purposes through research, as well as the objectives of education and service. In this role, we would understand the role of universities in a variety of functions contributing to the public interest. As institutions of knowledge formation in a knowledge or information economy, the university would be configured to use resources efficiently for the greatest level of output. If we focus on this role, the output productivity in terms of educated persons and knowledge formation relevant to the needs of the economy would be emphasized. If a model of private human capital formation is used, universities can be seen as producing a service commodity, the primary beneficiaries of which are the individuals who acquire a degree or professional credential. Finally, as quasi-independent or independent institutions, universities can also be seen as institutions of civil society. In this role, the democratic or at least collegial quality of decision-making is important, since universities make up one public forum that contributes to a democratic public sphere.

Universities, and the academic systems of tenure, promotion and peer review, serve as gatekeepers for what Innis (1951; 1972 [1951]) called "monopolies of knowledge." Research institutes, whether affiliated with universities, governments, non-profit organizations or industry advocacy groups, are also key sites of knowledge formation. Private non-profit foundations and professional associations provide key sites in civil society for credentialing, conference exchanges, and publication; these are often articulated with privately owned academic publishers that provide forums through publication of the results of peer review and evaluation. In addition, private knowledge-based industries, research consortia, university–private partnerships, and consulting firms are becoming an increasingly important producer, consumer, organizer, and owner of information, protected by emerging fields of law such as intellectual property rights. Hence, some analysts, such as Schement and Curtis (1997) and Mosco (1996), have noted the increasing privatization of information and knowledge systems. Although there are diverse knowledge formation strategies – public, private, market and non-market – the range of alternatives increasingly are constrained, clouded or underemphasized by a dominant rhetoric of free markets and intellectual property rights.

Conclusion

The university is a place – perhaps the most important place in modern Western society – for reflective discourse (Michael, 1986). That discourse then enriches our society through the instruction of students in their capacities as citizens and through advice and influence of public policy makers. In this chapter, we are concerned with how we talk about new media, not in the sense of what we should say but in terms of the conditions and the mechanisms for talk – what must be in place for effective discourse about new media to occur.

Considering the means for reflective discourse on the future of higher education

In higher education, the purposes of encouraging free and open inquiry are expressed in norms of academic freedom, tenure to provide the time and space necessary to undertake potentially unpopular research and voice unpopular ideas, and collegial and democratic governance by faculty and students. The extent to which these norms are actually instituted and practiced in each institutional setting varies considerably. Nevertheless, discourse can be constrained or opened in different ways related to institutional configuration and settings.

A serious effort to consider the means for a reflective discourse about new ICTs within the university is important for at least two reasons. First, insufficient means for reflection will affect what can be said. The sacrifice of reflection for the sake of speed and expediency can be expected to bring a corresponding decline, at least in accuracy and in argumentative and ethical coherence. We might also witness a decline in the self-monitoring required for responsible action directed toward the social good, because these things take time.

Second, if reflection suffers for the sake of short-term technological adoption and implementation, we can expect fewer people to be involved in decision-making. Despite the encouragement of the technologically literate, those with less experience and knowledge about technology will not be able to take part in the discourse at the same level as those conversant in both the technology and the issues.

One response to this concern over the pressures against reflective discourse concerning ICTs is that we should expect these things eventually to take care of themselves. In a sense, it is awkward to even advance our call in this technology-centered venue, filled with examples of innovation and scholarship that obviously are products of substantial reflection. But our hope is that we do not lose track of the fact that it is a relatively small community within the academy for whom the technology has a transparency that then allows those individuals to reflect on it, to talk about it and to imagine its possibilities and its constraints. Even for this community, technology moves quickly enough that its members constantly are reminded of the pressure – and often the failure – to keep current. For many of our colleagues in the academy, the constant changes and evolutions in technological artifacts, services and applications is bewildering. We simply cannot expect our normal measures of supporting reflective discourse to withstand such circumstances.

Recognizing the importance of our talk about the technology

If we cannot keep up with the technology, the question of how we talk about it is an interesting one. It is also important when we realize that it is through this talk we are developing a sense of what this technology is. Several theorists adopting a social shaping or social constructionist perspective toward technology have argued that discourse is a primary element through which technologies are constituted (Bijker, Hughes and Pinch, 1987; Jackson, 1996; Dutton, 1999). Even if one is not willing to grant the constitutive power of discourse, it is certainly reasonable to argue that at least we are forming a set of beliefs and common or collective understandings – a discourse – that can have some consequences for structuring institutions and societal relations (Giddens, 1984). If our discourse promotes a shallow understanding, we will be disadvantaged in arenas of research, governance or policy making. If the discourse is governed by certain ideologies, then action, choices and values will be constrained in ways that sustain certain patterns of power and domination that affect not only our abilities to truly conceptualize technology and its consequences for relationships, communication and society, but also what we can identify as potential paths we might take in making decisions about that technology and our uses of it.

Attending closely to the nature of the discourse surrounding ICTs reveals the great extent to which our talk revolves around the felt need to understand a technology, when that technology is constantly changing. Recognizing this, and acknowledging its potential problems for knowledge and understanding, leads us to a commitment to explore strategies for establishing spaces and places where alternative discourses might come to exist.

Note

1   The public university system in the US grew from legislation in the 1860s which granted federal lands to states to assist in establishing universities, with the goal of providing higher education at a reasonable cost in subject areas believed by the government to be critical to the development of society, such as agriculture and engineering. Studies in the humanities and social sciences were introduced subsequently.

22 Toward a digital academe

Guiding principles for innovations in online education

William H. Dutton et al.[1]

This final chapter concludes the book with a more prescriptive stance on key governance issues. It seeks to identify a set of guidelines that might increase the likelihood of a digital academe enhancing, rather than undermining, institutions of higher education and learning. The major lesson of this volume has been that there are many paths to online education and none of these is a sure win for access to high quality education. Educators are at the very early stages of charting the routes to a digital academe that achieve the opportunities – and avoid the pitfalls – identified by the many contributions to this book. These guidelines might help steer educators on the right course for their institution.

The need for guiding principles

This book has explored the many ways in which the Internet, Web and other new ICTs are helping to deliver a proliferating range of distance education courses and distributed learning activities in universities, corporate training, life-long learning and other educational arenas. As described and analyzed by contributors to this collection, individual faculty, departments, schools, university administrations and public agencies have launched a variety of ICT initiatives in distance education and distributed learning. In many cases, these have taken forward decades of experience in complementing and extending learning opportunities within the classroom and in remote locations. For example, the University of Southern California (USC) launched an educational radio program, entitled 'University of the Air', in 1934; moved to the production and distribution of educational television in the 1940s; and to an interactive – one-way video, two-way audio – instructional TV Network in 1972.[2]

However, past experience with educational broadcasting and distance education does not enable universities to stay at the forefront of innovation which exploits the potential of valuable technological advances in higher education and learning. A lack of innovation in these areas could actually undermine the role of established distance education providers as well as campus-based universities. In order to foster innovation while maintaining and enhancing academic quality, institutions of higher education need to follow a clear strategy designed to build and sustain an imaginative and effective long-term program for distance education and distributed learning. The primary aims of this strategy should be to improve the effectiveness of campus-based instruction and to reach new audiences for teaching and research, such as students whose location, career paths or other life circumstances mean they would otherwise be unable or unlikely to attend courses offered on a particular campus.

One of the key themes of this book has been the highlighting of the crucial role of social, economic and political factors in shaping the design and outcomes of technical and institutional changes tied to the deployment of ICT capabilities in higher education and learning. New technology has been essential to the opening up of many new services and facilities, but not on their own. ICTs are not a *deus ex machina* for education. Nor do they determine the outcomes of educational initiatives associated with their use. In fact, the designs and trajectories of this change are contingent on the contexts in which they occur. So there is limited value in continuing debate between the utopian and dystopian critics of new media in education. There are also limitations in forging any 'magic bullets' of universal 'best practice' advice, even though there are many commonalities of objectives and technologies across different institutions and activities. For example, most institutions are responding to similar perceptions of expanding technical capabilities and limitations.

A more promising focus of debate is on the identification of general guiding principles for the development of a digital academe. It is in that spirit that this chapter offers some general principles. These are based on a debate organized at one university,[3] USC, and research and literature on this subject, including the breadth and depth of experience and expertise represented in this book. These key guiding principles are summarized in the remainder of this chapter, as a starting point and helping hand for policy makers, managers of institutions, researchers, teachers and others involved in developing and implementing strategies for specific initiatives. Much more detail on the many issues raised can be found throughout this book.

A proposed set of guiding principles

The following are proposed general guidelines for initiatives aimed at building a digital academe that enhances higher education and learning:

Advance standards of excellence

Distance education courses and distributed learning activities should strive to meet or exceed the established academic standards for courses provided to on-campus students – whatever the campus. This should take into account the understanding that some courses or programs could be aimed at different kinds of people, ranging from high school students to life-long learners. The value of technical innovations in higher education and learning are relative to what they replace or augment within a particular educational setting with a specific set of teachers and students. ICTs do not automatically enhance the quality of distance or distributed learning. However, these initiatives can improve their likelihood of success by following a variety of strategies.

First, the developers should involve the very best teachers and researchers in key aspects of course design, delivery and evaluation, while ensuring that courses can benefit from the participation of a very wide array of individuals with diverse skills and interests. Course development is likely to become increasingly a team effort, but this does not mean that the most highly-qualified teachers and researchers should not play a primary role in the creation, selection and presentation of content.

In designing distance education and distributed learning courseware, teams should also use new ICTs, such as the Web, in ways that enhance the print and multimedia literacy of their students, improve their problem-solving and analytical skills, and raise the quality of existing courses and the overall quality of the curriculum offered to students. In distributed learning, for example, electronic media should supplement, rather than replace, face-to-face teaching and advising. In distance education, electronic media should enable two-way interactive access to teachers and learning materials that would otherwise be limited to one-way communication. Electronic multimedia should complement the reading of classic texts, for instance by gaining online access to an original manuscript.

In addition, educators should take advantage of the transparency of electronic courses, which can be open to the world, to design a process and set of tools for constructive student and peer evaluations of all course offerings. At the same time, educators can employ electronic course platforms to ensure the privacy of some activities, such as discussions among the instructor and class members. Teachers need to open and close doors to the classroom in ways that enhance the accountability and quality of the educational experience. ICTs do not force the classroom into the open, nor should administrative policy do so (Noble, 2001). But ICTs can be used by educators to reconfigure access to and from the classroom in ways that will benefit students.

Educationalists take a leading role in innovation

The state of the practice in online education is far from achieving the vision of its advocates. The technology and prevailing instructional techniques need to be advanced considerably to achieve the potential that many see in new media. It is essential that the very best teachers and researchers in higher education should take a leading role in the technological and institutional innovations that support distance education and distributed learning. Social and educational research should seek to contribute to the design and implementation of advancements in Web-based and multimedia technologies, that could be central to innovations in learning and education such as immersive immersive virtual reality, three-dimensional visualizations and simulations, as well as multimedia literacy. Techniques of teaching online need to receive every bit as much critical scrutiny as classroom teaching (Cole, 2000). Colleges and universities should not simply follow the calls for 'student-centered' learning, but play a role in the invention of new institutional and learning paradigms through critical research that informs the production and consumption of ICTs in higher education and learning.

Research and reach new audiences

Distance education programs should continually strive to reach new audiences and serve existing ones in more effective ways. The criteria for admission to distance education courses should be flexible enough to fit the rationale of particular offerings. For example, advanced placement courses might be offered to high school students, or any course might be open to the alumni or retired teachers of a university. Some courses might even be truly open, in the same spirit that Britain's Open University serves anyone seeking higher education. Greater worldwide access to educational offerings is one of the most enormous social and economic opportunities presented by the revolution in ICTs.

The use of new ICTs in distributed learning also opens up the opportunity for syllabi and other teaching and research materials to be accessible to a wider audience, locally and globally. Educators should encourage this access as a means to enhance the visibility of their teaching and research, and to attract the best students.

Enhance university-wide accountability and co-ordination

Aspects of distance education and distributed learning are inherently decentralized because they most depend on the creativity, expertise and initiative of individual teachers. However, a laissez-faire approach to distance education and distributed learning could pose risks to standards of excellence. There is a need, therefore, for accountability on the part of institutions of higher education and learning as a whole.

Colleges and universities should also use central co-ordination and policies to help ensure that the infrastructure used for the registration, financing, and advising of a geographically distributed student body is achieved well. They should co-ordinate a set of standard protocols for technology and educational excellence where they are warranted. Standards can play a positive role, such as illustrated by the Internet, which is based by a set of standards. The college or university should also seek to create a critical mass of activity, such as by establishing a strategic package of offerings and an electronic 'portal' to all online resources, including various departments and schools. This should be sufficient to:

1   attract resources and benefit from economies of scale and scope;
2   enhance the likelihood that the various individual offerings and initiatives add up to more than a sum of their parts; and
3   maximize the value of all distance education to the well-being of the college or university.

This means distance-education courses and distributed-learning resources must be appropriately recognized and credited to the institution responsible for them and must augment and not detract from other core teaching and research missions.

Manage copyright and intellectual property rights effectively

New ICTs reconfigure the relative power of different actors to control access to information – what has been called informational politics

(Dutton, 1999; Garnham, 1999). This is often viewed positively as a new opportunity for expanding access to educational opportunities. However, in commercial sectors, such as the recording industry, it is a threat to traditional business models. The increasing centrality of new media in higher education and learning has disrupted conventional assumptions about copyright by creating the potential for the content of teaching to be packaged for a larger audience. This new electronic El Dorado has made copyright and intellectual property right (IPR) a potential killer issue in the development of a digital academe. The faltering dot-com sector has tempered debate over copyright with a more realistic perspective on the costs and revenues of courseware, but the issue has not disappeared and requires resolution.

In the debate over how to properly manage and protect the copyright and other IPR associated with the online educational offerings of teaching faculty and institutions, there is the risk of a zero-sum mentality prevailing: seeking a win for one player in a game with multiple players, including students, content developers, teachers, course builders, designers, colleges and universities and other public and private education and learning ventures. Unless incentive structures can be devised for all players to win, initiatives in distance education and distributed learning will falter.

Failure to create innovative incentive structures within existing colleges and universities will favor the rise of new virtual universities, who build their organizations under a new set of rules. Therefore, it is essential for maintaining a diversity of educational options that faculty members, administrators and students invent a win-win-win formula for managing IPR. For example, some universities could separate the distance education products and services from the traditional IPR rights and responsibilities in colleges or universities, such as for syllabi and teaching materials used in on-campus instruction and distributed learning. Faculty members should be able to sign copyright agreements with a separate entity charged with the responsibility for providing distance education courses or for developing courseware that can be – in ways analogous to a textbook or video tape – used by other colleges or universities.

These agreements would operate in the same way as a traditional copyright and royalty agreement with an outside textbook publisher. Others argue that film production is a more appropriate analogy, due to the range of talent involved in producing courseware. Whatever the most appropriate analogy, colleges and universities need to explore new institutional arrangements that enable win-win approaches to managing copyright and distributing royalties.

Resolve conflicts of interest and commitment

A rise of distance education and distributed learning is likely to necessitate the formation of alliances with communication industries, venture-capital firms and other universities or educational institutions. These enterprises should be self-sufficient – on a profit or nonprofit basis – to avoid being subsidized by traditional on-campus courses. New business ventures and alliances carry a risk of losing the autonomy that underlies the academic freedom to enforce standards of academic rigor and to pursue scholarly inquiry wherever it leads (Press and Washburn, 2000). It is therefore paramount that mainstream, tenured faculty are involved in both the production and oversight of distance education, and that mechanisms are established to reduce real and perceived conflicts of interest. In the same spirit, policies should be developed to reduce conflicts of commitment, both real and perceived, by informing faculty and administrators of plans and activities at an early stage so that potential conflicts can be identified and resolved.

The stakes in this debate

The impact of new media in higher education and learning will be driven by how the principles outlined above are resolved. The role of online education remains open-ended and not determined by any inherent properties of emerging ICTs. Debate over the design of a digital academe must therefore move beyond the enthusiasts and critics of online education to include all educators, administrators and policy makers interested in the future of higher education and learning.

Notes

1 This chapter is based on a document prepared for discussion at an Open Forum organized by the University of Southern California's Academic Senate Task Force on Distance Education and Distributed Learning, held at the University's Annenberg School for Communication, University Park Campus, and the Doheny Eye Institute, Health Sciences Campus on 14 April 2000. The first author, who chaired the forum, thanks members of this task force for commenting on and contributing to the text of the report: John Crocker, Financial Aid; Visiting Professor Alain Dumort, School of International Relations; Professor Philip J. Ethington, College of Letters, Arts and Sciences; the late Professor Frederick George III, Keck School of Medicine; Professor Ellis Horowitz, School of Engineering; Professor Mark Kann, School of Letters, Arts & Sciences; Professor Ed Kazlauskas, Rossier School of Education; Retired Professor Jack M. Nilles, JALA International, Inc.; Professor Edwin McCann,

College of Letters, Arts & Sciences; Michael Renov, School of Cinema/Television. However, the opinions expressed here are those of the first author and do not necessarily represent those of the task force members or USC.

2   A chronology of USC events related to distance education or distributed learning is located at: www.usc.edu/academe/acsen/issues/distance_ed/ dl_chronology. html

3   The Task Force Report on which this is based in available online at: www.usc.edu/academe/acsen/issues/distance_ed/ddl-principles.html

Bibliography

Adelman, C. (2000) 'A parallel universe: certification in the Information Technology Guild', *Change*, vol. 32, no. 3, pp. 20–9.

AFT (2001) *A Virtual Revolution: Trends in the Expansion of Distance Education*, Washington, DC: American Federation of Teachers, May.

Agre, P. E. (1999) 'Information technology in higher education: the "global academic village" and intellectual standardization', *On the Horizon*, vol. 7, no. 5, pp. 8–11

Agre, P. (200) 'Infrastructure and institutional change in the networked university', *Information, Communication and Society*, 3(4): 494–507.

Allen, D. and Wilson, T. (1996) 'Information strategies in UK higher education institutions', *International Journal of Information Management*, no. 6, pp. 239–51.

Almeda, B. (1998) 'University of California Extension on-line: from concept to reality', *Journal of Asynchronous Learning Networks*, vol. 2, issue 2, pp. 1–20.

Alpert, D. (1985) 'Performance and paralysis: The organizational context of the American research university', *Journal of Higher Education,* vol. 56, no. 3, pp. 241–81.

Andersen, P. B., Holmqvist, B. and Jensen, J. F. (1993) *Computer as Medium*, New York: Cambridge University Press.

Anderson, B. (1983) *Imagined Communities: Reflection on the Origin and Spread of Nationalism*, London: Verso.

Anderson, L. (2001) 'News from campus: Duke Arm buys Pensare Software', *FT.com*, 18 June, globalarchive.ft.com

Anderson, T. and Haughey, M. (1998) *Networked Learning: The Pedagogy of the Internet*, Toronto and New York: Cheneliere/McGraw-Hill.

Apollo Group (1995) Public Relations release, 10 October.

Apollo Group, Inc. (2001) *Quarterly Report (Form 10-Q)*, US Securities and Exchange Commission, Washington, DC, filed 13 July.

Babson College (2000) *Babson College and Cenquest selected by Intel to develop custom MBA program for employees*, press release, 18 December, www.babsoninteractive.com/BabsonIntel.htm

Baer, W. S. (1998) 'Will the Internet transform higher education?', *The

Emerging Internet, Queenstown, MD: Institute for Information Studies, The Aspen Institute.

Baer, W. S. (2000) 'Competition and collaboration in online distance learning', *Information, Communication and Society*, vol. 3, no. 4, pp. 457–73.

Bannon, L. and Bødker, S. (1997) 'Constructing common information spaces', *Fifth European Conference on Computer Supported Cooperative Work*, The Netherlands: Kluwer Academic Publishers, pp. 81–96.

Barnard, J. (1997) 'The World Wide Web and higher education: the promise of virtual universities and online libraries', *Educational Technology*, vol. 37, no. 3, pp. 30–5.

Barnett, R. (2000) *Realizing the University in an Age of Supercomplexity*, Milton Keynes: Open University Press.

Bates, A. W. (1994) 'Distance education, educational technology', in Husen, T. and Postlethwaite, T. N. (eds) *The International Encyclopaedia of Education* (2nd edition), Oxford: Elsevier Science.

Bates, M. (1999) 'The invisible substrate of information science', *Journal of the American Society for Information Science*, vol. 50, no. 12, pp. 1185–205.

Bateson, G. (1972) *Steps to an Ecology of Mind*, New York: Ballantine.

Baumol, William J. (1967) 'Macroeconomics of unbalanced growth: the anatomy of urban crisis', *American Economic Review*, 57 (June 1967), pp. 415–26.

Bearman, C. T. (1986) 'Universities in the Information Age', in Neilson, W. A. W. and Gaffield, C. (eds) *Universities in Crisis: A Medieval Institution in the Twenty-First Century*, Ottawa: The Institute for Research on Public Policy, pp. 153–69.

Bell, D. (1999, 1973) *The Coming of Post-Industrial Society: A Venture in Social Forecasting*, New York: Basic Books.

Bell, T. H. (1988) 'Foreword', in Justiz, M. J. and Bjork, L. G. (eds) *Higher Education Research and Public Policy*, New York: Collier Macmillan Publishers, pp. v–ix.

Beniger, J. (1986) *The Control Revolution*, Cambridge, MA: Harvard University Press.

Benton Foundation (2000) *The E-Rate in America: A Tale of Four Cities*, online: www.benton.org/e-rate/4cities/pdf (July 2000).

Berg, M. and Timmermans, S. (1997) 'Orders and their Others: On the constitution of universalities in medical work'. Paper presented at the 'Actor Network and After' Conference, Keele University, UK, 10–11 July, 1997.

Besser, H. and Donahue, S. (1996) 'Introduction and overview', *Journal of the American Society for Information Science: Perspectives on distance independent education*, vol. 47, no. 11, pp. 801–4.

Bijker, W. E., Hughes, T. P. and Pinch, T. (1987) *The Social Construction of Technological Systems: New Directions in the Sociology and History of Technology*, Cambridge, MA: MIT Press.

Blankenship, L. (1993) *The cow ate my brain or A novice's guide to MOO programming, Part I*, September, online: www.cs.rdg.ac.uk/people/mkh/virtual_worlds/MOO/tutorials/mootutor1.html

Bloom, B. (1973) *Every Kid Can: Learning for Mastery*, Washington, DC: College/University Press.

Bloom, B. (1981) *All Our Children Learning: A Primer for Parents, Teachers, and Other Educators*, New York: McGraw Hill.

Bloom, B. (1984) 'The two sigma problem: the search for methods of group instruction as effective as one-to-one tutoring', *Educational Researcher*, 13: 4–15.

Bloom, B., Madaus, G. and Hastings, T. (1981) *Evaluation to Improve Learning*, New York: McGraw Hill.

Bloomer, M. (1998) 'Education for Studentship', *Knowledge and Nationhood*, London: Cassell, pp. 140–63.

Bloomfield, B. and Vurdubakis, T. (1994) 'Re-presenting technology: IT consultancy reports as textual reality constructions', *Sociology*, vol. 28, no. 2, pp. 455–77.

Blumenstyk, G. (1999) 'Distance learning at the Open University', *The Chronicle of Higher Education*, 23 July, pp. A35–7.

Blumenstyk, G. (1999a) 'In a first, the North Central Association accredits an on-line university', *The Chronicle of Higher Education*, 19 March, p. A27.

Blumenstyk, G. (2000) 'Company that owns the University of Phoenix plans for a major foreign expansion' *The Chronicle of Higher Education*, 11 August.

Blumenstyk, G. (2000a) 'DeVry Institutes wins accreditation for 2 online Bachelor's programs', *The Chronicle of Higher Education*, 16 August.

Blumenstyk, G. (2000b) 'Turning a profit by turning out professionals', *The Chronicle of Higher Education*, vol. 46, issue 18.

Blumenstyk, G. (2000c) 'U. of Phoenix sells $70-million worth of stock in its distance-education efforts', *The Chronicle of Higher Education*, 13 October.

Blumenstyk, G. (2000d) 'Expanding its reach in higher education, Kaplan buys Quest, a chain of commercial colleges', *The Chronicle of Higher Education*, 28 June.

BMBF (1998) 'Wissen weltweit nutzen. Pressemitteilung des BMBF zu den Siegern des Ideenwettbewerbs', online: www.medicdat.de/deutsch/projekt/bmbf/sieger.html (1 October 2001).

BMBF (2000) *Grund- und Strukturdaten 1999/2000*, Bonn: Bundesministerium für Bildung und Forschung, Referat Öffentlichkeitsarbeit, online: www.bmbf.de (1 September 2001).

BMBF (2000a) *New Media in Education Funding Programme*, Bonn: Bundesministerium für Bildung und Forschung, Referat Öffentlichkeitsarbeit, online: www.bmbf.de (12 September 2001).

BMBF (2001) 'Anytime, Anywhere – IT-gestütztes Lernen in den USA. Bericht zur Studienreise in die USA' 3–13 April 2001. Bundesministerium für Bildung und Forschung, online: www.bmbf.de (1 September 2001).

BMBF/BMWI (1999) *Innovation and Jobs in the Information Society of the 21st Century*, Bonn: Bundesministerium für Bildung und Forschung and Bundesministerium für Wirtschaft und Technologie, online: www.bmwi.de (20 September 2000).

Boland, R. and Tenkasi, R. (1995) 'Perspective making and perspective taking in communities of knowing', *Organization Science*, vol. 6, no. 4, pp. 350–72.

Bollag, B. (2000) 'The new Latin: English dominates in academe', *The Chronicle of Higher Education*, 8 September.

Bollag, B. (2001) 'Developing countries turn to distance education', *The Chronicle of Higher Education*, 15 June.

Bolter, J. D. (1991) *Writing Space: The Computer, Hypertext, and the History of Writing*, Hillsdale, NJ: Lawrence Erlbaum Associates, Inc.

Bonk, C. J. and Cummings, J. A. (1998) 'A dozen recommendations for placing the student at the center of Web-based learning', *Educational Media International*, vol. 35, no. 2, pp. 82–9.

Bonzi, S. (1993) *Proceedings of the 56th Annual Meeting of the American Society for Information Science*, October, Columbus, OH.

Borgman, C. L. (1996) 'Social aspects of digital libraries', Final Report to the National Science Foundation, UCLA-NSF *Social Aspects of Digital Libraries Workshop*, February 15–17, online: dlis.gseis.ucla.edu/DL/UCLA_DL_Report.html

Bork, A. (1999) 'The future of learning: an interview with Alfred Bork', *EDUCOM Review,* 34(4): 24–7, 48–50. Online: www.educause. edu/copyright.html (July 2000).

Bork, A. (2000a) 'Learning technology', *EDUCAUSE Review*, January/February: 74–81.

Bork, A. (2000b) 'Learning with the World Wide Web', *The Internet and Higher Education*, 2(2–3): 81–5.

Bork, A. (2001) 'Tutorial learning for the new century', *Journal of Science Education and Technology*, 10(1): 57–71.

Bork, A., Ibrahim, B., Levrat, B., Milne, A. and Yoshi, R. (1992). 'The Irvine-Geneva Course Development System', in R. Aiken (ed.) *Education and Society, Information Processing, 2,* Holland: Elsevier.

Bork, A. and Gunnarsdottir, S. (2001) *Tutorial Learning – Rebuilding Our Educational System*, New York: Kluwer Academic Systems.

Bowker, G. (1994), 'Information Mythology: The World of/as Information', in L. Bud-Frierman (ed.) *Information Acumen: The Understanding and Use of Knowledge in Modern Business*, London: Routledge, pp. 231–47.

Braman, S. (1998) 'The right to create: cultural policy in the fourth stage of the information society', *Gazette: The International Journal of Communication Studies*, pp. 77–91.

Bromley, H. and Apple, M. W. (1998) *Education/Technology/Power: Educational Computing as a Social Practice*, Albany, NY: SUNY Press.

Brown, S. and Capdevila, R. (1997) 'Perpetuum mobile: Substance, force and the sociology of translation', paper presented at the 'Actor Network and After' Conference, Keele University, UK, 10–11 July, 1997.

Brown, J. S. and Duguid, P. (1996) 'Fast forward: the university's digital future', *Change*, July/August, pp. 11–19.

Brown, J. S. and Duguid, P. (1996a) 'The social life of documents', *First Monday 1*, online: www.firstmonday.dk/issues/issue1/documents

Brown, J. S. and Duguid, P. (1998) 'Universities in the digital age', in Hawkins, B. L. and Battin, P. (eds) *The Mirage of Continuity: Reconfiguring*

Academic Resources for the 21st Century, Washington: Council on Library and Information Resources.

Brown, J. S. and Duguid, P. (2000) *The Social Life of Information*, Boston: Harvard Business School Press.

Brown, J. S., Collins, A. and Duguid, P. (1989) 'Situated cognition and the culture of learning', *Educational Researcher*, Jan–Feb, pp. 32–42.

Brunn, S. D. and Leinbach, T. R. (1991) (eds) *Collapsing Space and Time: Geographic Aspects of Communication and Information*, London: Harper Collins.

Buckingham Shum, S., Sumner, T. and Laurillard, D. (1996) 'On the future of journals: digital publishing and argumentation', *Adjunct Proceedings of HCI 96*, London (August).

Bulmahn, E. (2001) 'Zukunftsorientierte Bildung. Address of Secretary of Education' at *Education Fair 2001,* online: www.berlinews.de/archiv/1709. shtml (10 September).

Burge, E. J. (1994) 'Learning in computer conferenced contexts: The learners' perspective', *Journal of Distance Education*, vol. 9, no. 1, pp. 19–43.

Bush, V. (1945) 'As we may think', *The Atlantic Monthly*, vol. 176, pp. 101–8.

Business Week (2001) 'Giving it the old online try', 3 December, issue 16, pp. 77–8.

California State University (1999) *Access in Action: Extended University Annual Report*, 1997–1998, Los Angeles, California State University.

Callon, M. (1986) 'Some elements of a sociology of translation: the domestication of the scallops and the fishermen of St Brieuc Bay', in Law, J. (ed.) *Power, Action, Belief: A New Sociology of Knowledge*, London: Routledge and Kegan Paul.

Callon, M. (1986a) 'The sociology of an actor-network: the case of the electric vehicle', in Callon, M., Law, J. and Rip, A., *Mapping the Dynamics of Science and Technology*, London: Macmillan Press.

Campus Computing Project, The (2000) *The 2000 National Survey of Information Technology in US Higher Education*, www.campuscomputing.net

Carey, J. W. (1988) *Communications as Culture: Essays on Media and Society*, Boston: Unwin Hyman.

Carnevale, D. (1999) 'Professor says distance learning can increase colleges' income', *The Chronicle of Higher Education*, 13 October, pp. A27.

Carnevale, D. (2000) 'Two models for collaboration in distance education', *The Chronicle of Higher Education*, 19 May.

Carnevale, D. (2000a) 'San Diego State's Senate creates a detailed policy for distance courses', *The Chronicle of Higher Education*, 26 April.

Carnevale, D. (2000b) 'World Bank becomes a player in distance education', *The Chronicle of Higher Education*, 8 December.

Carnevale, D. (2001) 'Assessment takes center stage', *OnLine Learning, Chronicle of Higher Education*, April 13.

Carr, S. (2000) 'A for-profit subsidiary will market Cornell's distance programs', *The Chronicle of Higher Education*, 14 March.

Carr, S. (2000a) 'A new Web site aims to direct students to online courses, but price is steep', *The Chronicle of Higher Education*, 7 January.

Carrier, J. and Miller, D. (1998) (eds) *Virtualism: A New Political Economy*, Oxford: Berg.

Castells, M. (2000, 1996) *The Rise of the Network Society: The Information Age: Economy, Society and Culture, Volume 1*, 2nd edn, Oxford: Blackwell Publishers.

Castells, M. (2001) *The Internet Galaxy*, Oxford: Oxford University Press.

Castells, M., Flecha, R., Freire, P., Giroux, H. A., Macedo, D. and Willis, P. (1999) *Critical Education in the New Information Age*, New York and Oxford: Bowman & Littlefield Publishers, Inc.

Chandler, A. (1997) *The Visible Hand: The Managerial Revolution in American Business*, Cambridge: Harvard University Press.

Chandrasekaran (2001) 'US online education firms run into difficulties' on *Yahoo! News*, 12 July.

Chartrand, H. H. (1989) 'University research in the information economy: a clash of cultures', in Abu-Laban, B. (ed.) *University Research and the Future of Canada*, Ottawa: University of Ottawa Press.

Cherney, E. (2001) 'Thomson joins 16 Schools to start online university', *WSJ.com, The Wall Street Journal*, 20 August.

Child, J. (1972) 'Organization structure, environment and performance: the role of strategic choice', *Sociology*, vol. 6, no. 1, pp. 1–22.

Child, J. (1997) 'Strategic choice in the analysis of action, structure, organizations and environment', *Organization Studies*, vol. 18, no. 1, pp. 43–76.

Christensen, C. M. (1997) *The Innovators Dilemma*, Boston: Harvard Business School Press.

Cicchetti, D. V. (1991) 'The reliability of peer review for manuscript and grant submissions: a cross-disciplinary investigation', *Behavioral and Brain Sciences*, vol. 14, pp. 119–86.

Cole, R. A. (2000) (ed.) *Issues in Web-based Pedagogy: A Critical Primer*, Westport, CT: Greenwood Press.

Confederation of European Rectors' Conferences (1999) *Trends in learning structures in higher education in Europe*, Report to the European Commission.

Confessore, N. (1999) 'The virtual university', *The New Republic*, 4 October.

Cooper, G. and Woolgar, S. (1993) 'Software is society made malleable: the importance of conceptions of audience in software and research practice', *PICT Policy Research Paper no. 25*, Uxbridge, UK: Brunel University.

Council of Ministers of Education (1996) 'Resolution relating to educational multimedia software in the fields of education and training', *Official Journal of the EU*, 6 July.

Council of Ministers of Education (1997) 'Conclusions on education, information and communication technology and teacher-training for the future', *Official Journal of the EU*, 4 October.

Council of Ministers of Education (2001) 'Resolution on e-learning', *Official Journal of the EU*, 4 July, series C 204/3.

Crane, D. (1972) *Invisible Colleges: Diffusion of Knowledge in Scientific Communities*, Chicago: University of Chicago Press.

Cuban, L. (1986) *Teachers and Machines: The Classroom Use of Technology Since 1920*, New York: Teachers College Press.

Cunningham, S., Tapsall, S., Ryan, Y., Stedman, L., Bagden, K. and Flew, T. (1998) *New Media and Borderless Education: A Review of the Convergence between Global Media Networks and Higher Education Provision*, Australian Government, Department of Employment, Education, Training and Youth Affairs, Evaluations and Investigations Program, Higher Education Division (www.deetya.gov.au/highered/eippubs/eip97–22/eip9722.pdf).

Curry, M. R. (1996) *The Work in the World: Geographical Practice and the Written Word*, Minneapolis: University of Minnesota Press.

Czitrom, D. J. (1982) *Media and the American Mind: From Morse to McLuhan*, Chapel Hill: University of North Carolina Press.

Daniel, J. S. (1998) *Mega-Universities and Knowledge Media: Technology Strategies for Higher Education*, London: Kogan Page.

Daniel, J. S. (1999) 'Distance learning: the vision and distance learning: the reality. What works, what travels?' Conference presentation, *Leadership in the Knowledge Economy*, Boca Raton, Florida, 10–12 January.

Daniel, J. S. (1999a) 'Building in quality: the transforming power of distance learning', *Council for Higher Education Accreditation, Second Annual Conference*, San Diego, California, 2 February.

Daniel, J. S. (1999b) 'The rise of the mega university', in Leer, A., *Masters of the Wired World*, London: Pearson Education.

Daniel, J. S. (1999c) 'Innovation at scale in the delivery of learning and teaching: will the whole be greater than the sum of the parts?' Address at *12th International Meeting of University Administrators*, Edinburgh, 6 September.

Daniel, J. S. (2001) 'Evolution not an e-revolution in global learning', *Times Higher Educational Supplement*, 18 May, p. VIII.

Danziger, N., Dutton, W. H., Kling, R. and Kraemer, K. L. (1982) *Computers and Politics: High Technology in American Local Governments*, New York: Columbia University Press.

Darby, M. and Karnia, E. (1973) 'Free competition and optimal amount of fraud', *Journal of Law and Economics*, vol. 16, pp. 67–88.

Davenport, T. (1998) 'Putting the enterprise into the enterprise system', *Harvard Business Review*, 76. 4: 121–32.

Davis, J. R. and Huttenlocher, D. P. (1995) 'Shared annotations for cooperative learning', *Computer Support for Collaborative Learning (CSCL '95)*, Bloomington, IN: Lawrence Erlbaum Associates.

de Alva, J. K. (1999–2000) 'Remaking the academy in the age of information', *Issues in Science and Technology*, Winter, pp. 52–8.

Dede, C. (1996) 'Emerging technologies in distance education for business', *Journal of Education for Business*, vol. 71, no. 4, pp. 197–205.

Deibert, R. J. (1997) *Parchment, Printing, and Hypermedia: Communication in World Order Transformation*, New York: Columbia University Press.

Denning, P. J. (1996) 'The university's next challenges', *Communications of the ACM*, vol. 39, no. 5, pp. 27–31.

Dertouzos, M. (2001) *The Unfinished Revolution: Human-Centered Computers and What They Can Do for Us*, New York: Harper-Collins.

DfEE (Department for Education and Employment) (1998) *Sustaining Open Learning*, London: DfEE.

DfEE (1999) *Learning to Succeed White Paper*, cmnd No 4392, London: The Stationery Office Limited.

DfEE (2000) *Explanatory Notes to the Learning and Skills Act 2000*, PGA – 2000, Ch 21, London: The Stationery Office Limited.

DfES (Department for Education and Skills) (2001) *Learndirect Offers a Unique Service says Global Study – Wills*, Press release, 8 May (available at www.dfes.gov.uk).

Doheny-Farina, S. (1996) *The Wired Neighborhood*, New Haven: Yale University Press.

Downes, S. (1999) *What Happened at California Virtual University*, Threads www.atl.ualberta.ca/downes/threads/column041499.htm

Drucker, P. F. (1993) *Post-Capitalist Society*, Oxford and Boston: Butterworth-Heinemann.

Duart, J. M. and Sangra, A. (eds) (2000) *Aprender en la Virtualidad*, Barcelona: Gedisa Publ. & EDIUOC.

Dürr, H. P. (1997) 'Antwort auf Roman Herzogs Rede. Offener Brief der Vereinigung Deutscher Wissenschaftler', online: users.math.uni-potsdam.de/~oitner/ANHERZOG/anherzog.htm (20 August 2001).

Dutton, W. H. (1995) 'The ecology of games and its enemies', *Communication Theory*, vol. 5, no. 4, November, pp. 379–92.

Dutton, W. H. (ed.) (1996) with Malcolm Peltu, *Information and Communication Technologies – Visions and Realities*, Oxford and New York: Oxford University Press.

Dutton, W. H. (1999) *Society on the Line: Information Politics in the Digital Age*, Oxford: Oxford University Press.

Dutton, W. H. and Guthrie, K. (1991) 'An ecology of games: the political construction of Santa Monica's public electronic network', *Informatization and the Public Sector*, pp. 279–301.

Economist, The (2001) 'The Internet, untethered: a survey of the mobile Internet', 13 October, pp. 3–20.

ESRC (Economic and Social Research Council) (2001) 'A new research programme on information and communication technologies', *Prometheus*, vol. 19, no. 3, pp. 253–60.

European Association of Distance Teaching Universities (2000) *Wiring the ivory tower: linking European universities*, online: www.eadtu.nl (September).

European Commission (1996) 'Learning in the information society', *Communication to the European Parliament and the Council of Ministers*.

European Commission (2000) 'E-Europe, an information society for all', *Communication for the Special European Council of Lisbon*, 23 and 24 March.

European Commission (2001) 'The Educational Multimedia Task Force 1995–2001: Integrated Research Effort on Multimedia in Education and

Training', a series of reports available online: www.proacte.com/ infocentre/documents/eandt/index.asp

European Commission (2001a) 'E-learning: designing tomorrow's education', *Communication to the European Parliament and the Council of Ministers.*

Excelsior College (2000), *Two International Leaders in Distance Learning Join Forces to Expand Business and IT Programs Globally*, 18 January, online: www.excelsior.edu/exold/media/864.htm.

Farrell, G. M. (1999) 'Introduction' in Farrell, G. M. (ed.) *The Development of Learning: A Global Perspective*, London: The Commonwealth of Learning.

Feenberg, A. (1987) 'Computer conferencing and the humanities', *Instructional Science*, vol. 6, no. 2, pp. 169–86.

Feenberg, A. (1999) *Distance Learning: Promise or Threat?*, online: www.rohan.sdsu.edu/faculty/feenberg/TELE3.HTM

Finholt, T. A. and Olson, G. M. (1997) 'From laboratories to collaboratories: a new organizational form for scientific collaboration', *Psychological Science*, vol. 8, no. 1, pp. 28–37.

Fischer, G. and Stevens, C. (1991) 'Information access in complex, poorly structured information spaces', *Human Factors in Computing Systems (CHI '91)*, New Orleans, LA: ACM Press.

Fish, S. (1980) *Is there a Text in this Class? The Authority of Interpretive Communities*, Cambridge, MA: Harvard University Press.

Fisher, C., Dwyer, D. C. and Yocan, K. (1996) *Education and Technology: Reflections on Computing in Classrooms*, New York: Jossey-Bass Educational Series.

Flecha, R. (1999) 'New educational inequalities' in Castells, M., Flecha, R., Freire, P., Giroux, H. A., Macedo, D. and Willis, P., *Critical Education in the New Information Age*, New York and Oxford: Bowman & Littlefield Publishers, Inc. pp. 65–82.

Frank, R. H. and Cook, P. J. (1996) *The Winner-Take-All Society*, New York: Penguin Books.

Fransman, M. (1990) *The Market and Beyond: Cooperation and Competition in Information Technology in the Japanese System*, Cambridge: Cambridge University Press.

Freeman, C. (1996), 'The two-edged nature of technical change: employment and unemployment' in Dutton, W. H. (ed.) (1996a) *Information and Communication Technologies – Visions and Realities*, Oxford: Oxford University Press, pp. 19–36.

Freeman, C. (ed.) (1990) *The Economics of Innovation*, Aldershot, Hants: Edward Elgar.

Friedman, T. L. (1999) 'Next, it's E-ducation', *New York Times*, 17 November.

Furnas, G. W., Landauer, T. K., Gomez, L. M. and Dumais, S. T. (1987) 'The vocabulary problem in human-system communication', *Communications of the ACM 30(11)*, pp. 964–71.

Garnham, N. (1999) 'Information politics: the study of communicative power' in Dutton, W. H., *Society on the Line: Information Politics in the Digital Age*, Oxford: Oxford University Press, pp. 77–8.

Garson, G. D. (1986) 'The political economy of online education', *Social Science Computer Review*, vol. 14, no. 4, pp. 394–409.

Gasser, L. (1996) 'The integration of computing and routine work', *ACM Transactions on Office Information Systems*, 4: 205–25.

Gell, M. and Cochrane, P. (1996) 'Learning and education in an information society' in Dutton, W. H. (ed.) *Information and Communication Technologies: Visions and Realities*, Oxford: Oxford University Press, pp. 249–63.

Gellner, E. (1983) *Nations and Nationalism*, Ithaca, NY: Cornell University Press.

Gellner, E. (1983a) *Plough, Book and Sword: The Structure of Human History*, Chicago: University of Chicago Press.

Giddens, A. (1984) *The Constitution of Society*, Berkeley: University of California Press.

Giddens, A. (1998) *The Third Way: The Renewal of Social Democracy*, London: Polity Press.

Giles, L., Bollacker, K. and Lawrence, S. (1998) 'CiteSeer: an automatic citation indexing system', *Third ACM Conference on Digital Libraries*, Pittsburgh, PA: ACM Press, pp. 89–98.

Gladieux, L. E. and Swail, W. S. (1999) *The Virtual University & Educational Opportunity: Issues of Equity and Access for the Next Generation*, Washington, DC: The College Board, April, online: www.collegeboard.org

Goddard, A. D. and Gayward, P. H. (1994) 'MAC and the Oracle family: achievements and lessons learnt', *Axix*, vol. 1, no. 1, pp. 45–50.

Goddard, J. B., Charles, D., Pike, A., Potts, G. and Bradley, D. (1994) *Universities and Communities*, London: Committee of Vice-chancellors and Principals.

Goldman-Segall, R. (1995) 'Deconstructing the Humpty Dumpty myth: putting it together to create cultural meaning' in Barrett, E. and Redmond, M. (eds) *Contextual Media: Multimedia and Interpretation*, Cambridge, MA: MIT Press.

Goodlad, S. (ed.) (1983) *Economies of Scale in Higher Education*, Guildford, UK: Society for Research into Higher Education.

Gordin, D., Gomez, L.M., Pea, R. D. and Fishman, B. J. (1996) 'Using the World Wide Web to build learning communities in K-12', *Journal of Computer-Mediated Communications*, vol. 2, no. 3, online: www.ascusc.org/jcmc/vol2/issue3/gordin.html

Gordon, R. B. (1997) *The Texture of Industry*, Oxford: Oxford University Press.

Gore, A. (1991) 'Infrastructure for the Global Village', *Scientific American*, vol. 265, September, pp. 108–11.

Gottschalk, P. (1998) 'Cross national differences in the rise of earnings inequality: market and institutional factors', *Review of Economics and Statistics*, vol. 80, no. 4, pp. 489–503.

Granow, R. (2000) 'Studieren und lebenslanges Lernen im Netz und im Verbund. Bundesleitprojekt Virtuelle Fachhochschule', Unpublished Paper, Lübeck.

Green, K. C. (1997) 'Drawn to the light, burned by the flame?', *Money, Technology and Distance Education*, vol. 11, no. 5, pp. J1-J8.

Greenfield, P. M. (1984) *Mind and Media: The Effects of Television, Video Games, and Computers*, Cambridge, MA: Harvard University Press.

Gubernick, L. and Ebeling, A. (1997) 'I got my degree through e-mail', *Forbes*, 16 June, pp. 84–6.

Guernsey, L. (1998) 'NYU starts for-profit unit to sell on-line classes', *The Chronicle of Higher Education*, 16 October.

Guernsey, L. (1999) 'Click here for the Ivory Tower', *The New York Times on the Web*, 2 September.

Guzdial, M., Rick, J. and Kehoe, C. (2001) 'Beyond adoption to invention: teacher-created collaborative activities in higher education', *Journal of the Learning Sciences*, vol. 10, no. 3, pp. 265–79.

Hague, D. (1996) 'The firm as a university', *Demos Quarterly*, vol. 8, pp. 16–17.

Hague, D. (1996a) 'Knowledge goes out to market', *Times Higher Education Supplement*, 24 May.

Halliday, F. (1999) 'The chimera of the "International University"', *Foreign Affairs*, vol. 75, no. 1, pp. 99–120.

Halsey, A. H. (1992) *The Decline of Donnish Dominion*, Oxford: Oxford University Press.

Halsey, A. H., Trow, M. and Fulton, O. (1971) *The British Academics*, London: Faber and Faber.

Hammond, G., Quentin-Baxter, M., Drummond, P., Brown, T. and Jordan, R. (1997) *Student support and tutoring: a role for simple applications of computer mediated communication (CMC)*, Faculty of Medicine, University of Newcastle, undated (1997?), online: learning.support.ncl.ac.uk/sst-cmc/about/cti/

Handy, C. (1995) 'Trust and the virtual organization', *Harvard Business Review*, May-June, pp. 40–50.

Hara, N. and Kling, R. (1999) 'Student frustrations with a Web-based distance education course', *First Monday*, vol. 4, no. 12, December, online: www.firstmonday.dk/issues/issue4_12/index.html

Hara, N., Bonk, C. J. and Angeli, C. (2000) 'Content analysis of an on-line discussion in an applied educational psychology course', *Instructional Science*, vol. 28, pp. 115–52.

Harasim, L. M. (1987) 'Teaching and learning on-line: Issues in computer-mediated graduate courses', *Canadian Journal of Educational Communication*, vol. 16, no. 2, pp. 117–35.

Harris, M. (1997) 'Rethinking the Virtual Organization', in Jackson, P. and Van der Weilen, J. (eds) *From Telecommuting to the Virtual Organization*, London: Routledge, pp. 74–92.

Harris, M. and Corrigan, P. (1996) 'The university for industry', *New Statesman*, 20 December.

Harris, M. and Howells, J. (1996) 'Controls on the traffic of ideas', *Times Higher Education Supplement*, 7 June.

Harvey, D. (1991) *The Condition of Postmodernity: An Enquiry into the Origins of Cultural Change*, Oxford and New York: Blackwell, 1989.

Hayek, F. A. (1994) *The Road to Serfdom,* 50th Anniversary edn, Chicago: University of Chicago Press.

Hayes, W., Clarke, W. and Lorenz, C. (1985) *The Uneasy Alliance: Managing the Productivity-Innovation Dilemma*, Boston: Harvard Business School Press.

Haywood, T. (1999) *Only Connect: Shaping Networks and Knowledge for the New Millennium*, East Grinstead, England: Bowker-Saur.

Hechinger, J. (1999) 'Textbook publisher plans Web university', *Financial Express*, July, online: www.financialexpress.com/fe/daily/19990721/fec21078p.html

Heidegger, M. (1962) *Being and Time*, San Francisco: Harper.

Herzog, R. (1997) 'Durch Deutschland muß ein Ruck gehen'. Address of Federal President Roman Herzog, Berlin, 26 April, online: www.glidenet-global.de/herzog1.htm (8 September 2001).

Hesburgh, T. (1994), quoted in Templeton, J. M. *Looking Forward: The Next Forty Years*, New York: K. S. Giniger (Harper Business).

Hesse, B., Sproull, L., Kiesler, S. and Walsh, J. (1993) 'Returns to science computer networks in oceanography', *Communications of the ACM*, vol. 36, no. 8, pp. 90–101.

Hill, S., Harris, M. and Martin, R. (1997) 'Flexible technologies, markets and the firm: strategic choices and FMS' in McLoughlin, I. and Harris, M. (eds) *Innovation, Organizational Change and Technology*, London: International Thompson Business Press.

Hillman, J. (1996) *The University for Industry: Creating a National Learning Network*, London: IPPR.

Hiltz, S. R. (1998) *Teaching in a Virtual Classroom. Vol. 2: A Virtual Classroom on EIES: Final Evaluation Report*, Newark, NJ: New Jersey Institute of Technology.

Hoffmann, M., Sumner, T. and Wright, M. (2001) 'Supporting distributed participatory design with lightweight communication tools', *Technical Report*, Dept. of Computer Science, University of Colorado at Boulder.

Howell, D. (1994) 'The skills myth', *The American Prospect*, no 18, pp. 81–90, online: www.prospect.org/print/V5/18/howell-d.html

Howells, J. and Hine, J. (1993) *Innovative Banking: Competition and the Management of a New Network Technology*, London: Routledge.

Huffstutter, P. J. and Fields, R. (2000) 'A virtual revolution in teaching', *Los Angeles Times*, 28 April.

Humphrys, J. (2001) 'There goes another herd of A-level sheep to slaughter', *The Sunday Times*, 19 August.

Iacono, S. and Kling, R. (2001) 'Computerization movements: the rise of the Internet and distant forms of work' in Van Maanen, J. and Yates, J. (eds) *Information Technology and Organizational Change*, Newbury Park, CA: Sage, pp. 93–136.

IASS (Institute for Applied Social Sciences) (1998) 'The impact of ICT on the teacher', *Report to the European Commission*, Brussels: The European Commission.

ICDL (International Center for Distance Learning) (1995) *The Mega-Universities of the World: The Top Ten*, Milton Keynes: Open University.

IDC (International Data Corporation) (1999) *Online vs On-Site: To What Extent can Live Instruction be Replaced?* Framingham, MA: International Data Corporation.

Illich, I. (1971) *Deschooling Society*, 1st edn, New York: Harper & Row.

Innis, H. A. (1951) *The Bias of Communication*, Toronto: University of Toronto Press.

Innis, H. A. (1972) [1951] *Empire and Communications*, Toronto: University of Toronto Press.

Innis, H. A. (1995) *Staples, Markets and Cultural Change: Selected Essays*, Drache, D. (ed.) Montreal: McGill-Queen's University Press.

Institute for Higher Education Policy (1999) *What's the Difference? A Review of Contemporary Research on the Effectiveness of Distance Learning in Higher Education*, Washington, DC.

Irby, A. J. (1999) 'Postbaccalaureate certificates: higher education's growth market', *Change*, vol. 31, no. 2, pp. 36–41.

ITAP (Information Technology Advisory Panel to the Cabinet Office) (1982) *Report on Cable Systems*, London: HMSO.

Jackson, M. H. (1996) 'The meaning of "Communication Technology": the technology-context scheme' in Burleson, B. (ed.) *Communication Yearbook 19*, Beverly Hills: Sage, pp. 229–68.

Jaffee, D. (1998) 'Institutionalized resistance to asynchronous learning networks', *Journal of Asynchronous Learning Networks*, vol. 2, no. 2, online: www.aln.org/alnweb/journal/vol2_issue2/jaffee.htm

JIME, *Journal of Interactive Media in Education* (1996), online: www-jime.open.ac.uk/

JISC (Joint Information Systems Committee) (1995) An Information Strategy, online: www.jisc.ac.uk/pub/infstrat/

Joint Funding Council's Libraries Review (1993) *Report* (known as 'The Follett Report'), Bristol, UK: Higher Education Funding Council for England. Also online: www.ukoln.ac.uk/services/papers/follett/report/

Jones, G. R. (1997) *Cyberschools: an Education Renaissance*, Englewood, CO: Jones Digital Century, Inc.

Kartus, L. (2000) 'Gaining by degrees', *University Business*, vol. 3, no. 1, pp. 40.

Katz, R. N. and Rudy, J. A. (1999) (eds) 'Information technology in higher education: assessing its impact and planning for the future', *New Directions for Institutional Research*, no. 102, Summer, San Francisco, CA: Jossey-Bass, Inc.

Kay, A. C. (1991) 'Computers, networks, and education', *Scientific American*, vol. 265, no. 3, September, pp. 100–7.

Kenny, A. (1994) 'Digitized Beowulf takes library into the future', *Times Higher Education Supplement*, 13 May, pp. iv.

Kerres, M. (2001) 'Neue Medien in der Lehre: Von der Projektförderung zur systematischen Integration', online: www.ruhr-uni-bochum.de/kerres/articles/hochschulwesen-kerres-ef.pdf (1 September 2001).

Kerrey, B. (2000) 'The power of the Internet for learning: moving from promise to practice', *Report of the Web-based Education Commission,* Washington, DC.

Kidd, A. (1994) 'The marks are on the knowledge worker', *Human Factors in Computing Systems (CHI '94),* Boston, MA: ACM Press.

Kling, R. (1994) 'Reading all about computerization: how genre conventions shape non-fiction social analysis', *The Information Society,* vol. 10, no. 3, pp. 147–72, online: www.slis.indiana.edu/kling/read94a.html

Kling, R. (2000) 'Learning about information technologies and social change: the contribution of social informatics', *The Information Society,* vol. 16, no. 3, (July-Sept), pp. 217–32, online: www.slis.indiana.edu/TIS/articles/kling 16(3).pdf

Kling, R. and Courtright, C. (in press) 'Group behavior and learning, in electronic forums: a socio-technical approach', in Barab, S. and Kling, R., *Building Online Communities in the Service of Learning,* Cambridge: Cambridge University Press.

Kling, R. and Jewett, T. (1991) 'The dynamics of computerization in a social science research team: a case study of infrastructure, strategies, and skills', *Social Science Computer Review,* vol. 9, no. 2, Summer, pp. 246–75.

Kraut, R., Lundmark, V., Patterson, M., Kiesler, S., Mukhopadhyay, T. and Scherlis, W. (1998) 'Internet Paradox: A social technology that reduces social involvement and psychological well-being?', *American Psychologist,* vol. 53, no. 9, pp. 1017–31, online: http://www.apa.org/journals/amp/ amp5391017.html

Kuhn, T. S. (1996) *The Structure of Scientific Revolutions,* 3rd edn, Chicago: University of Chicago Press.

Lamberton, D. (1997) 'The knowledge-based economy: a Sisyphus model', *Prometheus,* vol. 15, no. 1, pp.73–81.

Latour, B. (1987) *Science in Action,* Cambridge, MA: Harvard University Press.

Latour, B. (1988) 'The politics of explanation: an alternative', in Woolgar, S. (ed.) *Knowledge and Reflexivity: New Frontiers in the Sociology of Knowledge,* London: Sage, pp. 155–76.

Latour, B. (1990) 'Drawing things together', in Lynch, M. and Woolgar, S. (eds) *Representations in Scientific Practice,* Cambridge, MA: MIT Press.

Latour, B. (1996) *Aramis or the Love of Technology,* Cambridge, MA: Harvard University Press.

Lave, J. (1991) 'Situated learning in communities of practice' in Resnick, L., Levine, J. and Teasley, S. (eds) *Perspectives on Socially Shared Cognition,* Washington, DC: American Psychological Association.

Lave, J. and Wenger, E. (1991) *Situated Learning: Legitimate Peripheral Participation,* Cambridge, UK: Cambridge University Press.

Law, J. (ed.) (1991) *A Sociology of Monsters,* London: Routledge.

Law, J. (1994) *Organising Modernity,* Oxford: Blackwell.

Lax, S. (ed.) (2001) *Access Denied in the Information Age,* London: Palgrave.

Leatherman, C. (1998) 'U. of Phoenix's faculty members insist they offer high-quality education', *The Chronicle of Higher Education*, 16 October.

Lehtinen, E. and Sinko, M. (1999) *The Challenge of ICT in Finnish Education*, Finland: Atena, Sitra edition.

Lievrouw, L. (1989) 'The invisible college reconsidered: bibliometrics and the development of scientific communication theory', *Communication Research*, vol. 16, no. 5, pp. 615–28.

Lipponen, L., Lakkala, M., Hakkarainen, K., Syri, J., Lallimo, J., Ilomki, L., Muukkonen, H. and Rahikainen, M. (1999) *Learning Through the Internet: A Review of Networked Learning*, Report to the European Commission, DCXXII, November,1999. Helsinki, Finland: University of Helsinki.

Lively, K. and Blumenstyk, G. (1999) 'Sylvan Learning Systems to start a network of for-profit universities overseas', *The Chronicle of Higher Education*, 29 January.

Lockwood, G. (1985) 'Universities as organizations' in Lockwood, G. and Davies, J. (eds) *Universities: The Management Challenge*, Windsor: NFER-Nelson Publishing.

MacDonald, J. and Mason, R. (1999) 'Information handling skills and resource based learning', Report to the Office of Technology Development, *Technical Report 101*, Institute of Educational Technology, The Open University (UK).

MacKenzie, D. and Wajcman, J. (1985) *The Social Shaping of Technology*, Milton Keynes: Open University Press.

Madrick, J. (1999) 'How new is the New Economy?', *New York Review of Books*, 23 September.

Mangan, K. S. (1999) 'Business enrollments boom at for-profit colleges', *The Chronicle of Higher Education*, vol. 46, issue 6.

Marchese, T. (1998) 'Not-so-distant competitors: how new providers are remaking the post-secondary market', *American Association for Higher Education Bulletin*, May, pp. 16–20.

Marion, A. and Hacking, E. (1998) 'Educational publishing and the World Wide Web', *Journal of Interactive Media in Education*, vol. 98, no. 2, online: www-jime.open.ac.uk/98/2

Marlino, M., Sumner, T., Fulker, D., Manduca, C. and Mogk, D. (2001) 'The Digital Library for Earth System Education: building community, building the Library', *Communications of the ACM*, vol. 44, no. 5 (Special issue on digital libraries – May), pp. 80–1.

Masunaga, H., Peterson, D. and Seymour, R. (1998) 'Effect of gerontology education: a 21-year report', *Educational Gerontology*, Jan-Feb, vol. 24, no. 1, pp. 79–89.

Maynard, J. (1971) *Some Microeconomics of Higher Education: Economies of Scale*, Lincoln: University of Nebraska Press.

McCormick, J. (2000) 'The new school', *Newsweek*, 24 April.

McGeehan, P. (1999) 'Unext.com, signs course deal with four more universities', *The Wall Street Journal*, 23 June.

McIsaac, M. S. and Gunawardena, C. N. (1996) 'Distance education' in

Johnassen, D. (ed.) *Handbook of Research for Educational Communications and Technology*, New York: Macmillan, pp. 403–37.

McKeachie, W. J. (1999) *Teaching Tips: Strategies, Research, and Theory for College and University Teachers*, 10th edn, Boston, MA: Houghton Mifflin Co.

McLoughlin, I. and Harris, M. (1997) *Innovation, Organizational Change and Technology*, London: International Business Press.

McNay, I. (1995) 'From the collegial academy to corporate enterprise: the changing cultures of universities', in Schuller, T. (ed.) *The Changing University?* Buckingham: Open University Press/SRHE.

Mendels, P. (1999) 'Hurdles for on-line education efforts', *New York Times on the Web*, 29 March.

Mendels, P. (1999a) 'On-line classes let small colleges expand offerings', *New York Times on the Web*, 18 August.

Mendels, P. (1999b) 'Study finds problems with web class', *The New York Times*, 22 September.

Merrill Lynch (1999) *The Book of Knowledge: Investing in the Growing Education and Training Industry*, 9 April, pp. 115.

Mesthene, E. G. (1969) 'The role of technology in society', reprinted in Teich (2000) *Technology and the Future*, 8th edn, Boston and New York: Bedford/St. Martin's, pp. 61–70.

Meyer, H. J. (1998) 'Noch heute gültige Wahrheiten. Humboldt könnte doch den Weg zu einer handlungsfähigen und handlungswilligen Universität weisen', *Frankfurter Allgemeine Zeitung*, 7 July, p. 11.

Michael, D. A. (1986) 'Universities in the Information Age' in Neilson, W. A. W. and Gaffield, C. (eds) *Universities in Crisis: A Medieval Institution in the Twenty-First Century*, Ottawa: The Institute for Research on Public Policy, pp. 195–213.

Michaels, J. W. and Smillie, D. (2000) 'Webucation', *Forbes Magazine*, 15 May.

Miles, I., Rush, H., Turner, K. and Bessant, J. (1988) *Information Horizons: The Long-Term Social Implications of New Information Technologies*, Aldershot, UK: Edward Elgar.

Mitchell, W. J. (1995) *City of Bits: Space, Place, and the Infobahn*, Cambridge, MA: MIT Press.

Mosco, V. (1996) *The Political Economy of Communication*, Thousand Oaks, CA: Sage.

Mulgan, G. J. (1991) *Communication and Control: Networks and the New Economies of Communication*, New York: Guilford.

Mutschler, D. in collaboration with Amor, P. and Laget, P. (1999) *Curriculum for the 21st Century: Technology in Education*, Washington DC: Delegation of the European Commission to the USA.

Myers, M. T. (2000) 'CyberU: what's missing', *The Washington Post*, 21 March.

National Center for Education Statistics (1998) *Issue brief: distance education in higher education institutions: incidence, audiences, and plans to expand*, online: nces.ed.gov/pubs98/98132.html

National Center for Educational Statistics (2001) *Projections of Education Statistics To 2011*, US Department of Education, NCES 01–083, August, pp. 25–6.

Negroponte, N. (1995) *Being Digital*, London: Hodder and Stoughton.

Newby, H. (1999) 'Higher education in the 21st century: some possible futures' discussion paper, London: CVCP (now Universities UK), March.

Newman, R. and Johnson, F. (1999) 'Sites of power and knowledge? Towards a critique of the virtual university', *British Journal of Sociology of Education*, vol. 20, no. 1, pp. 79–88.

Nicklin, J. L. (1995) 'They're all business', *The Chronicle of Higher Education*, 14 April.

Noam, E. M. (1995) 'Electronics and the dim future of the university', *Science*, vol. 270, 13 October, pp. 247–9.

Noble, D. (1998) 'Digital Diploma Mills, Part 1', *First Monday*, online: firstmonday.dk/issues/issue3_1/noble/index.html

Noble, D. (1998a) Digital Diploma Mills, Part 3, 'The Bloom is Off the Rose', online: communication.ucsd.edu/dl/ddm3.html

Noble, D. F. (1998b) 'Digital diploma mills: the automation of higher education', *Science as Culture*, vol. 7, no. 3, pp. 355–68.

Noble, D. F. (2001) *Digital Diploma Mills: The Automation of Higher Education*, New York: Monthly Review Press. Earlier editions have been available on *First Monday* 3.1 (www.firstmonday.dk/issues/issue3_1) Jan.

Noll, A. M. and Mays, J. (1971) 'Computer literacy: an education-technology initiative', Unpublished draft of staff report to Edward Jr., E. D, Science Advisor to President Richard Nixon, Washington, DC: Office of Science and Technology.

Norman, D. A. (1993) *Things That Make Us Smart*, Reading, MA: Addison-Wesley Publishing Company.

Odlyzko, A. M. (1995) 'Tragic loss or good riddance? The impending demise of traditional scholarly journals', *International Journal of Human-Computer Studies*, vol. 42, pp. 71–122.

Olivas, M. A. (1997) *The Law and Higher Education: Cases and Materials on Colleges in Courts*, 2nd edn, Durham, NC: Carolina Academic Press.

Olson, G. M., Atkins, D. E. et al. (1998) 'The Upper Atmospheric Research Collaboratory', *Interactions*, vol. 5, no. 3, pp. 48–55.

Organisation for Economic Co-operation and Development (2001) *E-learning: the Partnership Challenge*, Paris: OECD, Centre for Educational Research and Innovation.

Padilla, A. (1999), 'The University of Phoenix', in *On the Horizon*, 30 July.

Paepcke, A., Chang, C-C. K., Winograd, T. and Garcia-Molina, H. (1998) 'Interoperability for digital libraries worldwide', *Communications of the ACM 41U*, vol. 4, pp. 33–42.

Palattella, J. (1998) 'The British are coming, The British are coming', *University Business*, vol. 1, no. 3, p. 24.

Papert, S. (1980) *Mind-Storms: Children, Computers, and Powerful Ideas*, New York: Basic Books.

Parker, M. and Jary, D. (1995) 'The McUniversity: organization, management and academic subjectivity', *Organization*, vol. 2, no. 2, pp. 319–38.

Perkins, H. (1990) *The Rise of Professional Society: England Since 1880*, London: Routledge.

Perry, W. (1977) 'The Open University: history and evaluation of a dynamic innovation', *Higher Education*, New York: Jossey-Bass.

Peterson, D., Douglass, E., Seymour, R. and Wendt, P. (1997) *Aging Education and Training: Priorities for Grant Making Foundations*, Association for Gerontology in Higher Education, Washington, DC.

Peterson, D., Wendt, P. and Douglass, E. (1994) *Development of Gerontology, Geriatrics, and Aging Studies Programs in Institutions of Higher Education*, Association for Gerontology in Higher Education, Washington, DC.

Phelps, T. and Wilensky, R. (1996) 'Toward active, extensible, networked documents: multivalent architecture and applications', in *First ACM Conference on Digital Libraries*, Bethesda, MD: ACM Press, pp. 100–8.

Phipps, R. A., Harrison, K. V. and Merisotis, J. P. (1999) *Students at Private, For-profit Institutions, NCES 1999–178*, US Department of Education, National Center for Educational Statistics.

Phipps, R. and Merisotis, J. (1999) *What's the Difference? A Review of Contemporary Research on the Effectiveness of Distance Learning on Higher Education*, Washington, DC: The Institute for Higher Education Policy, April, online: www.ihep.com.

Picht, R. (2001) 'Renaissance durch Globalisierung? Europäische Wissensgesellschaften auf der Suche nach Bildung', *Merkur*, vol. 55, no. 3, pp. 211–21.

Polanyi, M. (1962) *Personal Knowledge: Towards a Post-Critical Philosophy*, Chicago: University of Chicago Press.

Pollock, N. (1998) *Working-Around a Computer System: Some Aspects of a Hybrid Sociology*, unpublished PhD thesis, University of Lancaster, UK.

Pollock, N. and Cornford, J. (2000) 'The theory and practice of the virtual university', *Ariadne*, issue 24, online: www.ariadne.ac.uk/issue24/virtual-universities/intro.html

Pollock, N. and Cornford, J. (2001) ERP Systems and the University as an 'Unique' Organization, Proceedings of the Critical Management Studies Conference, UMIST, 11–13 July, Manchester, online: www.mngt.waikato.ac.nz/ejrot/cmsconference/2001/papers-education.asp

Porter, T. M. (1994) 'Information, power and the view from nowhere' in Bud-Frierman, L. (ed.) *Information Acumen: The Understanding and Use of Knowledge in Modern Business*, London: Routledge.

Pouts-Lajus, S. and Riche-Magnier, M. (1998) *L'ecole a l'heure d'Internet – les enjeux du multimedia dans l'education*, Paris: Nathan edition.

Pouts-Lajus, S. and Riche-Magnier, M. (1999) 'L'enseignement ouvert et a distance en Europe: mythe et realites', *Revue internationale d'education*, vol. 23, Sevres, France.

Powell, W. W. and DiMaggio, P. J. (eds) (1991) *The New Institutionalism in Organizational Analysis*, Chicago: University of Chicago Press.

Press, E. and Washburn, J. (2000) 'The Kept University', *The Atlantic Monthly*, March, pp. 39–54.

Quinn, J. B. (1992) *Intelligent Enterprise*, New York: Free Press.

Ragsdale, R. G. (1988) *Permissible Computing in Education: Values, Assumptions, and Needs*, New York: Praeger.

Rahm, D. and Reed, B. J. (1998) 'Tangled webs in public administration: organizational issues in distance learning', *Public Administration and Management: An Interactive Journal*, vol. 3, no. 1.

Rao, R., Hearst, J. O. et al. (1995) 'Rich interaction in the digital library', *Communications of the ACM 38*, vol. 4, pp. 29–39.

Readings, B. (1996) *The University in Ruins*, Cambridge, MA and London: Harvard University Press.

Repenning, A., Ioannidou, A. and Ambach, J. (1998) 'Learn to communicate and communicate to learn', *Journal of Interactive Media in Education*, vol. 98, no. 7, online: www-jime.open.ac.uk/98/7

Resnick, P. and Varian, H. (1997) 'Recommender systems', *Communications of the ACM*, vol. 40, no. 3, pp. 56–58.

Rheingold, H. (1993) *The Virtual Community: Homesteading on the Electronic Frontier*, Reading, MA: Addison-Wesley.

Richards, T. (1993) *The Imperial Archive: Knowledge and the Fantasy of Empire*, New York: Verso.

Rifkin, J. (2000) *The Age of Access: The New Culture of Hypercapitalism Where All of Life Is a Paid-for Experience*, New York: Jeremy P. Tarcher/Putnam.

Ritzer, G. (1998) *The McDonaldization Thesis: Explorations and Extensions*, London: Sage.

Roberts, T. L. (1998) 'Are newsgroups virtual communities?', *Human Factors in Computing Systems (CHI '98)*, Los Angeles: ACM Press, pp. 360–7.

Robins, K. and Webster, F. (1989) *The Technical Fix: Education, Computers and Industry*, London: Macmillan Education Ltd.

Rochlin, G. I. (1997) *Trapped in The Net: The Unanticipated Consequences of Computerization*, Princeton, NJ: Princeton University Press.

Rose, E. (2000) *Hyper Texts: The Language and Culture of Educational Computing*, London, Ontario: The Althouse Press.

Ross, A. (2001) *Risks and Opportunities of Virtual Learning: The Experience of UOC*, online: www.uoc.es/Web/eng/index.html

Rossman, M. H. (1999) 'Successful online teaching using an asynchronous learner discussion forum', *Journal of Asynchronous Learning Networks*, vol. 3, no. 2, Nov., online: www.aln.org/alnweb/journal/jaln-vol3issue2.htm

Rudinow Saetnan, A. (1991), 'Rigid politics and technological flexibility', *Science, Technology and Human Values*, vol. 16, no. 4, pp. 419-47.

Runciman, W. G. (1983) *A Treatise on Social Theory, vol. 1*, Cambridge: Cambridge University Press.

Rusbridge, C. (1998) 'Towards the hybrid library', *D-Lib Magazine*, July/August.

Ryan, A. (1998) *Liberal Anxieties and Liberal Education*, New York: Hill and Wang.

Ryan, Y. (2000) 'The business of borderless education: US case studies and the HE response', Paper presented to the CVCP Conference *The Business of Borderless Education*, London, 28 March.

Sabel, C. (1991) 'Moebius strip organizations and open labour markets: some consequences of the reintegration of conception and execution in a volatile economy' in Bourdieu, P. and Coleman, J. (eds) *Social Theory For a Changing Society*, Boulder, CO: Westview.

Sambataro, M. (2000) 'Just-in-Time learning', *Computerworld*, 3 April.

Scardamelia, M. and Bereiter, C. (1994) 'Computer support for knowledge-building communities', *The Journal of the Learning Sciences*, vol. 3, no. 3, pp. 265–83.

Scharff, E. (1998) *CU-Write*, University of Colorado at Boulder, online: www.Colorado.EDU/kines/cuwrite/

Schatz, B., Mischo, W. et al. (1999) 'Federated search of scientific literature', *Computer*, vol. 32, no. 2, pp. 51–9.

Schement, J. R. and Curtis, T. (1997), *Tendencies and Tensions of the Information Age*, New Brunswick, NJ: Transaction Publishers.

Schiff, L. R., Van House, N. A. and Butler, M. (1997) 'Understanding complex information environments: a social analysis of watershed planning', *Second ACM Conference on Digital Libraries*, Philadelphia, PA: ACM Press.

Schiller, H. I. (1996) *Information Inequality: The Deepening Social Crisis in America*, New York and London: Routledge.

Schlager, M. S. and Schank, P. K. (1997) 'Tapped in: A new online teacher community concept for the next generation of Internet technology', *Computer Support for Collaborative Learning (CSCL '97)*, Toronto, Canada: ACM Press, pp. 230–41.

Schramm, W. (1977) *Big Media, Little Media: Tools and Technologies for Instruction*, Beverly Hills and London: Sage Publications.

Schroeder, R. (1996) *Possible Worlds: The Social Dynamic of Virtual Reality Technology*, Boulder, CO: Westview Press.

Schuller, T. (ed.) (1995) *The Changing University?* Buckingham: Open University Press/SRHE.

Schumpeter, J. A. (1939) *Business Cycles: a Theoretical, Historical and Structural Analysis*, New York: McGraw-Hill.

Scott, M. M. (1998) 'Intellectual property rights: A ticking time bomb in academia', *Academia*, vol. 84, no. 3, pp. 22–6.

Scribner, S. and Cole, M. (1981) *The Psychology of Literacy*, Cambridge: Harvard University Press.

Shapiro, A. L. (1999) *The Control Revolution*, New York: Century Foundation Book.

Shapiro, C. and Varian, H. (1998) *Information Rules: A Strategic Guide to the Network Economy*, Boston: Harvard Business School Press.

Sheehan, P. and Tegart, G. (1998) (eds) *Working for the Future: Technology and Employment in the Global Knowledge Economy*, Melbourne: Victoria University Press.

Shore, C. and Wright, S. (1999) *Audit Culture and Anthropology: Neo-liberalism in British Higher Education*, Unpublished mimeo, Goldsmiths College.

Silver, H. and Silver, P. (1997) *Students: Changing Roles, Changing Lives*, Milton Keynes: SRHE/Open University Press.

Slaughter, S. and Leslie, L. L. (1997) *Academic Capitalism: Politics, Policies and the Entrepreneurial University*, Baltimore: Johns Hopkins University Press.

Smith, A. and Webster, F. (eds) (1997) *The Postmodern University*, Buckingham: Open University Press/SRHE.

Soper, J. B. (1997) 'Integrating interactive media in courses: the WinEcon Software with Workbook Approach', *Journal of Interactive Media in Education*, vol. 97, no. 2, online: www-jime.open.ac.uk/97/2

Stanford Study (2001) *Distance Learning in Higher Education: Spain and the Universitat Oberta de Catalunya*, Stanford University, School of Education, online: www.stanford.edu/~kiky/UOC/

Star, S. L. and Ruhleder, K. (1996) 'Steps toward an ecology of infrastructure: design and access for large information spaces', *Information Systems Research*, vol. 7, no. 1, pp. 111–34.

Stefik, M. (1996) 'Letting loose the light: igniting commerce in electronic publication' in Stefik, M. (ed.) *Internet Dreams: Archetypes, Myths and Metaphors*, Cambridge, MA: MIT Press.

Strathern, M. (1997) '"Improving Ratings": audit in the British university System', *European Review*, vol. 5, no. 3, pp. 305–21.

Strosnider, K. (1997) 'For-profit university challenges traditional colleges', *The Chronicle of Higher Education*, 6 June.

Strosnider, K. (1998) 'For-profit higher education sees booming enrollments and revenues', *The Chronicle of Higher Education*, 23 January.

Sturken, M. and Cartwright, L. (2001) *Practices of Looking: An Introduction to Visual Culture*, Oxford: Oxford University Press.

Sumner, T. and Buckingham Shum, S. (1998) 'From documents to discourse: shifting conceptions of scholarly publishing', in *Human Factors in Computing Systems (CHI '98)*, Los Angeles: ACM Press, pp. 95–102.

Sumner, T. and Domingue, J. et al. (1998) 'Enriching representations of work to support organisational learning', *First Interdisciplinary Workshop on Building, Maintaining, and Using Organizational Memories (OM-98)*, Brighton, UK, online: www.aifb.uni-karlsruhe.de/WBS/ECAI98OM

Sumner, T. R. and Dawe, M. (2001) 'Looking at digital library usability from a reuse perspective', *ACM/IEEE Joint Conference on Digital Libraries (JCDL '01)*, (Roanoke, Virginia (June 24–8), pp. 416–25.

Sumner, T., Buckingham Shum, S., Wright, M., Bonnardel, N., Chevalier, A. and Piolat, A. (2000) 'Redesigning the peer review process: a developmental theory-in-action' in Dieng, R., Giboin, A., Karsenty, L. and De Michelis, G. (eds) *Designing Cooperative Systems: The Use of Theories and Models*, Amsterdam: IOS Press, pp. 19–34.

Sumner, T., Yates, S., Buckingham Shum, S. and Perrone, J. (1998) 'Managing persistent discourse: organizational goals and digital texts', *Technical Report KMI-TR-62*, Knowledge Media Institute, The Open University (UK). Available HTTP: kmi.open.ac.uk/techreports/papers/kmi-tr-62.pdf

Taub, J. (2000) 'This campus is being simulated', *The New York Times Magazine*, 19 November.

Tehranian, M. (1996) 'The end of university?', *The Information Society*, vol. 12, pp. 441–7.

Teich, A. H. (2000) *Technology and the Future*, 8th edn, Boston and New York: Bedford/St. Martin's.

Terveen, L., Selfridge, P. and Long, M. D. (1993) 'From "Folklore" to "Living Design Memory"', *Human Factors in Computing Systems (Interact '93 and CHI '93)*, Amsterdam: ACM Press, pp. 15–22.

Times Higher Education Supplement (2001) Editorial, 13 July, p. 14.

Toffler, A. (1970) *Future Shock*, New York: Random House.

Trigg, M. (2001) 'Apollo's rocket ride', *MotleyFool.com*, 25 June.

Triplett, J. E. (1999), 'The Solow productivity paradox: what do computers do to productivity?', *Canadian Journal of Economics*, vol. 32, no. 2, online at www.csls.ca/jrn/v32n2_04.pdf

Turkle, S. (1984) *The Second Self: Computers and the Human Spirit*, New York: Simon and Schuster.

UNext.com (1999) 'Who We Are', www.unext.com/company_overview/whoweare.html

University of Illinois (1999) 'Teaching at an internet distance: the pedagogy of online teaching and learning' *Report of a 1998–1999 University of Illinois Faculty Seminar*, online www.vpaa.uillinois.edu/tid/report

US Department of Commerce (1998) *Falling Through the Net II: New Data on the Digital Divide*, Washington DC: US Department of Commerce.

US Department of Education (1999) *Preparing Tomorrow's Teachers to Use Technology*, Washington DC: US Department of Education.

Veltman, K. (1997) 'Frontiers in electronic media', *Interactions*, vol. 4, no. 4, pp. 32–64.

Vygotsky, L. S. (1962) *Thought and Language*, Cambridge, MA: MIT Press.

Vygotsky, L. S. (1978) *Mind in Society*, Cambridge, MA: Harvard University Press.

Weber, M. (1972) *Wirtschaft und Gesellschaft. Grundriss der verstehenden Soziologie*, provided by J. Winckelmann, 5th edn, Tübingen: Mohr.

Wegerif, R. (1998) 'The social dimension of asynchronous learning networks', *Journal of Asynchronous Learning Networks*, vol. 2, no. 1, online: www.aln.org/alnweb/journal/vol2_issue1/wegerif.htm

Wehler, H. U. (1989) 'Von der Reformära bis zur industriellen und politischen Deutschen Doppelrevolution', *Deutsche Gesellschaftsgeschichte*, vol. 2, Munich: C. H. Beck.

Wiesenberg, F. and Hutton, S. (1995) 'Teaching a graduate program using computer mediated conferencing software', paper presented at the *Annual Meeting of the American Association for Adult and Continuing Education*, November, Kansas City, MU.

Wildavsky, A. (1983) 'Information as an organizational problem', *Journal of Management Studies*, vol. 20, no. 1, pp. 28–40.

Williams, F. (1982) *The Communications Revolution*, Beverly Hills and London: Sage Publications.

Williams, R. and Edge, D. (1996) 'The social shaping of technology', in Dutton. W. H. (ed.) *Information and Communication Technologies – Visions and Realities*, Oxford: Oxford University Press, pp. 69–86.

Winner, L (1998) *Automatic Professor Machine*, online: www.rpi.edu/~winner/apm1.html (June 6, 1999).

Woody, T. (1999) 'Ivy Online', *The Standard*, 22 October, online: www.thestandard.net/article/display/0,1151,7122,00.html

Woolgar, S. (1996) 'Technologies as cultural artifacts', in Dutton, W. H. (ed.) *Information and Communication Technologies – Visions and Realities*, Oxford: Oxford University Press, pp. 87–102.

Woolgar, S. and Cooper, G. (1999) 'Do artefacts have ambivalence?: Moses' bridges, winner's bridges and other urban legends, in SandTS', *Social Studies of Science*, 29, 3: pp. 433–49.

Wulf, W. A. (1993) 'The collaboratory opportunity', *Science*, 13 August, pp. 854–5.

Yakimovicz, A. D. and Murphy, K. L. (1995) 'Constructivism and collaboration on the Internet: case study of a graduate class experience', *Computers and Education*, vol. 24, no. 3, pp. 203–9.

Yates, N. (1997), 'Millions visit Mars – on the Internet', *Los Angeles Times*, 14 July, pp. A16.

Yates, S. J. and Perrone, J. L. (1998) 'Politics on the Web', *International Conference on Internet Research and Information in the Social Sciences*, Bristol, UK, online: www.sosig.ac.uk/iriss/papers/paper46.htm

Young, J. R. (1999) 'Universities create on-line education portal', *The Chronicle of Higher Education*, 25 June.

Young, M. (1996, 1994) *The Rise of the Meritocracy*, New Brunswick and London: Transaction Publishers.

Zuckerman, H. and Merton, R. K. (1971) 'Patterns of evaluation in science: institutionalisation, structure, and functions of the referee system', *Minerva*, vol. 9, no. 1, pp. 66–100.

Index

academic capitalism 216
academic collaborations 182
academic freedom 108; loss 331
academic identity 182
academic institutions: for-profit
  subsidiaries 179
academic staff: deskilling 216
academic/for-profit collaboration:
  models 172–80
accelerated change 320
acceleration: countering 322–4
accountability: liability 272
accountability and co-ordination 329
accreditation status: virtual university
  117
accrediting standards 92
active recruitment 304
Actor Network Theory 235–6
actor-networks: building 302
administration: managerial dimensions
  17
administrative services and marketing
  model 174–5
administrative systems 310–13
affordable accessibility 142
Allen, D.: and Wilson, T. 223
alliances: formation 331
applications: network boundary 154
Applied Sciences: virtual university
  206–14
archives: digital resource 135
asynchronous format: problems 78
asynchronous instruction 98
asynchronous text-based
  communication 80
audience: conception 25; researching

and reaching 328–9; targeting
  specific 14
authorship: boundaries 147–8
"Automatic Professor Machine" 303

B3002 project 44
Bates, A.W. 79
Baumol's disease 263
Bearman, C.T. 320
Bell, D. 256
bench-marking 294
Berg, M.: and Timmermans, S. 243
Blair, T. 3
Bonk, C.J.: and Cummings, J.A. 73–4
Bork, A. 10
Bowker, G. 247
branding: value 221
British Broadcasting Corporation
  (BBC) 189–90
broadband access 46
brokerage 294; role 218
Brown, J.S.: and Duguid, P. 137
bundled pricing 102
business: proven opportunities 292
business model: new 94
Business Process Re-engineering 23
business-to-business supply chain
  258

Caliber Learning Network Inc. (USA)
  202
California State Polytechnic University
  195
Californian Virtual University 291
Callon, M. 235
Cambridge University 47

campus: virtual 117; wired 23; wired and wireless 12
capital formation: importance 264–6
Cardean University: alliances 177–8
Cartwright, L.: and Sturken, M. 54
Castells, M. 2, 216, 217, 226–9, 262
Catalan language 123
Catalonia: Internet-based education 121–3; Open University 121–6
central steering committee 210
chalk-talk 21
Chartrand, H.H. 322
Christensen, C.M. 96
Chronicle of Higher Education 270
classmates: interaction 58
classroom: dominant teaching technique 36; traditional metaphor of 65
clearing house: approach 199–203; online 179
Cochrane, P.: and Gell, M. 216
cognitive skills 257; demand 265
collaboratories: online communities 150–1
"collapsing time and space" 320
collective memory 14
colleges: for-profit 94–8
collegial self-management: traditions 308
commercial enterprises 293
commercial exploitation 212
communication: instruction 81–4
communication medium: influence 323
communication technologies: implications of new 323
communities: gated 137–8; interacting 136; of practice 137
community colleges 88
competing institutions: distance-learning course 112
competition: intensified 215; new 93–9; responding 105
competitive environment 111
computers: early use 9; literacy 12; networked 263
conferencing system 309
consultants 124
consumption: ICTs 13
content: approaches 15–16; creation 298; developer and/or instructor

model 178–9; development and instruction 175
continuing education 97; just-in-time 98
continuous evaluation 124
copyright 329–30
corporate contracts: distance learning 114
corporation employees 97
correspondence schools 36
correspondence teaching 188
cost/quality relationship 90
costs 133; research 90; university 102; virtual university 212
course: components 59
course communication: socio-technical complexity 84
course content: insufficient 77
course management: groupware 10; software 11, 30
courseware 5
credentialing: agencies 99; alternative 99; higher education 92; of value 93
credentialing power: reputational 92
critiques: neo-liberal and radical 224–6
culture: adaptation 133; development 267; diversity 298; objects 275–6; property 284
Cummings, J.A.: and Bonk, C.J. 73–4
Cunningham, S.: et al. 303, 304
curriculum: centrally designed 98; job opportunities 95; rapid development 95
Cyber Culture course 314
cybergraduation 117

Daniel, Sir J. 44, 47, 220
Dartmouth v. Woodward (1819) 271
decentralization 163
degree: costs 188; credit structure 191; programs 211
developing countries: distance learning 102
development: personal and professional 13
digital communications 62
digital diploma mill 41, 303
digital divide 2, 297
Digital Document Discourse Environment (D3E) 144–5
digital environment 220

digital imaging 8
digital libraries 150
discovery software 9
"disruptive technologies" (Christensen) 93–4
distance education 19, 36, 38, 329; dedicated or incorporated 186; distributed learning 5–7; funding 193; Internet-enabled 62–3; new media 290–9; private or public 186; ring-fencing 194; six models 187–204, *187*; strategic or non-strategic 186; university provision 185–205; value of reach 43–4
distance higher education 45–8
distance learning 40, 111–14, 132–3, 263; autonomous budgets 195; catalyst for competition 99–102; course material development 194; developing countries 102; global market 221; interactive tutorials 128–34; Internet advantages 171; Internet-mediated 97, 102; scalability 101; schemes 43; teacher training 192
distress: dealing with 78–80; student 64, 66–72
distributed learning 1, 111–14, 329; development 109; distance education 5–7
Doctor of Philosophy (PhD): distance learning 193; programs 90
document framework: contextually-enriched 139–41
document-annotation systems 149
Douglas, Justice W.O. 278
Duguid, P.: and Brown, J.S. 137

e-commerce 258
e-learning sector 290–1
e-mail 36, 70–2, 309; asynchronous 72; conversations 71; glut 82; problems with reliance 71
e-university (UK) 46
ecology: new media 31–2
economic divides: reinforcing 29–30
economy: constraints 269; resources and constraints 25
education: autonomy 270; competitors 102; continuing 97; demand in

gerontology 56–7; disabilities 279; fluid and fixed experiences 39–40; historical perspective 36; inclusion of general 95; market consolidation 104; new climate 292; online 1; quality 89; socio-economic benefits 298; software 209; technical convergence 27; traditional experience 40–1; undergraduate 89; virtual 35
education and learning: tele-access 7–13
education-service: software 197
educational choices: enrichment 299
educational delivery: technologies 255–6
educational innovation: early advocates 21
educational institutions: changing geography 17
educational intranets: interoperability 126
educational organization: virtualized forms 217
educational technology: diffusion 297
"edutainment" 26
elderly: expanding population 56
Electronic Tutor Marked Assignments (ETMAs) 309
electronics: conferencing 226; course transparency 328; information packaging 11; networking 10–11; portal 329; service delivery 1; services 7
employees: corporation 97
end of knowledge 216
endowments 91
engineering schools 36
enriched document lifecycle 141
enterprise: benefits 238; mantra 239–42
Enterprise Resource Planning Systems (ERP) 233
enthusiasm 191
entry barriers 92
environment: changing competitive 24; online case studies 51–2
Europe 290
European Association of Distance Teaching Universities (EADTU) 294
excellence: advancing standards 330–1; increased focus 107

expenditure per student: quality
    measure 110
export potential: development 225

faculty: evaluation 95; multi-tiered 118;
    quality 90; unbundling role 100
Fathom.com: for-profit partnership 180
federal and state programs 208–9
feedback: lack of 72; lack of prompt
    73; prompt unambiguous 82
FernUniverstät Hagen 207
Ferrate, Dr. G. 121, 123
financial and production models 186
fingertip effect 23
firm: and academic institution model
    175–7; changing nature 262–3
First Amendment: abandonment 282;
    denial of rights 285; right 279
Fish, S. 136
flagship projects 208
flexibility 317
focus groups 234
for-profit colleges: enrollment growth
    96
for-profit firms 172
for-profit institutions: direct providers
    100
for-profit instructional models 181–2
for-profit subsidiaries: academic 179
formal infrastructure 316
fossil fuels: economic growth 260
funding: virtual university 212

gated communities 137–8
gatekeepers: reconfiguring 30–1
Gell, M.: and Cochrane, P. 216
Gellner, E. 265
general training: provision 267
geographic constraints 101
geographic limitations 93
geographical location 277
German language: online courses 212
Germany 206–14, 256
gerontology: demand for education
    56–7; Master of Arts 56–61; Web-
    based Master of Arts 57
Gerontology Center: Ethel Percy
    Andrus 57
Gerontology Library: 'Library Works'
    online services 58

goods to knowledge production 257–8
Gordon, R. 260
Gottschalk, P. 264
governance 165; Faculty 111;
    networked university 163–5; shared
    108
government: education responsibility
    271
government agencies (USA) 99
government intervention 269
government regulations 19
government sponsorship 191
graduation: cyber 117
groupware: course management 10
growth: scalable 229
Gunawardena, C.N.: and McIssac, M.S.
    73

Hague, D. 216
Harley Davidson 53
Harvard Business School: case studies
    50–5; executive education programs
    51
Haywood, T. 48
Herzog, R. 206
Hesburgh, T. 129
heterogeneous engineering 302, 314–15
higher education: change 41–3;
    competitive 87–115; credentialing
    92; diversity 180; flexible 198; future
    326; German system 207; increased
    competition 27–8, 114–15;
    information and communication
    technologies (ICTs) 3; market 159;
    modular 'a la carte' 188; new media
    1–32; new technology 318–27;
    productivity raising 255;
    restructuring 268–89; techno-
    organizational form 215; trends
    292–5; virtual model 116–18;
    virtuality 301–16; winner-take-all
    110
Higher Education Statistics Agency
    (HESA) 305
Hillman, J. 219
holistic approach: strength 148
Howell, D. 264
human factor management 44
hypertext: development 9

Illich, I. 128
incentive structures 21
individual learning account 228
industry organizations 99
information: control of interpretation
    139; electronic packaging 11;
    flexibility 237; socioeconomic class
    270; tele-access 8; value 260
information age: and university 324–5
information and communication
    technologies (ICTs) 13; educational
    delivery 291; governance 18–20;
    higher education 3; impact in
    learning 26; impact on productivity
    258; multidisciplinary research and
    publications 319; reflective
    discourse 326; social shaping 20;
    support of tele-access 4; teaching
    machines 23
information infrastructures: investment
    292
information knowledge: public sphere
    284–5
information networks 226
information overload 14, 261
information processing: history 240
information skills: transferable 266
Information Skills module 314
information society 206, 322;
    distracting concept 267; production
    of knowledge 256–7; theory or
    ideology 253–67
information systems 233
information technology 268–89;
    education 297–9; networked 155–6;
    role 160–1
information-skills requirements 265
informational mantra 248
Informational Mythology (Bowker) 236
informational substrate 162
informationalism 217, 226
Innis, H. 323–4
innovation 328; pains 81; premium 260
institutional arrangements: re-
    imagination 16
institutional boundaries: blurring 27
institutional contexts and choices
    185–205
institutional transparency 19
institutions: political systems 185

instruction: ambiguous 76–8;
    communication 81–4
instructional approach: enhancement
    14
instructional competencies: raising 84
instructional delivery 160
instructional material: ownership 63
instructors: coaxing 83; expectations 77
intellectual capacity 276–7
intellectual goods: commodification
    216
intellectual lineage: tracing 138
intellectual property rights (IPR) 21,
    182, 210, 276, 325, 329–30
interactive tutorials: distance learning
    128–34
international competition 207
Internet 6, 31, 35; advancing
    technologies 292; complementary
    facilities 294; high costs of use 46;
    learning communities 151;
    library supplement 36; re-
    inforcing education 298; wireless
    access 12
Internet Interdisciplinary Institute
    (IN3) 125–6
Internet-based education: Catalonia
    121–3
Internet-enabled distance education
    62–3
Internet-mediated distance learning 97,
    102
interpersonal communication 265
interpersonal skills 257; demand 265
invisible colleges: research 156
Irvine–Geneva system 131
isolation: student 64

job opportunities: curriculum 95
Johnson, F.: and Newman, R. 303
joint curricula 210
Jones International University (USA)
    40, 116–20, 293
*Journal of Interactive Media in
    Education* (JIME) 141–8; archive
    design 145–6

Kentucky Commonwealth Virtual
    University (USA) 201
knowledge: monopoly 324, 325; social

productivity 262; utilities 219; value 276
knowledge formation strategies 325
knowledge networks 151
knowledge products: facilitating interactions 138
Knowledge Society 253
Knowledge TV (USA) 200
knowledge workers: changing role 262–3
knowledge-based economy: transition 305
knowledge-building environments 149
Kuhn, T.S. 146

labor-saving technologies 259
language: diversity 298
Latour, B. 140
Lave, J. 137
learndirect network: University for Industry 217–19
learning: community 79; distributed 1; individualized economical 16; non-linear 100; non-sequential 51–3; on demand 228; tutorial-based 129–34
learning communities: Internet 151
learning consortia 230
learning content: homogenization 230
Learning Development Services 314
learning material: right to 225
learning support: mature students 6
learning technologies 62
lectures: video 132
legitimate peripheral participation 137
Leicester University (UK) 192–5
liability: accountability 272
lifelong learning 89, 95, 130; market 299; revenue streams 170
lifetime employment 108
local knowledge 316
local order 247
location tools: resources 138
London University 46

Management & Administrative Computing system (MAC) 233; replacing by Enterprise 238–9
managerial dimensions: administrative 17
mantra: significance of 239

market making 219
market place: network 28
marketing: aggressive 119
marketing and administrative services model 174–5
Massachusetts Institute of Technology 47
Masters in Business Administration (MBA) 176
mature students 43; learning support 6
McIssac, M.S.: and Gunawardena, C.N. 73
McNay, I. 306, 308
McRae, H. 253–4
media messages: culture 29
medical schools 103
mega-universities 5, 220
metacampus 126
Methodological Resources program 123
military: simulations 10
mission: bundled-function 106; focus 105–7
multi-pass: reviewing strategies 147
multi-source methodology: importance 81
multidisciplinary participants: dialogue 146–7
multimedia 263; centrally-prepared materials 98; created in partnership 54–5; post of producer 55; thin 51
multimedia courseware: investment 164
mutual support 79

name-brand degrees: economic value 105
national educational system 206
National Information Infrastructure (NII) (USA) 3
National Technological University (NTU) (USA) 200
Negroponte, N. 257
Nettuno 47
network: applications boundary 154; effects 164; enterprise 217; market place 28; personal 40
network society: virtual learning 215–30
networked bureaucracy 223
networked information revolution 152–3

networked information technology 153, 155–6
networked university 17; governance 163–5; infrastructure and institutional change 152–65
networking 294; electronic 10–11
new courses: creation 108
new media: ecology 31–2
New Media in Education Program 209–13
new media employment: organizational forms 16–18
Newman, R.: and Johnson, F. 303
night working 69–70
Noble, D. 41, 42, 216–17, 224, 303
non-linear learning 100
non-prestigious universities 88
non-sequential learning 51–3
non-traditional students: recruitment 304

oligopolies: development 263
on-campus education: innovations 112
online approach: challenges 59
online clearing houses 179
online communities: collaboratories 150–1
online courses: academic paradigm 295; German language 212; labor-intensive 83; problems 172; student distress 66–72; students' experience 63; technology driven 295; validation procedures 315
online education 1; cost 126; future 24; guiding principles 328–34
online enrollment 211
online environment case studies 51–2
online interaction: instructor and student 196
online learning 169–82
online programs: launching 293
online resources 33–52
Open University (Catalonia) 121–6
Open University (UK) 5, 40, 44, 98–9, 187–9, 192, 226, 228, 309; bureau professionalism 227; development and delivery 189–90; international expansion 189; as networked bureaucracy

227; technology-based learning 219–20
Open University (USA) 99
open-entry policy 190
organizational form: new media employment 16–18
organizational model: flexible 125
organizational structure 134

parochialism 243
participant observation 234
participation: legitimate peripheral 161
partnership models 299
pedagogical model 124–5
pedagogy: Web-based 22
personal network 40
physical model: university 241
Polanyi, M. 54
political systems: institutions 185
Porter, T. 316
post-secondary education 170–2
postgraduate programs 192
postmodern university 216
price/value relationship 104
pricing: bundled 102
private enterprise 225
private sector: university partnerships 322
private strategic model 198–9, 203–4
private university: public mission 123
production and financial models 186
production of knowledge: information society 256–7
productivity growth: rates 258–9
productivity and innovation: balance 229–30
productivity innovation dilemma 221
productivity and technological change in education 259–61
productivity-innovation dilemma 222–4
professional skills 162
professors 124
profit motive 204
profit sharing 114
programs: access 58; closure 111; multi-lingual 119
promotional bias: positive 63
Public Broadcasting Service (PBS) (USA) 200
public funds: accountability 305

public incorporated strategic model 192–5
public mission: private university 123
public non-strategic model 195–9
public/private strategic model 199–203
public sphere: information technology 284–5; participation 269; university as 277
public strategic model 192–5
public-sphere functions: abandonment 286
publishing toolkit: generic 144
purchasing systems 246

R1.edu 202
recreating the institution 312–14
relationship: price/value 104
religious affinity: universities 272
research: globally distributed groups 157; invisible colleges 156; methods 65–6, 302; reduction of grant support 103–4; state of the art link to 149; teaching synergies 106
research universities: revenue streams 110; stability 89–93; threats to 105
resource relevance: judgement 139
resource sources: relationship 111
restructuring: in situ 304
retrieval: community-based 142
revenue streams: research university 110
revenues: tuition 103
Richards, T. 271
Roemer v. Maryland Public Works Board (1976) 272
rule by committee: heritage 308

sabbaticals: effectiveness 109
scalable growth 221, 229
scholarly archives: integration 151
scholarly review: new forms 16
scholarship: concept 136; disinterested 222; promoting through design 135–51; supporting 136; transformation 135–6
schools: moving online 295–6
Schramm, W. 6
Science in Action (Latour) 235
search engine 73, 138
seed money 123
September 11 (2001) 8

service delivery: culture 224; electronics 1
shared texts 137
sheltered workshop 241
Siegel, D. 51
simulations 130
skills shortages: importance of 264–6
social filter: provision 267
social forecasting 256
social infrastructure 91
social isolation 14
social productivity: knowledge 262
socio-technical complexity: course communication 84
socioeconomic class: information 270
sociology 303
'soft money' 103
software: course management 30
Solow paradox 258
space constraints 101
space and time barriers 321
spatialization 320
standardization: dangers 157–8; incentives 153–5; pressure 310
standardized procedures: rejection 316
state and federal programs 208–9
strategic alliances 125
strategic consortia 225
strategic focus 110
strategic partners 229
student: dismissal 279; target market 186
student admission system: automation 245–6
student competencies: raising 84
student distress 64; instructors' misperception 80; online course 66–72
student isolation 64
student perspective: understanding 72–80
student satisfaction: emphasis 109–10
student-centered learning 22
student-centered thinking 292
students: part-time 107; rights of speech 279–80; South East Asia 193
students and teachers: conceptions 13
study centers: encounters 207
Sturken, M.: and Cartwright, L. 54
summer schools 309

support infrastructure 172

targeting: working professional 56–61
taxpayer support 91
teacher training 60; distance learning 192
teacher-centered learning 22
teachers: facilitators 23; qualifications 188; role 296–7
teachers and students: conceptions 13
teaching: asynchronous delivery 229; evaluation 109; load measurement 211; material 124; redefinition of roles 112; relief 106; research synergies 106; skills development 108; vertically integrated 100
technical capabilities and limitations 329
technical educational convergence 27
technical support 60
techno-organizational form: higher education 215
technological change and productivity in education 259–61
technological limitations 22
technological problems 74–6
technology: assessing appropriateness 320; benefits of advanced 83; decreasing cost 292; disruptive 101; enhancing discourse 318–27; hard and soft 44–5; home grown system 174; labor-saving 259; learning 62; mix 186, 190; new 94; rebuild around 313; sustaining 101; tele-access 12
technology vendor model 173–4
tele-access 3, 31; education and learning 7–13; information 8; information and communication technologies (ICTs) 4; learning by virtually doing 9–10; people 10–11; services 11; technologies 12
tele-education 36
thin multimedia 51
third way 219
Timmermans, S.: and Berg, M. 243
traditional practices: constraints 20–1
training: teacher 60
training services: brokerage 293
transfer credits 112

tuition: revenues 103
tutorial: learning 129–34
tutorial action 124
tutorial education (UK) 43
tutorial learning units 131; design 131; evaluation 132; implementation 132; project management 131
tutors 124; co-option of part time 191

Ufi Ltd 218–22, 226–30
undergraduate education 89
undergraduate research 106
Unext.com 202
United Kingdom (UK): e-university 46; Leicester University 192–5; Open University 5, 40; technology-based learning 219–20; university expansion 304; university procedural ritual 42
United States of America (USA): Caliber Learning Network Inc. 202; California State Polytechnic University 195; Californian Virtual University 291; government agencies 99; Jones International University virtual university 116–20; Kentucky Commonwealth Virtual University 201; Knowledge TV 200; National Information Infrastructure (NII) 3; National Technological University (NTU) 200; Open University 99; policy initiatives 290–9; Public Broadcasting Service (PBS) 200; research universities 87–115; Supreme Court and higher education 269–77; University of Phoenix 198; Western Governors University 201
Universitas 21 consortium 178
universities: American research 87–115; autonomy 269, 281, 322; behavior parameters 274; bookstore 37; campus 155; core functions 292; culture *collegium* 306; economic activity 283; economics 273; expansion (UK) 304; for-profit entities 283; future roles 266–7; informational substructure and professional skills 161–3; informational view 232–48; Internet

Service Providers (ISPs) 282; land and property 275; as models for firms 263; nation-state goals 272; networked 17; non-prestigious 88; old to new model 242–4; payments to 274–5; planning and practice 204–5; producers of a service commodity 325; religious affinity 272; rest of the world 160–1; sense of identity 306–17; special status 273; system preservation 115; teaching 158, 305; transformations 286; *see also* virtual university
University for Industry: learndirect network 217–19
University of Phoenix (USA) 198
university–private sector partnership 322
user workarounds: systems 247

value: labor theory 261–2
vendor corporations 99
Venezuela 236
vertical bureaucracy 217
vested interests 244
Veterans' Administration (VA) 273
video 36; -conferencing technologies 314; interviews 53; lectures 132; links 161; technology 8
virtual campus 117, 215; debate 216–17; platform 123
virtual corporation 224
Virtual Development Academy 119
virtual field trip problems 66–9
virtual learning: network society 215–30
virtual library 125
virtual model: higher education 116–18; university 241
virtual structure 210

virtual transparency 30
virtual university 2, 6, 14, 234; accreditation status 117; Applied Sciences 206–14; building 308–15; definition 302; foundation 118; ignored 294; Jones International University (USA) 116–20; living in 244–8
virtuality: implications 9, 302–3
virtualized diploma mills 216
virtualized learning material 221
'Vision Simulator' 59
visions of learning: future goals 128
visual literacy 53–4
vocational training 223
voice input systems 130
Vygotsky, L.S. 131

wealth: new 260; shifting 260
Web-based courses 281; ethnographic study 62–84
Web-enhanced learning 47
weightless economy: capitalism 261–2
Western Governors University (USA) 201
white-collar work 265
Wieler, S. 264
Wilson, T.: and Allen, D. 223
Winner, L. 303
wired campus 23, 318
wireless: Internet access 12
workflow process diagrams 311
working professionals 161; targeting 56–61
World Wide Web 6, 164; changes 37; failures 44; individual elements 52; optimization 119

zone of proximal development 131